Biomaterials for Oral Health

Editors

JACK L. FERRACANE
CARMEM S. PFEIFER
LUIZ E. BERTASSONI

DENTAL CLINICS OF NORTH AMERICA

www.dental.theclinics.com

October 2017 • Volume 61 • Number 4

ELSEVIER

1600 John F. Kennedy Boulevard • Suite 1800 • Philadelphia, Pennsylvania, 19103-2899

http://www.dental.theclinics.com

DENTAL CLINICS OF NORTH AMERICA Volume 61, Number 4
October 2017 ISSN 0011-8532, ISBN: 978-0-323-54660-7

Editor: John Vassallo; j.vassallo@elsevier.com
Developmental Editor: Kristen Helm

Dental Clinics of North America (ISSN 0011-8532) is published quarterly by Elsevier Inc., 360 Park Avenue South, New York, NY 10010-1710. Months of issue are January, April, July, and October. Business and Editorial Offices: 1600 John F. Kennedy Boulevard, Suite 1800, Philadelphia, PA 19103-2899. Periodicals postage paid at New York, NY and additional mailing offices. Subscription prices are $288.00 per year (domestic individuals), $569.00 per year (domestic institutions), $100.00 per year (domestic students/residents), $350.00 per year (Canadian individuals), $737.00 per year (Canadian institutions), $422.00 per year (international individuals), $737.00 per year (international institutions), and $200.00 per year (international and Canadian students/residents). International air speed delivery is included in all *Clinics* subscription prices. All prices are subject to change without notice. **POSTMASTER:** Send address changes to *Dental Clinics of North America*, Elsevier Health Sciences Division, Subscription Customer Service, 3251 Riverport Lane, Maryland Heights, MO 63043. **Customer Service (orders, claims, online, change of address): Elsevier Health Sciences Division, Subscription Customer Service, 3251 Riverport Lane, Maryland Heights, MO 63043. Tel: 1-800-654-2452 (U.S. and Canada). Fax: 314-447-8029. E-mail: journalscustomerservice-usa@elsevier.com (for print support); journalsonlinesupport-usa@elsevier.com (for online support).**

Reprints. For copies of 100 or more, of articles in this publication, please contact the Commercial Reprints Department, Elsevier Inc., 360 Park Avenue South, New York, NY 10010-1710. Tel.: 212-633-3874; Fax: 212-633-3820; E-mail: reprints@elsevier.com.

The *Dental Clinics of North America* is covered in *MEDLINE/PubMed (Index Medicus)*, *Current Contents/Clinical Medicine*, *ISI/BIOMED* and *Clinahl*.

Contributors

EDITORS

JACK L. FERRACANE, PhD
Professor and Chair, Division Director of Biomaterials and Biomechanics, Department of Restorative Dentistry, Oregon Health & Science University, Portland, Oregon, USA

CARMEM S. PFEIFER, DDS, PhD
Associate Professor, Division of Biomaterials and Biomechanics, Department of Restorative Dentistry, Oregon Health & Science University, Portland, Oregon, USA

LUIZ E. BERTASSONI, DDS, PhD
Assistant Professor, Division of Biomaterials and Biomechanics, Departments of Restorative Dentistry and Biomedical Engineering, OHSU Center for Regenerative Medicine, OHSU School of Medicine, OHSU School of Dentistry, Portland, Oregon, USA

AUTHORS

DWAYNE D. AROLA, PhD
Departments of Materials Science and Engineering, Oral Health Sciences, and Restorative Dentistry, University of Washington School of Dentistry, Seattle, Washington, USA

AVATHAMSA ATHIRASALA, MS
Division of Biomaterials and Biomechanics, Department of Restorative Dentistry, OHSU School of Dentistry, Portland, Oregon, USA

YUXING BAI, DDS, PhD
Professor, Department of Orthodontics, School of Stomatology, Capital Medical University, Beijing, China

ANA BEDRAN-RUSSO, DDS, MS, PhD
Associate Professor, Department of Restorative Dentistry, University of Illinois at Chicago College of Dentistry, Chicago, Illinois, USA

LUIZ E. BERTASSONI, DDS, PhD
Assistant Professor, Division of Biomaterials and Biomechanics, Departments of Restorative Dentistry and Biomedical Engineering, Center for Regenerative Medicine, OHSU School of Medicine, OHSU School of Dentistry, Portland, Oregon, USA

SUNIL KUMAR BODA, PhD
Mary and Dick Holland Regenerative Medicine Program, Department of Surgery-Transplant, University of Nebraska Medical Center, Omaha, Nebraska, USA

DESPOINA BOMPOLAKI, DDS, MS, FACP
Diplomate, American Board of Prosthodontics, Fellow, American College of Prosthodontists, Assistant Professor, Department of Restorative Dentistry, OHSU School of Dentistry, Portland, Oregon, USA

MARCO C. BOTTINO, DDS, PhD
Department of Cariology, Restorative Sciences, and Endodontics, University of Michigan School of Dentistry, Ann Arbor, Michigan, USA

RICARDO M. CARVALHO, DDS, PhD
Division of Biomaterials, Department of Oral Biological and Medical Sciences, Faculty of Dentistry, The University of British Columbia, Vancouver, British Columbia, Canada

SHANSHAN GAO, PhD, MD, DDS
State Key Laboratory of Oral Diseases, National Clinical Research Center for Oral Diseases, West China Hospital of Stomatology, Sichuan University, Chengdu, China

JORGE GARAICOA, DDS, MS
Assistant Professor, Department of Restorative Dentistry, OHSU School of Dentistry, Portland, Oregon, USA

JASON A. GRIGGS, PhD, FADM
Professor and Chair, Biomedical Materials Science, Associate Dean for Research, The University of Mississippi Medical Center School of Dentistry, Jackson, Mississippi, USA

J. ROBERT KELLY, DDS, PhD
Professor, Department of Biomedical Engineering, University of Connecticut Health Center, Farmington, Connecticut, USA

ARIENE A. LEME-KRAUS, DDS, MS, PhD
Senior Researcher, Department of Restorative Dentistry, University of Illinois at Chicago College of Dentistry, Chicago, Illinois, USA

ADRIANA P. MANSO, DDS, MSc, PhD
Department of Oral Biological and Medical Sciences, Division of Biomaterials, Faculty of Dentistry, The University of British Columbia, Vancouver, British Columbia, Canada

RADI MASRI, DDS, MS, PhD
Department of Endodontics, Prosthodontics, and Operative Dentistry, University of Maryland School of Dentistry, Baltimore, Maryland, USA

JACQUES E. NÖR, DDS, PhD
Department of Cariology, Restorative Sciences, and Endodontics, University of Michigan School of Dentistry, Ann Arbor, Michigan, USA

DIVYA PANKAJAKSHAN, PhD
Department of Biomedical and Applied Sciences, Indiana University School of Dentistry, Indianapolis, Indiana, USA

CARMEM S. PFEIFER, DDS, PhD
Associate Professor, Division of Biomaterials and Biomechanics, Department of Restorative Dentistry, Oregon Health & Science University, Portland, Oregon, USA

RICHARD B.T. PRICE, BDS, DDS, MS, PhD
Professor, Department of Dental Clinical Sciences, Dalhousie University, Halifax, Nova Scotia, Canada

AMIT PUNJ, BDS, DMD, FACP
Diplomate, American Board of Prosthodontics, Fellow, American College of Prosthodontists, Assistant Professor and Associate Director of Clinical Restorative Dentistry, Department of Restorative Dentistry, OHSU School of Dentistry, Portland, Oregon, USA

MARK A. REYNOLDS, DDS, PhD
Professor, Department of Endodontics, Periodontics, and Prosthodontics, University of Maryland School of Dentistry, Baltimore, Maryland, USA

ERICA C. TEIXEIRA, DDS, MS, PhD
Associate Professor, Department of Operative Dentistry, The University of Iowa College of Dentistry and Dental Clinics, Iowa City, Iowa, USA

GREESHMA THRIVIKRAMAN, PhD
Division of Biomaterials and Biomechanics, Department of Restorative Dentistry, OHSU School of Dentistry, Portland, Oregon, USA

CHELSEA TWOHIG, DDS
Division of Biomaterials and Biomechanics, Department of Restorative Dentistry, OHSU School of Dentistry, Portland, Oregon, USA

CRISTINA M.P. VIDAL, DDS, MS, PhD
Assistant Professor, Department of Operative Dentistry, The University of Iowa College of Dentistry and Dental Clinics, Iowa City, Iowa, USA

MICHAEL D. WEIR, PhD
Assistant Professor, Department of Endodontics, Periodontics, and Prosthodontics, University of Maryland School of Dentistry, Baltimore, Maryland, USA

HOCKIN H.K. XU, PhD
Professor, Department of Endodontics, Periodontics, and Prosthodontics, University of Maryland School of Dentistry, Center for Stem Cell Biology & Regenerative Medicine, University of Maryland School of Medicine; Department of Mechanical Engineering, University of Maryland, Baltimore County, Baltimore, Maryland, USA

HAI ZHANG, DMD, PhD
Department of Restorative Dentistry, University of Washington School of Dentistry, Seattle, Washington, USA

KE ZHANG, DDS, PhD
Assistant Professor, Department of Orthodontics, School of Stomatology, Capital Medical University, Beijing, China; Department of Endodontics, Periodontics, and Prosthodontics, University of Maryland School of Dentistry, Baltimore, Maryland, USA

NING ZHANG, DDS, PhD
Associate Professor, Department of Orthodontics, School of Stomatology, Capital Medical University, Beijing, China; Department of Endodontics, Periodontics, and Prosthodontics, University of Maryland School of Dentistry, Baltimore, Maryland, USA

YU ZHANG, PhD
Associate Professor, Department of Biomaterials and Biomimetics, NYU College of Dentistry, New York, New York, USA

Contents

Preface: Biomaterials for Oral Health   xi

Jack L. Ferracane, Carmem S. Pfeifer, and Luiz E. Bertassoni

The Tooth: Its Structure and Properties   651

Dwayne D. Arola, Shanshan Gao, Hai Zhang, and Radi Masri

> This article provides a brief review of recent investigations concerning the structure and properties of the tooth. The last decade has brought a greater emphasis on the durability of the tooth, an improved understanding of the fatigue and fracture behavior of the principal tissues, and their importance to tooth failures. The primary contributions to tooth durability are discussed, including the process of placing a restoration, the impact of aging, and challenges posed by the oral environment. The significance of these findings to the dental community and their importance to the pursuit of lifelong oral health are highlighted.

Bioactive Dental Composites and Bonding Agents Having Remineralizing and Antibacterial Characteristics   669

Ke Zhang, Ning Zhang, Michael D. Weir, Mark A. Reynolds, Yuxing Bai, and Hockin H.K. Xu

> Current dental restorative materials are typically inert and replace missing tooth structures. This article reviews efforts in the development of a new generation of bioactive materials designed to not only replace the missing tooth volume but also possess therapeutic functions. Composites and bonding agents with remineralizing and antibacterial characteristics have shown promise in replacing lost minerals, inhibiting recurrent caries, neutralizing acids, repelling proteins, and suppressing biofilms and acid production. Furthermore, they have demonstrated a low cytotoxicity similar to current resins, with additional benefits to protect the dental pulp and promote tertiary dentin formation.

Advanced Scaffolds for Dental Pulp and Periodontal Regeneration   689

Marco C. Bottino, Divya Pankajakshan, and Jacques E. Nör

> No current therapy promotes root canal disinfection and regeneration of the pulp-dentin complex in cases of pulp necrosis. Antibiotic pastes used to eradicate canal infection negatively affect stem cell survival. Three-dimensional easy-to-fit antibiotic-eluting nanofibers, combined with injectable scaffolds, enriched or not with stem cells and/or growth factors, may increase the likelihood of achieving predictable dental pulp regeneration. Periodontitis is an aggressive disease that impairs the integrity of tooth-supporting structures and may lead to tooth loss. The latest advances in membrane biomodification to endow needed functionalities and technologies to engineer patient-specific membranes/constructs to amplify periodontal regeneration are presented.

An Overview of Dental Adhesive Systems and the Dynamic Tooth–Adhesive Interface   **713**

Ana Bedran-Russo, Ariene A. Leme-Kraus, Cristina M.P. Vidal, and Erica C. Teixeira

From the conception of resin–enamel adhesion to today's contemporary dental adhesive systems, clinicians are no longer afraid of exploring the many advantages brought by adhesive restorative concepts. To maximize the performance of adhesive-based restorative procedures, practitioners must be familiar with the mechanism of adhesion, clinical indications, proper handling, the inherent limitations of the materials, and the biological challenges. This review provides an overview of the current status of restorative dental adhesives, their mechanism of adhesion, mechanisms of degradation of dental adhesive interfaces, how to maximize performance, and future trends in adhesive dentistry.

Polymer-based Direct Filling Materials   **733**

Carmem S. Pfeifer

After a brief review of current restorative materials and classifications, this article discusses the latest developments in polymer-based direct filling materials, with emphasis on products and studies available in the last 10 years. This will include the more recent bulk fill composites and self-adhesive materials, for which clinical evidence of success, albeit somewhat limited, is already available. The article also introduces the latest cutting-edge research topics on new materials for composite restorations, and an outlook for the future of how those may help to improve the service life of dental composite restorations.

Light Curing in Dentistry   **751**

Richard B.T. Price

The ability to light cure resins "on demand" in the mouth has revolutionized dentistry. However, there is a widespread lack of understanding of what is required for successful light curing in the mouth. Most instructions simply tell the user to "light cure for xx seconds" without describing any of the nuances of how to successfully light cure a resin. This article provides a brief description of light curing. At the end, some recommendations are made to help when purchasing a curing light and how to improve the use of the curing light.

Dental Impression Materials and Techniques   **779**

Amit Punj, Despoina Bompolaki, and Jorge Garaicoa

Dental impression making is the process of creating a negative form of the teeth and oral tissues, into which gypsum or other die materials can be processed to create working analogues. Contemporary dentistry generates new information every year, and digital dentistry is becoming established and influential. Although dentists should stay abreast of new technologies, some of the conventional materials and time-tested techniques remain widely used. It is important to review the impression-making process to ensure that practitioners have up-to-date information about how to safely and effectively capture the exact form of the oral tissues to provide optimal patient management.

Dental Ceramics for Restoration and Metal Veneering 797

Yu Zhang and J. Robert Kelly

> A survey of the development of dental ceramics is presented to provide a better understanding of the rationale behind the development and clinical indications of each class of ceramic material. Knowledge of the composition, microstructure, and properties of a material is critical for selecting the right material for specific applications. The key to successful ceramic restorations rests on material selection, manufacturing technique, and restoration design, including the balancing of several factors, such as residual stresses, tooth contact conditions, tooth size and shape, elastic modulus of the adhesives and tooth structure, and surface state.

Dental Cements for Luting and Bonding Restorations: Self-Adhesive Resin Cements 821

Adriana P. Manso and Ricardo M. Carvalho

> Self-adhesive resin cements combine easy application of conventional luting materials with improved mechanical properties and bonding capability of resin cements. The presence of functional acidic monomers, dual-cure setting mechanism, and fillers capable of neutralizing the initial low pH of the cement are essential elements of the material and should be understood when selecting the ideal luting material for each clinical situation. This article addresses the most relevant aspects of self-adhesive resin cements and their impact on clinical performance. Although few clinical studies are available to establish solid evidence, the information presented provides guidance in the dynamic environment of material development.

Biomaterials for Craniofacial Bone Regeneration 835

Greeshma Thrivikraman, Avathamsa Athirasala, Chelsea Twohig,
Sunil Kumar Boda, and Luiz E. Bertassoni

> Functional reconstruction of craniofacial defects is a major challenge in craniofacial sciences. The advent of biomaterials is an alternative to standard autologous/allogenic grafting procedures to achieve successful bone regeneration. This article discusses classes of biomaterials currently used in craniofacial reconstruction. Also reviewed are clinical applications of biomaterials as delivery agents for sustained release of stem cells, genes, and growth factors. Recent promising advancements in 3D printing and bioprinting techniques that may be promising for future clinical treatments for craniofacial reconstruction are covered. Relevant topics in the bone regeneration literature exemplifying the potential of biomaterials to repair bone defects are highlighted.

Dental Implants 857

Jason A. Griggs

> Systematic reviews of literature over the period between 2008 and 2017 are discussed regarding clinical evidence for the factors affecting survival and failure of dental implants. The factors addressed include publication bias, tooth location, insertion torque, collar design, implant-abutment connection design, implant length, implant width, bone augmentation, platform switching, surface roughness, implant coatings, and the use of ceramic materials in the implant body and abutment.

DENTAL CLINICS OF NORTH AMERICA

FORTHCOMING ISSUES

January 2018
Oral Cancer
Eric T. Stoopler and Thomas P. Sollecito,
Editors

April 2018
Dental Public Health
Michelle M. Henshaw and Astha Singhal,
Editors

July 2018
**Imaging Technologies in the
Dento-Maxillofacial Region**
Rujuta Katkar and Hassem Geha, *Editors*

RECENT ISSUES

July 2017
Evidence-Based Pediatric Dentistry
Donald L. Chi, *Editor*

April 2017
Clinical Microbiology for the General Dentist
Arvind Babu Rajendra Santosh and
Orrett E. Ogle, *Editors*

January 2017
Endodontics: Clinical and Scientific Updates
Mo K. Kang, *Editor*

ISSUE OF RELATED INTEREST

Oral and Maxillofacial Surgery Clinics of North America
February 2017 (Vol. 29, No. 1)
Emerging Biomaterials and Techniques in Tissue Regeneration
Alan S. Herford, *Editor*
Available at: www.oralmaxsurgery.theclinics.com

Preface

Biomaterials for Oral Health

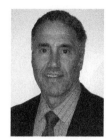 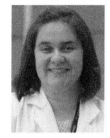 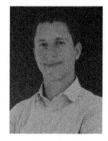

Jack L. Ferracane, PhD   Carmem S. Pfeifer, DDS, PhD   Luiz E. Bertassoni, DDS, PhD

Editors

Biomaterials for use in the maintenance of oral health are developing at a rapid pace. While the dental practitioner will continue to use synthetic biomaterials to provide care that includes the prevention, restoration, and replacement of lost or missing oral tissues, the future promises exciting new developments. In the future, the desire for a biomaterial to be inert and nonharmful to the patient, while still relevant and necessary, will no longer be considered sufficient. New materials, currently being introduced, under development, or simply envisioned, are expected to be bioactive, in that they will be intended to interact in some positive way with the oral environment. These materials will provide a wide range of diverse functions, including the routine inhibition of bacterial biofilm formation, remineralization of lost dentin and enamel, and the regeneration of diseased pulp, bone, and soft tissues.

This issue provides a review of current biomaterials in use by the dental profession for the purpose of delivering optimal oral health care. Topics include a review of tooth structure, and specifically, its resistance to fracture, a discussion of important considerations in the complex process of light curing of dental resin-based materials, the exploding field of bioactive materials for remineralizing teeth and inhibiting oral bacteria, as well as exciting new materials and strategies designed to promote the regeneration of the dentin-pulp complex and other craniofacial structures. Articles also include the continuing improvements in resin-based dental adhesives and restorative composites with the promise of enhanced durability and longevity. In addition, the issue provides a review of existing impression materials as contrasted with new methods for imaging oral structures for producing prosthetic devices, improved dental ceramics for tooth reconstruction including the expanding use of CAD-CAM technology, and new developments in dental cements for securing prosthetic devices to existing tooth structure. Finally, strategies for the development of bone augmentation materials and a review of the clinical performance of dental implants are discussed.

Dent Clin N Am 61 (2017) xi–xii
http://dx.doi.org/10.1016/j.cden.2017.07.001
0011-8532/17/© 2017 Published by Elsevier Inc.

dental.theclinics.com

The dental practitioner of the future will continue to be exposed to less "traditional" materials and methods in their daily practice. Rapid and significant advances in science and technology will provide real products and methods that were only dreamed about just a few short years ago. The intent of this compilation is to review the current state-of-the-art in biomaterials for oral health, while introducing the developments that will continue to transform the field and the practice of dentistry.

Jack L. Ferracane, PhD
Department of Restorative Dentistry
Oregon Health & Science University
2730 Southwest Moody Avenue
Portland, OR 97201, USA

Carmem S. Pfeifer, DDS, PhD
Department of Restorative Dentistry
Oregon Health & Science University
2730 Southwest Moody Avenue
Portland, OR 97201, USA

Luiz E. Bertassoni, DDS, PhD
Department of Restorative Dentistry
Oregon Health & Science University
2730 Southwest Moody Avenue
Portland, OR 97201, USA

E-mail addresses:
ferracan@ohsu.edu (J.L. Ferracane)
pfeiferc@cohsu.edu (C.S. Pfeifer)
bertasso@ohsu.edu (L.E. Bertassoni)

The Tooth

Its Structure and Properties

Dwayne D. Arola, PhD[a,b,c,]*, Shanshan Gao, PhD, MD, DDS[d], Hai Zhang, DMD, PhD[c],
Radi Masri, DDS, MS, PhD[e]

KEYWORDS

• Aging • Dentin • Durability • Enamel • Fatigue • Fracture • Tubules

KEY POINTS

- The tooth's durability is reduced by the introduction of damage in dentin or enamel, which can occur in the cutting of preparations and etching, and as a result of cyclic contact.
- There is a substantial reduction in the fatigue and fracture resistance of both dentin and enamel with increasing patient age, which should be considered in the treatment plan.
- Exposure of dentin to acidic environments reduces its fatigue strength and reduces the tooth's durability. Exposure to biofilm and aggressive or over-etching should be avoided.

INTRODUCTION

It seems appropriate to begin this review of the structure and properties of the tooth from the foundation provided by previous noteworthy reviews. For instance, Pashley[1] reviewed the microstructure of dentin, and the variations in tubule density and dimensions, from the deep to the peripheral regions. He discussed their influence on fluid movement within the lumens, that is, the fluid dynamics, as well as contributions of the smear layer developed during cutting to dentin permeability. Results from that body of work established the importance of the smear layer to adhesive dentistry and have guided the development of products to treat dentin sensitivity.

This work was supported in part by the National Institute of Dental and Craniofacial Research of the National Institutes of Health (NIDCR NIH) under award numbers R01DE016904 (PI D.D. Arola), and R01DE015306. The content is solely the responsibility of the authors and does not necessarily represent the official views of the National Institutes of Health.

[a] Department of Materials Science and Engineering, University of Washington School of Dentistry, Roberts Hall, 333, Box 352120, Seattle, WA 98195-2120, USA; [b] Department of Oral Health Sciences, University of Washington School of Dentistry, Seattle, WA 98195-2120, USA; [c] Department of Restorative Dentistry, Box 357456, University of Washington School of Dentistry, Seattle, WA 98195-7456, USA; [d] State Key Laboratory of Oral Diseases, National Clinical Research Center for Oral Diseases, West China Hospital of Stomatology, Sichuan University, Renmin South Road, Chengdu, 610041, China; [e] Department of Endodontics, Prosthodontics and Operative Dentistry, University of Maryland School of Dentistry, 650 West Baltimore Street, 4th Floor, Suite 4228, Baltimore, MD 21201, USA
* Corresponding author. Department of Materials Science and Engineering, University of Washington School of Dentistry, Roberts Hall, 333, Box 352120, Seattle, WA 98195-2120.
E-mail address: darola@uw.edu

Dent Clin N Am 61 (2017) 651–668
http://dx.doi.org/10.1016/j.cden.2017.05.001
0011-8532/17/© 2017 Elsevier Inc. All rights reserved.

Marshall and colleagues[2] also reviewed the structure and properties of dentin and placed emphasis on adhesive bonding due to the transition taking place in restorative materials. That review provided a comprehensive discussion of sclerotic and transparent dentin, as well as demineralized, remineralized, and hypermineralized forms. These altered forms exhibit distinct microstructures, which are important to acid etching and bonding.[3,4] The importance of location and tubule orientation to the mechanical behavior of dentin were also highlighted, as well as the need for adopting site-specific descriptions of properties that could be developed using instrumented indentation.

Kinney and colleagues,[5] presented a comprehensive review of the structure and mechanical behavior of dentin, the first after decades. That review serves as the bible on the mechanical behavior of dentin and now guides the way we think about the tooth as a loadbearing structure. More emphasis was placed on the importance of the collagen and its contribution to the elastic properties and viscoelastic behavior of dentin. This review also started the discussion of flaws in dentin, including their contributions to the strength and fatigue behavior. Kinney and colleagues[5] proposed that a fracture mechanics approach should be adopted to describe the strength of dentin, especially when considering the importance of changes in microstructure associated with the altered forms.

The last decade has brought greater interest in and understanding of the tooth's durability. Therefore, the objective of this article is to discuss the structure and properties most relevant to tooth durability, with an emphasis on their importance to clinical practice.

DAMAGE AND FLAWS

The mechanical forms of tooth failure originate at defects, which could be intrinsic or extrinsic, for example, as a result of treatment or induced during function. Defects within the tooth structure reduce its capacity to bear loads, thereby reducing its resistance to the forces of mastication.

Cracks in teeth facilitate tooth fracture[6,7]; but how do they develop? This question is being debated in the fields of endodontics and prosthodontics. In endodontics, the concern is whether flaws are introduced during instrumentation of the canal and if they are the cause of vertical root fractures. Some studies have reported that damage is introduced during instrumentation of the canal,[8–10] whereas others have shown there is no difference in the number of microcracks within instrumented teeth versus controls (ie, without instrumentation).[11–13] This debate is ongoing and has yet to address the residual strength of a tooth with defects.

Recent investigations have explored whether the introduction of cavity preparations and adhesive bonding reduce the tooth's durability. For instance, laser cutting preparations were shown to introduce cracks in dentin[14] that reduce the strength. However, Sehy and Drummond[15] could not identify visible or microscopic cracking in dentin after performing bur treatments. Majd and colleagues[16] evaluated the influence of bur cutting and an abrasive air jet treatment on the fatigue strength of coronal dentin. Despite an increase in surface roughness with respect to control surfaces and development of a smear layer, flaws or cracks were not evident in the prepared surfaces and there was no change to the static strength. However, both treatments caused a significant reduction in the fatigue strength of dentin, with bur cutting resulting in nearly 40% reduction in the fatigue limit.

More recently, Majd and colleagues[17] explored the influence of cutting direction on the fatigue strength of tooth structure. Treatments involved cutting of coronal dentin using a medium-grit diamond in parallel and transverse cutting directions with respect to the direction of cyclic tensile stress. A reduction in static strength of approximately

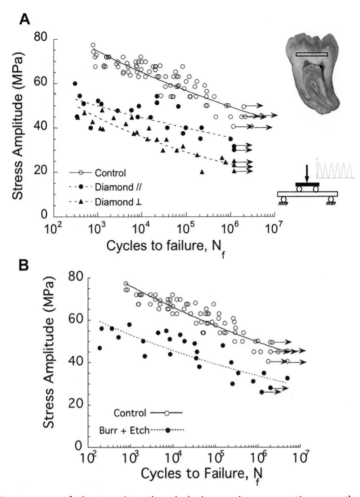

Fig. 1. Importance of damage introduced during cavity preparations on the fatigue strength of coronal dentin. The control in these 2 diagrams consists of beams of coronal dentin prepared with diamond slicing wheels and with average surface roughness of less than 0.2 μm. (*A*) Comparison of the fatigue strength after cutting treatments with medium diamond abrasive and water spray irrigation. Results are shown for cutting parallel (*//*) and perpendicular (⊥) to the length of the beam, which is important to the orientation of damage. Data points with arrows represent beams that did not fail and the test was discontinued. (*B*) Comparison of the fatigue strength distribution of the control with dentin beams subjected to a bur cutting treatment followed by a 15 second etch with 37.5% gel. Cutting was performed with a 6-flute tungsten carbide straight fissure bur and commercial air turbine with water spray irrigation. (*Adapted from* [*A*] Majd B, Majd H, Porter JA, et al. Degradation in the fatigue strength of dentin by diamond bur preparations: importance of cutting direction. J Biomed Mater Res B Appl Biomater 2016;104(1):39–49, with permission; and [*B*] Lee HH, Majd H, Orrego S, et al. Degradation in the fatigue strength of dentin by cutting, etching and adhesive bonding. Dent Mater 2014;30(9):1067, with permission.)

20% resulted from cutting in each direction. Results from cyclic loading (**Fig. 1**A) showed that the cutting caused a significant reduction in fatigue strength; the largest decrease (nearly 60%) resulted from cutting in the perpendicular direction. The messages from these studies are that (1) the process of cutting dentin with either carbide or diamond abrasive burs introduces flaws within dentin and (2) although these flaws are not visible, they undergo growth as a result of cyclic loading until reaching a length that enables failure. The results also indicate that the fatigue strength of dentin is very sensitive to the presence of flaws.[18] Due to the substantial reduction in fatigue strength by diamonds, they should not be used in the cutting of dentin. Because diamonds are regularly used in the clinic, this deserves immediate attention.

Etching generally follows cutting of the cavity preparation. That process could alter the surface generated by cutting. Lee and colleagues[19] explored whether etching and adhesive bonding improved the durability of dentin after cutting. The fatigue strength distribution of dentin subjected to bur treatment followed by etching for 15 seconds, with that of flaw-free controls is shown in **Fig. 1**B. Etching does not improve the fatigue strength after bur cutting. That study also showed that etching alone, sans cutting, caused a reduction in fatigue strength and that application of a resin adhesive afterward did not improve the fatigue strength.[19] Hence, the processes used in placing bonded restorations introduce flaws that reduce the tooth's durability.

Damage may also be introduced in enamel as a result of cutting and the placement of restorations. However, the microstructure of enamel resists the growth of this damage (see later discussion). Cyclic contact is also a source of damage. Indeed, due to the improvements in clinical success of dental ceramics, contact between these engineered materials and natural tooth structure is increasingly common. Damage to the opposing natural tooth enamel is a relevant concern.

Gao and colleagues[20] recently evaluated the damage resulting from cyclic contact of enamel with ceramic restorations. Results from cyclic loading experiments are presented in terms of a contact load-life diagram in **Fig. 2**A. As expected, there is a decrease in number of cycles to failure (ie, life) with increasing contact load. This outcome reflects the importance of occlusal adjustment to avoid concentration of contact stress and its magnitude. Furthermore, enamel does not exhibit a fatigue limit; that is, all cyclic loads caused damage and there is no minimum load that the enamel can bear an infinite number of cycles. An example of the contact fatigue damage due to cyclic loading at a maximum load of 400 N is shown in **Fig. 2**B. The indentations exhibited 2 separate families of cracks, including cylindrical cracks within the contact area and radial cracks extending outside the contact region. Both the length and number of radial cracks increased with the magnitude of contact loads. The cracks also developed at contact stresses well below those necessary for damage under static indentations.[21] The changes in surface roughness and damage could facilitate bacterial adhesion, bacterial penetration, or even tooth fracture. Contact fatigue damage in the opposing enamel should be considered in the future development of materials for crown replacement. Clearly, greater clinical focus on opposing tooth structure to crowns and their prognosis is warranted.

IMPORTANT COMPONENTS OF STRUCTURE

The durability of the tooth depends on the structure and properties of the individual tissues. Shahmoradi and colleagues[22] recently presented an interesting review of the structure and properties of the cementum, dentin, and enamel. The present effort is focused on the dentin and enamel, in essence, the loadbearing tissues and aspects important to their durability.

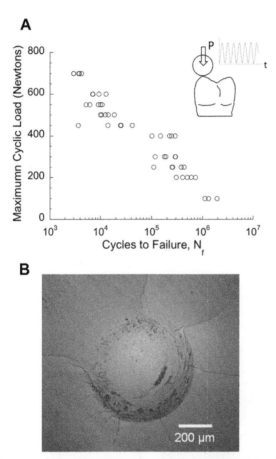

Fig. 2. Contact damage of enamel resulting from cyclic loading. (*A*) Load-life diagram for cyclic contact of cuspal enamel described in terms of the maximum contact load and the number of cycles to failure. Failure was defined by an increase in maximum indentation depth that exceeded that in the first cycle by 15 μm. (*B*) Typical contact damage pattern resulting from cyclic loading. Note the large number of circumferential cracks inside the contact zone and the radial cracks extending from the contact periphery. This particular damage pattern resulted from cyclic contact with maximum load of 400 N and after a total of 160 k cycles. P, load; t, time; N_f, cycles to failure (*Adapted from* Gao SS, An BB, Yahyazadehfar M, et al. Contact fatigue of human enamel: experiments, mechanisms and modeling. J Mech Behav Biomed Mater 2016;60:440–43; with permission.)

Dentin and enamel are regarded as hierarchical materials due to the multiple length scales of the microstructural elements. At the largest length scale, the most distinct feature of the structure of dentin is the tubules. The tubules serve many functions, including hydration of the tooth, a conduit for transduction of physical signals to sensory responses, and as an anchor in adhesive bonding.[23] This network of channels extends radially outward from the pulp toward the dentin enamel junction (DEJ) and cementum. The tubule density and diameter are lowest at the DEJ and increase with proximity to the pulp.[1,2] Although this basic microstructure is well recognized, the potential importance of factors such as ethnic background, environment, diet, and so forth are generally ignored.

A recent study addressed this concern by comparing the microstructure of coronal dentin from age-matched pairs of donor teeth from the United States (US) and Colombia (CO), South America.[24] There was a significant reduction in the lumen density with depth ($P \leq .05$) for both donor groups and no significant difference ($P > .05$) in the tubule density between them. However, there were differences evident in the diameter of the lumens. **Fig. 3**A compares representative micrographs of peripheral dentin from the teeth of donors living in the US and CO. The average lumen diameters of the coronal dentin within the deep, middle, and peripheral regions of the 2 donor groups are compared in **Fig. 3**B. For the US group, there was a significant decrease in lumen diameter from the deep to the peripheral dentin, with average lumen diameters decreasing from approximately 1.8 µm to equal to or less than 1 µm. However, there was no significant change in the lumen diameter with depth for the CO donors. The largest difference between the 2 groups was evident in the peripheral dentin (see **Fig. 3**A), in which the average lumen diameter of tissue from the CO donors was more than 40% greater.

A

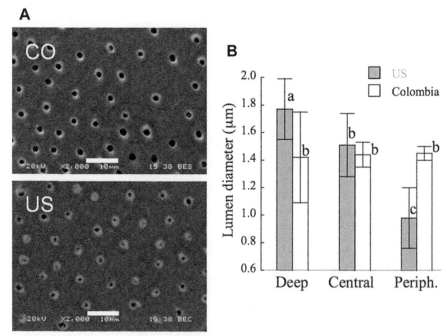

Fig. 3. A comparison of the structure of coronal dentin obtained from donor teeth of residents from CO and the US. The 2 groups consist of age-matched young donors with 18 ≤ age ≤ 35 years. (*A*) Micrographs obtained from scanning electron microscopy of peripheral dentin obtained from representative donor teeth of residents from the US and CO. (*B*) The distribution of tubule lumen diameter of coronal dentin in the deep, central, and peripheral (Periph) regions. The column height represents the average and the caps indicate the standard deviation. Columns with different letters are significantly different (*P* ≤ 05). Note the consistent diameter of the 3 locations of the Colombian teeth. ([*A*] *Adapted from* Ivancik J, Naranjo M, Correa S, et al. Differences in the microstructure and fatigue properties of dentin between residents of North and South America. Arch Oral Biol 2014;59(10):1005, with permission; and [*B*] *From* Ivancik J, Naranjo M, Correa S, et al. Differences in the microstructure and fatigue properties of dentin between residents of North and South America. Arch Oral Biol 2014;59(10):1005, with permission.)

For both donor groups, the measures of microstructure were within the ranges previously reported for tubule density[25] and tubule diameter.[26] Nevertheless, a similar study of teeth from Brazilian donors reported a constant lumen diameter over the crown depth.[27] There are two consequences of these findings to consider. First, dentin bond strength is a function of both tubule density and tubule dimensions.[28,29] Thus, reported spatial variations in bond strength related to dentin microstructure, and the choice of products based on this expectation, may not be applicable to all patient groups. Second, based on the correlations between microstructure and properties of dentin,[30–32] the differences in microstructure could be relevant to tooth durability.

The investigation performed by Ivancik and colleagues[24] also compared the fatigue crack growth resistance of dentin for the US and CO groups. For the US donor teeth, the fatigue crack growth resistance decreased significantly from the peripheral to the deep dentin. In contrast, there were no significant differences in the crack growth resistance of dentin between the three depths for the CO donors. These results are highly relevant to the propensity for fracture of restored teeth. For instance, for shallow restorations extending only into peripheral dentin, there is greater probability for fatigue crack growth to facilitate tooth fractures in the teeth of CO patients due to the lower resistance to cyclic crack growth. For restorations extending into the deep dentin, there is a greater probability of fatigue crack growth and consequent tooth fracture in the patients of the US. In essence, the concept of extension for prevention would be more detrimental in the teeth of US patients. A previous investigation reported significant differences in the fatigue crack growth resistance of dentin obtained from donor teeth of residents of the US and China but did not include a detailed assessment of the microstructure.[33] Based on the implications to tooth durability, this topic should be explored in further detail. It should also be considered in the future development of biomimetic restorative materials.

The most dominant feature of the enamel at the microscopic scale is the enamel rods. Each rod consists of an assembly of apatite nanocrystalline needle-like structures that are aligned parallel to each other and maintained as a cohesive unit by the noncollagenous proteins. This description is a simplification, and more detailed treatments are presented elsewhere.[34–36] The enamel rods extend from the DEJ to the occlusal surface of the tooth. Adjacent to the occlusal surface within the outer enamel, the rods extend inwards in a nearly parallel arrangement. In the inner enamel (approaching the DEJ), the rods are assembled in subunit bands. Each band of rods follows a slightly opposed path that results in a complex decussating structure[37] This structure is responsible for the Hunter-Schreger bands (HSBs) evident in visual inspections of the enamel that result from the variations in reflected light with rod orientation.[23]

The discovery of HSBs in tooth enamel was reported more than 2 centuries ago. However, Lynch and colleagues[38] recently presented an interesting evaluation of HSB distributions in human teeth that showed that the packing densities were greatest in regions where the functional or occlusal loads were largest. They implied that the HSB packing densities and patterns are important to adhesive bond strengths to enamel, abfraction lesions, and even the cracked tooth syndrome. That is consistent with recent evaluations concerning the fracture resistance of enamel[39–42] (see later discussion).

Over the past decade, there has been an increasing emphasis on the importance of the organic phase, which operates at the nanoscale to contribute to the properties of dentin and enamel. Recent work has provided a better understanding of the proteoglycans and their contributions to the mechanical behavior of dentin.[43–45] These matrix proteins are noncollagenous structures that have been largely overlooked in the past. The proteoglycans serve as linkages between the collagens fibrils[46] and secure the collagenous network together. Recent work on the mechanical behavior of enamel has been focused on the importance of the matrix proteins. The proteins constitute between 1% and 2% of the total composition and are primarily located at the interface of the enamel rods. The proteins are important in modulating stress in the enamel of the tooth crown[35] and play roles in the elastic and viscoelastic behavior.[22]

The proteins and their viscoelastic behavior are considered responsible for the toughness of mineralized tissues.[47] Thus, damage or denaturation of the noncollagenous proteins in dentin and enamel are expected to decrease tooth durability. Indeed, the loss of enamel proteins by tooth whitening[48,49] or by treatment with potassium hydroxide[50] causes a significant reduction of the fracture toughness. Considering that both whitening treatments[51–53] and radiation therapy for oral cancers[54] cause degradation of the enamel proteins, this is an important issue to dentistry that requires further investigation.

PROPERTIES OF IMPORTANCE

The properties of primary relevance to tooth durability are those defining the fatigue and fracture behavior. There have been several reviews in the last decade concerning the fatigue behavior of hard tissues of the tooth.[33,55,56] Therefore, the emphasis here is placed on recent findings and their importance to the practitioner.

If flaws are introduced within dentin as a result of the cavity preparation (see previous discussion), the largest degradations in properties will be realized in the resistance to cyclic loading and fatigue. Dentin exhibits anisotropy, with lower resistance to fatigue failure when the cyclic stresses are directed parallel to the axis of the tubules. Cracks within coronal dentin prefer to grow perpendicular to the tubules.[57] This characteristic of the fatigue behavior is among the primary contributions to cusp fractures in restored teeth; that is, cracks initiate near stress concentrations (eg, the line angles of the preparation) and then extend perpendicular to the tubules. The anisotropy in fatigue resistance is actually due to the orientation of the collagen fibrils in the intertubular dentin and their ability to resist crack growth via extrinsic toughening.

Another recent finding concerning the durability of dentin is the importance of tubule density. A comparison of the fatigue crack growth resistance of coronal dentin from the deep, central, and peripheral regions is shown in **Fig. 4**A. There is a significant decrease in the fatigue crack growth resistance with increasing proximity to the pulp cavity. Specifically, cyclic crack growth in deep dentin will occur at stresses approximately 40% lower than those required for peripheral dentin.[58] In addition, cracks in deep dentin undergo cyclic extension at incremental rates of between 100 to 1000 times faster than in peripheral dentin. There are equivalent spatial variations in the fracture toughness of coronal dentin with depth.[32,59,60] Overall, these findings indicate that the probability of restoration failure by tooth fracture increases with penetration of the caries beyond the DEJ and significantly with the depth of the preparation into dentin. Early detection is critical for many reasons.

Fatigue is equally important to the enamel but has received limited attention. Results of contact fatigue suggest that the enamel is not resistant to cyclic loading.[20] An estimate of the fatigue limit of outer (near-occlusal) enamel was recently reported in an assessment of adhesive bond durability.[61] For cyclic tensile stresses directed perpendicular to the rods, the apparent fatigue limit of the enamel was approximately 9 MPa. That value is less than 25% of the fatigue limit of coronal dentin[62] and less than one-tenth the apparent ultimate tensile strength of enamel.[21] Thus, cyclic loads that cause

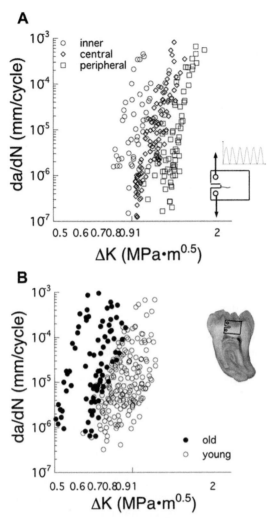

Fig. 4. The importance of location and age on the fatigue crack growth resistance of coronal dentin. (A) Responses obtained for cyclic crack growth occurring in-plane with the dentin tubules. These responses are for young dentin (≤30 years) and stratified according to depth, including close to the pulp (inner), the midcoronal region (central), and close to the DEJ (peripheral). (B) Comparison of cyclic crack growth in the dentin of teeth from young (≤30 years) and old (≤55 years) donors. These responses are for cyclic crack growth occurring perpendicular to the dentin tubules. (*Adapted from* [A] Ivancik J, Neerchal NK, Romberg E, et al. The reduction in fatigue crack growth resistance of dentin with depth. J Dent Res 2011;90(8):1033, with permission; and [B] Ivancik J, Majd H, Bajaj D, et al. Contributions of aging to the fatigue crack growth resistance of human dentin. Acta Biomater 2012;8(7):2740, with permission.)

stresses transverse to the enamel rods are highly likely to induce fatigue cracks within the enamel.

Considering its low fatigue strength, why do all teeth with visible cracks in the tooth crown not undergo fracture? Although the DEJ has been credited with preventing cracks from continuing into the dentin,[63,64] recent studies concerning the crack growth resistance of enamel[40,41,65] support an alternative explanation. Specifically, these studies have shown that the fracture toughness of enamel increases with crack length. For cracks extending from the occlusal surface toward the DEJ, the crack growth resistance can undergo an increase by a factor of 3 or more (**Fig. 5A**). On entering the decussated enamel, the crack encounters a concert of mechanisms operating at many length scales to resist crack growth. As such, cracks that reach the DEJ have limited energy to propagate further. Consequently, it is generally not necessary to restore a tooth with visible enamel cracks because they have been arrested by the underlying microstructure. Perhaps contrary to previous views, the DEJ itself is actually the second line of defense against crack propagation from enamel into dentin.[66] There is also some evidence that cracks in the occlusal enamel can actually undergo healing as a result of crack closure forces promoted by the enamel proteins that extend between the enamel rods.[67] These forces result in a reduction in the crack opening width and a decrease in overall length with time.

There has been some debate whether cracks in teeth initiate from the occlusal surface or from the enamel tufts at the DEJ.[68,69] Recent work has shown that cracks extending from the DEJ undergo a limited increase in toughness ($\sim$30%) in comparison with nearly a 400% increase for cracks extending from the occlusal surface.[40] It seems that the microstructure of enamel has evolved to be most effective at resisting crack growth from the occlusal surface. This is an exciting observation and could potentially inspire the design of the next generation of materials for tooth crown replacement. The design of enamel suggests that materials for crown replacement should be designed with greater toughness, and perhaps with graded microstructure, to resist crack growth from both the occlusal surface and interior, rather than with uniform properties throughout.

Cracks on the tooth's surface must undergo a combination of growth toward the DEJ (ie, longitudinally along the rods) and about the occlusal surface (ie, transverse to the rods). Using bovine incisors, Bechtle and colleagues[41] found that the resistance to fracture is greatest in the transverse orientation. However, in a similar evaluation of human enamel,[42] the crack growth resistance was essentially the same in both directions. Results showed that the most important contributor to the crack growth resistance was the degree of decussation that the crack encountered. Inner enamel, which possesses the highest percentage of decussation, achieved the largest increase in crack growth resistance with extension. These results complement those of Lynch and colleagues[38] concerning the importance of HSBs in enamel and convey that regions with the largest packing density (ie, complexity in the decussation pattern) exhibit the largest resistance to crack growth. Clearly, these results indicate that preserving the decussated enamel is critical to maintaining the tooth's durability.

AGING

There are changes in the structure of dentin and enamel with age that are relevant to the tooth's durability. In dentin, there is a gradual reduction in the diameter of the tubule lumens with age due to their progressive filling with mineral.[70] This process begins in the third decade of life, and continues until the lumens become completely filled,[55] at which point the tissue is considered sclerotic.[23] As a consequence, there is an increase in the mineral content of dentin with age.[59]

The changes in microstructure of dentin with age cause a degradation in the fatigue and fracture properties.[71] For example, there is a substantial reduction in the fatigue strength. Over a span of age from loose definitions of young ($\leq$30 years) to old ($\leq$55 years), the decrease in fatigue strength of coronal dentin is approximately 50%.[61]

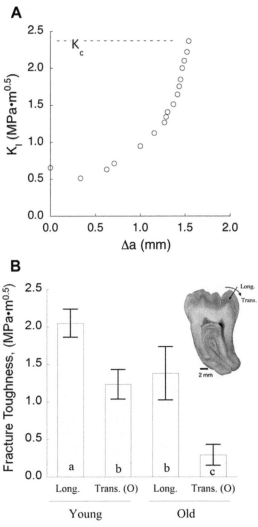

Fig. 5. Characteristics of the crack growth resistance of enamel. (*A*) The increase in resistance to fracture of enamel with crack extension. These data were obtained from crack growth in the longitudinal direction of cuspal enamel (ie, from the occlusal surface toward the DEJ). The fracture toughness of the specimen (Kc), was identified from the last point of stable crack extension preceding bulk fracture. (*B*) The fracture toughness of the enamel from third molars for cracks extending from the occlusal surface to the DEJ (longitudinal) versus growth with buccal-lingual orientation (transverse). The columns represent the average values with standard deviations. Columns with different letters are significantly different. ([*A*] *Data from* Bajaj D, Arola D. Role of prism decussation on fatigue crack growth and fracture of human enamel. Acta Biomater 2009;5(8):3045–56; and [*B*] *Adapted from* Yahyazadehfar M, Zhang D, Arola D. On the importance of aging to the crack growth resistance of human enamel. Acta Biomater 2016;32:269; and Bajaj D, Arola D. Role of prism decussation on fatigue crack growth and fracture of human enamel. Acta Biomater 2009;5(8):3046; with permission.)

The reduction seems to be less extensive for the midcoronal third of the root,[71] which suggests that there are spatial variations in aging. One limitation to this interpretation is that few studies have explored aging of radicular dentin. Nevertheless, this decrease in fatigue strength increases the sensitivity to defects introduced during cavity preparations.

If a crack is introduced in dentin as a result of the cavity preparation, then the fatigue crack growth resistance and fracture toughness become critical to tooth durability. A comparison of cyclic crack growth in coronal dentin from a selection of young and old donor teeth[57,72] is shown in **Fig. 4**B. These results show that there is a decrease in resistance to cyclic crack growth with age, and an increase in the incremental rate of growth by nearly 100 times. Regardless of age, the direction of lowest fatigue crack growth resistance is perpendicular to the lumens and the degradation by aging is most severe in the peripheral dentin.[57] Consistent with the changes in fatigue crack growth resistance, there is a reduction in the fracture toughness of dentin with aging.[59,73,74] Thus, the occlusal force borne by the restoration in teeth of senior patients should be reduced, or the contact area increased, to reduce the stress from mastication to prevent fracture.

The principal cause for the age-related degradation in properties of dentin is still unclear. In a recent multivariate analysis of the reduction in flexure strength of dentin with age, Shinno and colleagues[75] reported that the changes were correlated with increasing advanced glycation end (AGE) product content and increasing mineral density. AGEs are intrafibrillar and interfibrillar nonenzymatic crosslinks that develop through glycation.[76] There is an accumulation of AGEs in dentin collagen with age and the density of AGEs is greatest in collagen near the dentin tubules.[77] Because this process causes a decrease in strength and fracture resistance of human bone with age, an equivalent response would be expected in dentin. Further exploration of the mechanisms of aging in dentin is needed.

There are also changes to the structure and properties of enamel with age. Anecdotal evidence shows that the density of cracks and craze lines in the enamel increases with age. The hardness and elastic modulus of enamel increase with age[78,79] and both contribute to an increase in the indentation brittleness.[80] This suggests that there is greater propensity for cracks and contact damage to develop in the teeth of senior patients.

Once cracks are identified in the surface of teeth, it is common to question whether they warrant treatment. From a mechanical point of view, the answer depends on the crack length and the relative crack growth resistance of the tissue. A comparison of the fracture toughness in two directions of cuspal enamel from the teeth of young (age $\leq$25 years) and old (age $\geq$55 years) donor teeth are shown in **Fig. 5**B.[81] For the longitudinal direction, the fracture toughness decreased by approximately 35% over the age span from the young and old groups. For the transverse direction of crack extension, the fracture toughness of the old enamel (0.25 MPa•m[0.5]) was nearly 70% lower than that obtained from the young teeth. Contrary to the crack growth toughening observed in young enamel (see **Fig. 5**A), the process is negligible in old enamel.[81] This finding provides further evidence of why cracks are more frequently identified in the surfaces of teeth of seniors. Due to the reduction in fracture toughness, cracks are much more detrimental in the teeth of seniors and may warrant greater attention.

What are the mechanisms contributing to the changes in mechanical properties? There is an increase in the mineral density of enamel with aging,[82,83] and a decrease in the volume of protein matrix. This reduction can occur progressively as a result of the variations in oral cavity pH.[23] It can also result from restorative or cosmetic dental procedures such as teeth whitening[51,84,85] that damage or denature the enamel proteins. Indeed, a recent evaluation concerning the mechanical behavior of enamel after whitening showed that bleaching resulted in an average 40% decrease in the fracture toughness after treatment by carbamide peroxide or hydrogen peroxide treatments.[49] These results suggest that whitening treatments could cause an accelerated aging of the enamel, which could be tremendously detrimental at later stages of life or after accumulated treatments.

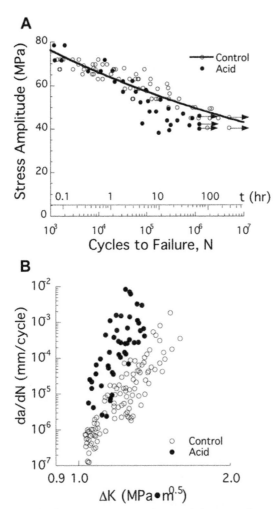

Fig. 6. Degradation in the fatigue resistance of coronal dentin with exposure to an acidic environment. (*A*) Stress life fatigue behavior. The data points with arrows represent beams that did not fail and the test was discontinued. Note that a significant degradation in fatigue strength occurs after only 4 hours of acid exposure. (*B*) Fatigue crack growth resistance of midcoronal dentin. (*A, B*) The control was evaluated in a neutral environment (pH = 7) and the acid condition consisted of exposure to a lactic acid solution with pH = 5. ([*A*] *Adapted from* Do D, Orrego S, Majd H, et al. Accelerated fatigue of dentin with exposure to lactic acid. Biomaterials 2013;34(34):8652, with permission; and [*B*] *From* Orrego S, Xu H, Arola D. Degradation in the fatigue crack growth resistance of human dentin by lactic acid. Mater Sci Eng C Mater Biol Appl 2017;73:720, with permission.)

ORAL ENVIRONMENT

A recurrence of caries at the tooth margin may result from the acid production of biofilms and is considered the primary reason for the replacement of restorations.[86,87] Acidic environments resulting from biofilm activity could also increase the probability of tooth fractures due to synergism between chemical and mechanical mechanisms of degradation. This is a relatively new area of exploration.

The importance of pH variations in the oral environment on the fatigue strength of dentin were recently evaluated by Do and colleagues.[88] A comparison of fatigue life diagrams for coronal dentin evaluated in neutral and a lactic acid environment with a pH of 5 is shown in **Fig. 6**A. Exposure to the acidic conditions caused a significant reduction in fatigue strength and nearly 30% reduction in the fatigue limit. Surprisingly, the reduction in fatigue strength began after only 4 hours of exposure to the lower pH.

The influence of lactic acid exposure on the fatigue crack growth resistance was also recently evaluated by Orrego and colleagues.[89] A comparison of the fatigue crack growth responses of midcoronal dentin exposed to neutral and lactic acid conditions (pH = 5) is shown in **Fig. 6**B. The acidic conditions caused a nearly 10-fold increase in the incremental rate of cyclic crack extension. The study also showed that the degradation by acid exposure increased from the peripheral to the midcoronal dentin and that resin adhesive penetration within the lumens had no influence on the fatigue resistance. Therefore, exposing dentin to acidic environments contributes to the development of caries but also increases the chance of tooth fractures via fatigue-related failure and at lower mastication forces. The results of Lee and colleagues[19] showed that even a 15-second phosphoric acid etching treatment caused a reduction in the fatigue strength of dentin, which ultimately reduces the tooth's durability. This new understanding suggests that it may be prudent to explore the use of less aggressive acid etches for adhesives, or adhesives with the capacity to repair this damage. Alternatively, if bonding continues to be the mainstay of restorative dentistry, the development of nonacidic adhesives could be a viable approach.

SUMMARY

A review of the structure and properties of the tooth is presented with an emphasis on its durability. New findings indicate that the tooth's durability is reduced by cracks and other forms of damage that are introduced during restorative processes and that result from cyclic contact fatigue with opposing teeth, and especially with ceramic crowns. The potential for growth of this damage depends on the fatigue and fracture resistance of the dentin and enamel, as well as their spatial variations in the tooth. Removal of the decussated enamel and the extension of restorations into the deep dentin are detrimental to durability and not simply due to the reduction in tooth structure. Furthermore, there is greater understanding of the decreases in damage tolerance of dentin and enamel as a consequence of aging and by exposure to acid conditions. The knowledge in this area is growing and will be critical in making future improvements in restorative practices, as well as in extending the definition of lifelong oral health.

REFERENCES

1. Pashley DH. Dentin: a dynamic substrate-a review. Scanning Microsc 1989;3(1): 161–74 [discussion: 174–6].
2. Marshall GW Jr, Marshall SJ, Kinney JH, et al. The dentin substrate: structure and properties related to bonding. J Dent 1997;25(6):441–58.

3. Perdigao J, Swift EJ Jr, Denehy GE, et al. In vitro bond strengths and SEM evaluation of dentin bonding systems to different dentin substrates. J Dent Res 1994;73(1):44–55.
4. Tay FR, Pashley DH. Resin bonding to cervical sclerotic dentin: a review. J Dent 2004;32(3):173–96.
5. Kinney JH, Marshall SJ, Marshall GW. The mechanical properties of human dentin: a critical review and re-evaluation of the dental literature. Crit Rev Oral Biol Med 2003;14(1):13–29.
6. Arola D, Huang MP, Sultan MB. The failure of amalgam dental restorations due to cyclic fatigue crack growth. J Mater Sci Mater Med 1999;10(6):319–27.
7. Lubisich EB, Hilton TJ, Ferracane J. Cracked teeth: a review of the literature. J Esthet Restor Dent 2010;22(3):158–67.
8. Shemesh H, Bier CA, Wu MK, et al. The effects of canal preparation and filling on the incidence of dentinal defects. Int Endod J 2009;42(3):208–13.
9. Adorno CG, Yoshioka T, Jindan P, et al. The effect of endodontic procedures on apical crack initiation and propagation ex vivo. Int Endod J 2013;46:763–8.
10. Bürklein S, Tsotsis P, Schäfer E. Incidence of dentinal defects after root canal preparation: reciprocating versus rotary instrumentation. J Endod 2013;39(4):501–4.
11. Arias A, Lee YH, Peters CI, et al. Comparison of 2 canal preparation techniques in the induction of microcracks: a pilot study with cadaver mandibles. J Endod 2014;40(7):982–5.
12. De-Deus G, Silva EJ, Marins J, et al. Lack of causal relationship between dentinal microcracks and root canal preparation with reciprocation systems. J Endod 2014;40(9):1447–50.
13. De-Deus G, Belladonna FG, Souza EM, et al. Micro-computed tomographic assessment on the effect of proTaper next and twisted file adaptive systems on dentinal cracks. J Endod 2015;41(7):1116–9.
14. Staninec M, Meshkin N, Manesh SK, et al. Weakening of dentin from cracks resulting from laser irradiation. Dent Mater 2009;25(4):520–5.
15. Sehy C, Drummond JL. Micro-cracking of tooth structure. Am J Dent 2004;17(5):378–80.
16. Majd H, Viray J, Porter JA, et al. Degradation in the fatigue resistance of dentin by bur and abrasive air-jet preparations. J Dent Res 2012;91(9):894–9.
17. Majd B, Majd H, Porter JA, et al. Degradation in the fatigue strength of dentin by diamond bur preparations: importance of cutting direction. J Biomed Mater Res B Appl Biomater 2016;104(1):39–49.
18. Arola D. Fatigue testing of biomaterials and their interfaces. Dent Mater 2017;33(4):367–81.
19. Lee HH, Majd H, Orrego S, et al. Degradation in the fatigue strength of dentin by cutting, etching and adhesive bonding. Dent Mater 2014;30(9):1061–72.
20. Gao SS, An BB, Yahyazadehfar M, et al. Contact fatigue of human enamel: experiments, mechanisms and modeling. J Mech Behav Biomed Mater 2016;60:438–50.
21. Chai H. On the mechanical properties of tooth enamel under spherical indentation. Acta Biomater 2014;10(11):4852–60.
22. Shahmoradi M, Bertassoni LE, Elfallah HM, et al. Fundamental structure and properties of enamel, dentin and cementum. Advances in Calcium Phosphate Biomaterials. 2014;2(17):511–47.
23. Nanci A. Ten Cate's oral histology: development, structure, and function. 8th edition. Mosby-Year Book Inc; St Louis, MO, 2012.
24. Ivancik J, Naranjo M, Correa S, et al. Differences in the microstructure and fatigue properties of dentine between residents of North and South America. Arch Oral Biol 2014;59(10):1001–12.

25. Garberoglio R, Brännström M. Scanning electron microscopic investigation of human dentinal tubules. Arch Oral Biol 1976;21(6):355–62.
26. Schilke R, Lisson JA, Bauss O, et al. Comparison of the number and diameter of dentinal tubules in human and bovine dentine by scanning electron microscopic investigation. Arch Oral Biol 2000;45(5):355–61.
27. Coutinho ET, Moraes d'Almeida JR, Paciornik S. Evaluation of microstructural parameters of human dentin by digital image analysis. Mater Res 2007;10(2):153–9.
28. Carvalho RM, Fernandes CA, Villanueva R, et al. Tensile strength of human dentin as a function of tubule orientation and density. J Adhes Dent 2001;3(4):309–14.
29. Giannini M, Carvalho RM, Martins LR, et al. The influence of tubule density and area of solid dentin on bond strength of two adhesive systems to dentin. J Adhes Dent 2001;3(4):315–24.
30. Mannocci F, Pilecki P, Bertelli E, et al. Density of dentinal tubules affects the tensile strength of root dentin. Dent Mater 2004;20(3):293–6.
31. Arola D, Ivancik J, Majd H, et al. On the microstructure and mechanical behavior of radicular and coronal dentin. Endod Top 2009;20:30–51.
32. Montoya C, Arango-Santander S, Peláez-Vargas A, et al. Effect of aging on the microstructure, hardness and chemical composition of dentin. Arch Oral Biol 2015;60(12):1811–20.
33. Arola D, Bajaj D, Ivancik J, et al. Fatigue of biomaterials: Hard tissues. Int J Fatigue 2010;32(9):1400–12.
34. Robinson C, Kirkham J, Shore R. Dental enamel: formation to destruction. Boca Raton (FL): CRC Press; 1995. p. 151–2.
35. He LH, Swain MV. Understanding the mechanical behaviour of human enamel from its structural and compositional characteristics. J Mech Behav Biomed Mater 2008;1(1):18–29.
36. An B, Wang R, Zhang D. Role of crystal arrangement on the mechanical performance of enamel. Acta Biomater 2012;8(10):3784–93.
37. Macho GA, Jiang Y, Spears IR. Enamel microstructure–a truly three-dimensional structure. J Hum Evol 2003;45(1):81–90.
38. Lynch CD, O'Sullivan VR, Dockery P, et al. Hunter-Schreger Band patterns in human tooth enamel. J Anat 2010;217(2):106–15.
39. Bajaj D, Nazari A, Eidelman N, et al. A comparison of fatigue crack growth in human enamel and hydroxyapatite. Biomaterials 2008;29(36):4847–54.
40. Bajaj D, Arola D. Role of prism decussation on fatigue crack growth and fracture of human enamel. Acta Biomater 2009;5(8):3045–56.
41. Bechtle S, Habelitz S, Klocke A, et al. The fracture behaviour of dental enamel. Biomaterials 2010;31(2):375–84.
42. Yahyazadehfar M, Bajaj D, Arola DD. Hidden contributions of the enamel rods on the fracture resistance of human teeth. Acta Biomater 2013;9(1):4806–14.
43. Bertassoni LE, Orgel JP, Antipova O, et al. The dentin organic matrix–limitations of restorative dentistry hidden on the nanometer scale. Acta Biomater 2012;8(7):2419.
44. Bertassoni LE, Swain MV. The contribution of proteoglycans to the mechanical behavior of mineralized tissues. J Mech Behav Biomed Mater 2014;38:91–104.
45. Bertassoni LE, Kury M, Rathsam C, et al. The role of proteoglycans in the nanoindentation creep behavior of human dentin. J Mech Behav Biomed Mater 2015;55:264–70.
46. Goldberg M, Takagi M. Dentine proteoglycans: composition, ultrastructure and functions. Histochem J 1993;25(11):781–806.

47. Ji B, Gao H. Mechanical properties of nanostructure of biological materials. J Mech Phys Solids 2004;52(9):1963–90.
48. Elfallah HM, Bertassoni LE, Charadram N, et al. Effect of tooth bleaching agents on protein content and mechanical properties of dental enamel. Acta Biomater 2015;20:120–8.
49. Elfallah HM, Swain MV. A review of the effect of vital teeth bleaching on the mechanical properties of tooth enamel. N Z Dent J 2013;109(3):87–96.
50. Yahyazadehfar M, Arola D. The role of organic proteins on the crack growth resistance of human enamel. Acta Biomater 2015;19:33–45.
51. Jiang T, Ma X, Wang Y, et al. Investigation of the effects of 30% hydrogen peroxide on human tooth enamel by Raman scattering and laser-induced fluorescence. J Biomed Opt 2008;13(014019):1–9.
52. Zimmerman B, Datko L, Cupelli M, et al. Alteration of dentin-enamel mechanical properties due to dental whitening treatments. J Mech Behav Biomed Mater 2010;3(4):339–46.
53. Lubarsky GV, Lemoine P, Meenan BJ, et al. Enamel proteins mitigate mechanical and structural degradation in mature human enamel during acid attack. Mater Res Express 2014;1(2):1–20.
54. Reed R, Xu C, Liu Y, et al. Radiotherapy effect on nano-mechanical properties and chemical composition of enamel and dentin. Arch Oral Biol 2015;60(5): 690–7.
55. Arola D. Fracture and aging in dentin. In: Curtis R, Watson T, editors. Dental biomaterials: imaging, testing and modeling. Cambridge (United Kingdom): Woodhead Publishing; 2007. p. 314–42.
56. Kruzic JJ, Ritchie RO. Fatigue of mineralized tissues: cortical bone and dentin. J Mech Behav Biomed Mater 2008;1:3–17.
57. Ivancik J, Majd H, Bajaj D, et al. Contributions of aging to the fatigue crack growth resistance of human dentin. Acta Biomater 2012;8(7):2737–46.
58. Ivancik J, Neerchal NK, Romberg E, et al. The reduction in fatigue crack growth resistance of dentin with depth. J Dent Res 2011;90(8):1031–6.
59. Ivancik J, Arola DD. The importance of microstructural variations on the fracture toughness of human dentin. Biomaterials 2013;34(4):864–74.
60. Montoya C, Arola D, Ossa EA. Importance of tubule density to the fracture toughness of dentin. Arch Oral Biol 2016;67:9–14.
61. Yahyazadehfar M, Mutluay MM, Majd H, et al. Fatigue of the resin-enamel bonded interface and the mechanisms of failure. J Mech Behav Biomed Mater 2013;21: 121–32.
62. Arola D, Reprogel RK. Effects of aging on the mechanical behavior of human dentin. Biomaterials 2005;26(18):4051–61.
63. Imbeni V, Kruzic JJ, Marshall GW, et al. The dentin-enamel junction and the fracture of human teeth. Nat Mater 2005;4(3):229–32.
64. Bechtle S, Fett T, Rizzi G, et al. Crack arrest within teeth at the dentinoenamel junction caused by elastic modulus mismatch. Biomaterials 2010;31(14): 4238–47.
65. Yilmaz ED, Schneider GA, Swain MV. Influence of structural hierarchy on the fracture behaviour of tooth enamel. Philos Trans A Math Phys Eng Sci 2015;373(2038) [pii:20140130].
66. Yahyazadehfar M, Ivancik J, Majd H, et al. On the mechanics of fatigue and fracture in teeth. Appl Mech Rev 2014;66(3):0308031–3080319.
67. Rivera C, Arola D, Ossa A. Indentation damage and crack repair in human enamel. J Mech Behav Biomed Mater 2013;21:178–84.

68. Chai H, Lee JJ, Constantino PJ, et al. Remarkable resilience of teeth. Proc Natl Acad Sci U S A 2009;106(18):7289–93.
69. Myoung S, Lee J, Constantino P, et al. Morphology and fracture of enamel. J Biomech 2009;42(12):1947–51.
70. Porter AE, Nalla RK, Minor A, et al. A transmission electron microscopy study of mineralization in age-induced transparent dentin. Biomaterials 2005;26(36): 7650–60.
71. Kinney JH, Nalla RK, Pople JA, et al. Age-related transparent root dentin: mineral concentration, crystallite size, and mechanical properties. Biomaterials 2005; 26(16):3363–76.
72. Bajaj D, Sundaram N, Nazari A, et al. Age, dehydration and fatigue crack growth in dentin. Biomaterials 2006;27(11):2507–17.
73. Koester KJ, Ager JW 3rd, Ritchie RO. The effect of aging on crack-growth resistance and toughening mechanisms in human dentin. Biomaterials 2008;29(10): 1318–28.
74. Nazari A, Bajaj D, Zhang D, et al. Aging and the reduction in fracture toughness of human dentin. J Mech Behav Biomed Mater 2009;2(5):550–9.
75. Shinno Y, Ishimoto T, Saito M, et al. Comprehensive analyses of how tubule occlusion and advanced glycation end-products diminish strength of aged dentin. Sci Rep 2016;6:19849.
76. Bailey AJ. Molecular mechanisms of ageing in connective tissues. Mech Ageing Dev 2001;122:735–55.
77. Miura J, Nishikawa K, Kubo M, et al. Accumulation of advanced glycation end-products in human dentine. Arch Oral Biol 2014;59(2):119–24.
78. Park S, Wang DH, Dongsheng Z, et al. Mechanical properties of human enamel as a function of age and location in the tooth. J Mater Sci Mater Med 2008;19(6):2317–24.
79. Zheng Q, Xu H, Song F, et al. Spatial distribution of the human enamel fracture toughness with aging. J Mech Behav Biomed Mater 2013;26:148–54.
80. Park S, Quinn JB, Romberg E, et al. On the brittleness of enamel and selected dental materials. Dent Mater 2008;24(11):1477–85.
81. Yahyazadehfar M, Zhang D, Arola D. On the importance of aging to the crack growth resistance of human enamel. Acta Biomater 2016;32:264–74.
82. Bertacci A, Chersoni S, Davidson CL, et al. In vivo enamel fluid movement. Eur J Oral Sci 2007;115(3):169–73.
83. He B, Huang S, Zhang C, et al. Mineral densities and elemental content in different layers of healthy human enamel with varying teeth age. Arch Oral Biol 2011;56(10):997–1004.
84. Efeoglu N, Wood D, Efeoglu C. Microcomputerised tomography evaluation of 10% carbamide peroxide applied to enamel. J Dent 2005;33(7):561–7.
85. Wang X, Mihailova B, Klocke A, et al. Side effects of a non-peroxide-based home bleaching agent on dental enamel. J Biomed Mater Res A 2009;88(1):195–204.
86. Sakaguchi RL. Review of the current status and challenges for dental posterior restorative composites: clinical, chemistry, and physical behavior considerations. Dent Mater 2005;21(1):3–6.
87. Featherstone JD. The continuum of dental caries e evidence for a dynamic disease process. J Dent Res 2004;83(Spec Iss C):C39e42.
88. Do D, Orrego S, Majd H, et al. Accelerated fatigue of dentin with exposure to lactic acid. Biomaterials 2013;34(34):8650–9.
89. Orrego S, Xu HHK, Arola DD. Degradation in the fatigue crack growth resistance of human dentin by lactic acid. Mater Sci Eng C Mater Biol Appl 2017;73:716–25.

Bioactive Dental Composites and Bonding Agents Having Remineralizing and Antibacterial Characteristics

Ke Zhang, DDS, PhD[a,b], Ning Zhang, DDS, PhD[a,b],
Michael D. Weir, PhD[b], Mark A. Reynolds, DDS, PhD[b],
Yuxing Bai, DDS, PhD[a,*], Hockin H.K. Xu, PhD[b,c,d,*]

KEYWORDS

- Bioactive composites • Bonding agents • Antibacterial monomers
- Remineralization • Calcium phosphate nanoparticles • Silver nanoparticles
- Oral biofilms • Caries inhibition

KEY POINTS

- Secondary caries is a primary reason for restoration failures. It is beneficial to develop a new generation of bioactive composites and bonding agents with therapeutic functions.
- Calcium phosphate nanoparticles in composites and adhesives can remineralize existing lesions and inhibit future caries from occurring.
- Antibacterial resins can suppress biofilms and acid production. Protein-repellent resins can make it more difficult for bacteria to attach to the surface of dental materials.
- Combining multiple bioactive agents synergistically can lead to much greater reductions in oral biofilms than using a single agent, while also achieving remineralization.
- The new antibacterial and remineralizing dental materials not only possess cytotoxicity similar to existing dental monomers and resins but also can induce milder pulpal inflammation and facilitate the healing of dentin-pulp complex in animal models.

Disclosure statement: There is no conflict of interest for all authors.
Many of the studies cited in this article were supported by NIH R01DE17974 (HX), National Natural Science Foundation of China grant 81400540 (KZ), and a seed fund (HX) from the University of Maryland School of Dentistry.
[a] Department of Orthodontics, School of Stomatology, Capital Medical University, 4 Tiantanxili Street, Beijing 100050, China; [b] Department of Endodontics, Periodontics and Prosthodontics, University of Maryland School of Dentistry, Baltimore, MD 21201, USA; [c] Center for Stem Cell Biology & Regenerative Medicine, University of Maryland School of Medicine, 655 West Baltimore Street, Baltimore, MD 21201, USA; [d] Department of Mechanical Engineering, University of Maryland, Baltimore County, 1000 Hilltop Cir, Baltimore County, MD 21250, USA
* Corresponding authors. University of Maryland School of Dentistry, 650 West Baltimore Street, EPOD, Baltimore, MD 21704.
E-mail addresses: byuxing@263.net (Y.B.); hxu@umaryland.edu (H.H.K.X.)

Dent Clin N Am 61 (2017) 669–687
http://dx.doi.org/10.1016/j.cden.2017.05.002
dental.theclinics.com

INTRODUCTION

Dental caries is a prevalent disease worldwide and composites have become increasingly popular for restoring teeth damaged by caries, largely because of their esthetics.[1–7] Composite compositions and properties have been substantially improved, yielding longer clinical lifetimes.[8–14] Nonetheless, recurrent caries along the tooth-composite interfaces remains a predominant reason for failure and replacement of restorations.[15,16] A study showed that for class I composite restorations, secondary caries was the cause in 113 out of 129 cases of failure (88%), followed by fracture.[17] Another study showed that for class II restorations, secondary caries was a primary cause for failure (73.9%), followed by lost restorations (8.0%) and material fracture (5.3%).[18] Contributing factors to composite restoration failures include

1. Composites tend to accumulate more biofilms than other restorative materials.[19] "The percentage mutans streptococci of total colony-forming units (CFU) count in plaque was higher on composite (mean 13.7) and amalgam (mean 4.3) than on glass-ionomer (mean 1.1) restorations,"[20] "Resin composites inherently enhance bacterial growth," [21] and "There is a potential impact of composite resins on the ecology of microorganisms in the dental plaque biofilm" due to an increased biofilm buildup on composites.[22]
2. The composite-tooth bonded interface is the weak link of the restoration, often forming microgaps and allowing microleakage over time in vivo, providing a site for bacterial invasion that may lead to recurrent caries.[23–25]

To overcome these problems, efforts have been devoted to developing a new generation of bioactive dental materials containing additives that have remineralizing and antimicrobial capabilities.

DENTAL COMPOSITES AND ADHESIVES WITH REMINERALIZING PROPERTIES

Dental resins containing calcium phosphate (CaP) filler particles were developed with remineralizing capabilities.[26–30] The CaP particle sizes ranged from about 1 μm to 55 μm in traditional CaP-containing resins.[26–28] These composites released supersaturating levels of calcium (Ca) and phosphate (P) ions and were shown to remineralize tooth lesions in vitro.[26,27] One study showed that whisker-reinforced CaP composite, which was proposed for use in atraumatic restorative treatments, remineralized natural dentin and dentin with artificial caries.[31] To improve the load-bearing properties, a stronger barium-glass filler was also incorporated into a composite containing amorphous CaP (ACP), yielding improvement in flexural strength and elastic modulus, with no adverse influence on ion release profiles.[32]

One drawback of traditional CaP composites was that they were mechanically weak, with flexural strength about half that of unfilled resin.[26,27] A material with such a low strength was not acceptable for use as a restorative.[26] More recently, nanoparticles of CaP (NACP) of sizes of about 100 nm were synthesized via a spray-drying technique and loaded into dental resins.[29,30] The CaP nanocomposite achieved Ca and P ion releases similar to those of traditional CaP-containing composites, while possessing much greater mechanical properties.[29,30]

In an in vitro study,[33] enamel was first demineralized, then a composite containing NACP was used to remineralize the enamel lesions. A cyclic demineralization (pH 4) and remineralization (pH 7) regimen showed that NACP nanocomposite achieved an enamel remineralization that was 4-fold that of a commercial fluoride-releasing composite control.[33] This was likely because NACP neutralized the acid and raised the pH during demineralization, and enhanced remineralization by providing Ca and P ions.

Another study investigated the caries-inhibition effect of NACP composite via an in situ model in 25 human participants.[34] NACP composite substantially reduced caries formation in situ under oral biofilms that were supplied with sucrose 8 times per day to allow the biofilms to produce acids. The enamel mineral loss at the margins around NACP composite was only one-third of the mineral loss around the control composite (**Fig. 1**).[34] The mechanism for this caries reduction was likely the neutralizing effect of NACP on acids released by the biofilms, thereby protecting the tooth structures from demineralization. However, a major limitation of CaP-containing resins was that the Ca and P ion release was short-term, typically lasting for only a couple of months, which limits their commercialization potential. Recently, this shortcoming was

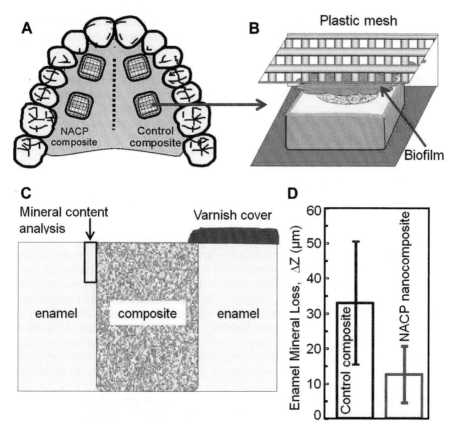

Fig. 1. Human in situ caries inhibition via NACP composite. (*A*) One hundred bovine enamel slabs of 5 × 5 × 2 mm were obtained. A cavity of 2 mm in diameter and 1.5 mm in depth was prepared and restored with a composite. Twenty-five volunteers wore palatal devices each containing 4 slabs: 2 filled with NACP nanocomposite on one side and 2 filled with control composite on the other side. (*B*) A plastic mesh with 1 mm space protected the biofilms in situ. (*C*) Enamel slabs were cut to sections for microradiography. (*D*) Enamel mineral loss around NACP nanocomposite was reduced to nearly one-third of that around control composite (*P*<.05). ([*A, B, C*] *From* Melo MA, Weir MD, Rodrigues LK, et al. Novel calcium phosphate nanocomposite with caries-inhibition in a human in situ model. Dent Mater 2013;29(2):233, with permission; and [*D*] *Adapted from* Melo MA, Weir MD, Rodrigues LK, et al. Novel calcium phosphate nanocomposite with caries-inhibition in a human in situ model. Dent Mater 2013;29(2):237, with permission.)

overcome with the development of novel rechargeable CaP-containing resins (see later discussion).

Besides composites, NACP have also been incorporated into dental adhesives.[35] NACP mass fractions of up to 40% were mixed into an adhesive without decreasing the dentin bond strength.[35] After acid-etching the dentin and during bonding, the small sizes of NACP allowed them to flow with the adhesive into dentinal tubules. Scanning electron microscopy (SEM) examination revealed many resin tags with numerous NACP infiltrated into the tubules. The NACP could release Ca and P ions to remineralize the remnants of lesions in the prepared tooth cavity, as well as neutralize acids and raise the local pH in the case of marginal gap formation and microleakage with bacterial invasion at the margins.[36] Indeed, a NACP composite was able to quickly raise the pH from a cariogenic pH of 4 to a safe pH of greater than 6, while other restorative materials, including a glass ionomer cement, failed to raise the pH to higher than 4.[36] Therefore, CaP-containing dental composites and adhesives with improved mechanical properties and remineralizing capabilities are promising candidates to combat recurrent caries.

With the purpose of enhancing the bonded interface durability, a study investigated the effect of NACP and an antibacterial monomer on dentin bonding after biofilm degradation.[37] The bonding agent and composite contained NACP, as well as other antibacterial agents. Twin resin-dentin bonded interface specimens were prepared using extracted human teeth. Flexural strength was evaluated after 1-day and 7-day water-storage and 7-day biofilm challenges. Cyclic loading of specimens was performed after 1-day water-storage and 7-day biofilm challenge using a universal testing system with a 4-point bending configuration. The results showed that biofilm challenge significantly reduced the flexural strength and fatigue resistance of the resin-dentin interface of the control group. However, the antibacterial and remineralizing materials were able to reduce the cariogenic impact of the biofilm, thereby improving the mechanical strength and fatigue resistance of the dentin-resin bonded interface.[37]

Besides NACP, sol-gel processed bioactive glasses (BAGs) that release calcium and phosphate ions have also been incorporated into dental restorative materials. Such experimental materials have also been tested for their antimicrobial effect against *Streptococcus sobrinus* (ATCC33478), *S mutans* (ATCC25175), and *Enterococcus faecalis* (ATCC19433).[38] Bacterial suspensions were independently incubated with BAG in particulate form (<3 μm) for 4 and 24 hours. Viability was determined by CFUs. At 4 hours, all BAG groups produced an order of magnitude reduction in all 3 types of bacteria. After 24 hours, all BAG groups produced a significant reduction in *S sobrinus* colonies but no further reduction in *S mutans*. BAG groups also significantly reduced *E faecalis* compared with the control. At 4 hours, an increase in the pH was noted for the BAG groups (to pH 9) that could also have contributed to the bactericidal effect.[38] In addition, a separate study examined the effect of BAG incorporation in a composite on bacterial biofilms penetrating into marginal gaps of simulated tooth fillings in vitro during cyclic mechanical loading.[39] The results showed that the average depth of bacterial penetration into the marginal gap for the BAG group was significantly less than that without BAG. Hence, dental composite incorporating BAG may be promising to hinder the development and propagation of recurrent caries at the tooth-restoration interfaces.[39]

In addition to composites and adhesives, several calcium silicate cements are commercially available for direct and indirect pulp-capping treatment. Biodentine (Septodont, Lancaster, PA, USA) is used for pulp capping, permanent dentin restorations, temporary enamel restorations, and so forth. It contains tricalcium silicate, dicalcium silicate, and calcium carbonate as fillers, polycarboxylate as a water-reducing agent, and calcium chloride as an accelerator. Biodentine has a relatively rapid setting time of 9 to 12 minutes, which helps minimize potential premature dissolution of the cement. Furthermore, effective sealing is obtained via micromechanical interlocking of crystals in the dentin tubules. Like other calcium silicate cements, Biodentine exhibits significant calcium ion release and the ability to increase the local pH. Biodentine can induce the formation of dentin bridges and the repair of pulpal tissues. In addition, an alternate approach is to combine the ion-releasing, sealing, and dentin-repairing aspects of calcium-silicate cements with light-cured resin systems. Materials such as TheraCal (BISCO Dental Products, Schaumburg, IL, USA) contain calcium silicate, fumed silica, and photopolymerizable methacrylate resins, and can be used for direct and indirect pulp capping and as a liner under other restorative materials. TheraCal is effective at sealing the dental pulp area and has a rapid setting time due to light-curing properties. The rapid setting time is important because it prevents premature dissolution of unset material, which can occur with traditional calcium silicate cements. Another commercial product, ACTIVA (Pulpdent, Watertown, MA, USA), has been used as a base or liner, as well as in bulk fill, post, and core build up procedures. ACTIVA consists of a resin-modified glass ionomer, a proprietary bioactive ionic resin, a rubberized resin, and is photopolymerizable. This composition allows for the release of calcium, phosphate, and fluoride; enhances wear-resistance and fracture-resistance; protects against microleakage; and has antibacterial properties. In addition, an antibacterial methacryloyloxydodecylpyridinium bromide (MDPB)-based bonding agent, Clearfil Protect Bond (Kuraray Dental, New York, NY, USA), is also available for clinical use. Therefore, new bioactive materials are gradually being commercialized as the dental industry finds these antibacterial and remineralizing functions worthy of pursuit.

RECHARGEABLE COMPOSITE AND ADHESIVE WITH LONG-TERM CALCIUM OR PHOSPHATE ION RELEASE

A major drawback of CaP composites is that the Ca and P ion release lasts for only weeks to months, and then diminishes over time.[26–30] However, to have practical implications in vivo, the CaP-containing restoration needs to be effective for much longer than a few months and, in fact, must continue to release Ca and P ions to suppress enamel and dentin demineralization for many years. Therefore, it would be highly desirable for the CaP composite to be able to repeatedly recharge and re-release Ca and P ions, thereby providing these ions indefinitely with long-term caries-inhibition capability.

Recently, an experimental rechargeable CaP dental composite was developed.[40] Three NACP nanocomposites were tested using resins including

1. Bisphenol A glycidyl dimethacrylate (BisGMA) and triethylene glycol dimethacrylate (TEGDMA)
2. Pyromellitic glycerol dimethacrylate (PMGDM) and ethoxylated bisphenol A dimethacrylate, together referred to as PE group
3. BisGMA, TEGDMA, and Bis[2-(methacryloyloxy)ethyl] phosphate (BisMEP).

BisGMA and TEGDMA were frequently used in dental resins. PMGDM and BisMEP were selected because both are acidic adhesive monomers and may chelate with Ca and P ions from a recharge solution to achieve the recharge capability. For each group, the Ca and P ion release was first exhausted, then the exhausted specimens were recharged to measure the re-release for 7 days as 1 cycle. This was then repeated for 6 cycles as described in **Fig. 2**A. The results (**Fig. 2**B) showed that the ion recharge capability was the greatest for PE group. For each recharge cycle, the

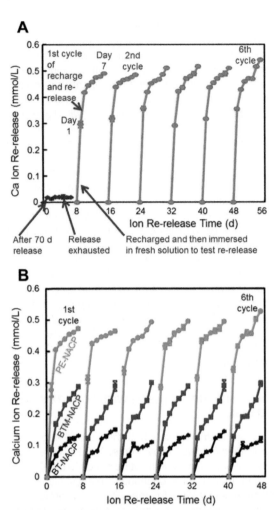

Fig. 2. Rechargeable NACP composite for long-term Ca and P ion release. (*A*) NACP composite was immersed in a pH 4 solution for 70 days to exhaust the ion release (*lower left arrow*). Then the specimens were immersed in a new pH 4 solution to confirm that the ion release was exhausted (*lower middle arrow*). Specimens were recharged in a recharge solution, then tested for ion re-release for 7 days (third *arrow* at the bottom of A). This constituted the first recharge and re-release cycle. This process was repeated for 6 cycles. (*B*) Three NACP nanocomposites with 6 cycles of recharge and re-release, showing no decrease in ion release with increasing recharge cycles (*P*>.1). (*From* Zhang L, Weir MD, Chow LC, et al. Novel rechargeable calcium phosphate dental nanocomposite. Dent Mater 2016;32(2):288, with permission; and Zhang L, Weir MD, Chow LC, et al. Novel rechargeable calcium phosphate dental nanocomposite. Dent Mater 2016;32(2):289; with permission.)

ion re-release reached similarly high levels, showing that the ion re-release did not decrease with increasing the number of recharge cycles.[40]

In addition, a rechargeable CaP bonding agent was also developed with the purpose of suppressing recurrent caries at the bonded tooth-restoration interfaces.[41] The Ca and P ion release from the adhesive resin remained high and did not decrease with increasing the number of recharge and re-release cycles. After the third recharge cycle, specimens without any further recharge exhibited a continuous Ca and P ion release for 2 to 3 weeks.[41] Therefore, it seemed to be possible to recharge the restoration only once per week to have sustained ion re-release for at least a week. These results demonstrated the potential for sustained Ca and P ion release for an NACP nanocomposite and NACP adhesive to potentially achieve a long-term caries-inhibition capability.

ANTIBACTERIAL DENTAL COMPOSITES AND BONDING AGENTS

Dental caries is one of the most common bacterial infections in humans and is a dietary carbohydrate-modified bacterial infectious disease.[42] Tooth demineralization is caused by acid generated by bacterial biofilms (dental plaque) in the presence of fermentable carbohydrates.[43] One approach to this problem has been the development and synthesis of antibacterial quaternary ammonium methacrylates (QAMs) and their incorporation into resins for use in dental restorative systems.[44-49] Pioneering work by Imazato and colleagues[50] yielded MDPB, which could be copolymerized and covalently bonded in the resin matrix, thus becoming immobilized to provide long-term contact-inhibition against oral bacteria.[51] A commercially available MDPB-containing bonding agent, Clearfil Protect Bond, was shown to possess potent antibacterial activity against S mutans, Lactobacillus casei, and Actinomyces naeslundii, and was able to eradicate residual bacterial inside dentinal tubules of prepared tooth cavities.[50] In addition, several other antimicrobial formulations were also developed, including a methacryloxylethyl cetyl dimethyl ammonium chloride containing adhesive,[52] quaternary ammonium polyethylenimine, nanoparticles for antimicrobial dental composites,[53] antibacterial glass ionomer cements,[54] and antibacterial nanocomposites and bonding agents incorporating a quaternary ammonium dimethacrylate.[55-57] Besides composites, bonding agents are important in adhering resin-based restorations to tooth structures.[24,58] Previous studies have greatly enhanced the bonding agent compositions and procedures, leading to greater tooth-restoration bond strengths.[24,59-63] To reduce caries at the tooth-restoration margins, antibacterial bonding agents were formulated.[50-52] They can kill the residual bacteria in the prepared tooth cavity, and inhibit new bacteria at the tooth-restoration interfaces when marginal leakage occurs.[44,50,51] Several meritorious antibacterial bonding agents containing QAMs were shown to effectively suppress bacteria attachment and substantially reduce biofilm growth.[44,50,51,56,57,64,65]

QAM resins possess positively charged quaternary amine N⁺, which can interact with the negatively charged membrane of bacteria, leading to membrane disruption and cytoplasmic leakage.[53] It is postulated that long-chained quaternary ammonium compounds can be especially effective by inserting into the bacterial membrane, resulting in physical disruption and bacteria death.[66] One study developed antimicrobial glass ionomer materials that showed stronger antimicrobial activity with increasing alkyl chain length (CL).[54] A recent study on bonding agents demonstrated that the oral biofilm viability and CFU counts were substantially decreased with increasing alkyl CL.[67] This was also shown in a dental composite in which a dental plaque microcosm biofilm model using human saliva was used to evaluate the antibacterial activity.[68] QAM incorporation did not compromise the flexural strength and elastic modulus of the NACP nanocomposites. Increasing the CL from 3 to 16 greatly enhanced the antibacterial activity of NACP nanocomposite, and a nanocomposite with CL16 reduced the biofilm CFU counts of total microorganisms, total streptococci, and mutans streptococci by 2 orders of magnitude (**Fig. 3**).[68] The NACP

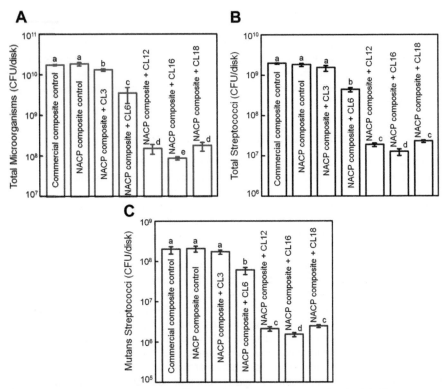

Fig. 3. Dental plaque microcosm biofilm model with CFU counts of 2-day biofilms on composites: (*A*) total microorganisms, (*B*) total streptococci, and (*C*) mutans streptococci (mean ± SD; n = 6). In each plot, values with dissimilar letters are significantly different from each other (*P*<.05). The 2 control composites had the highest CFU counts. Increasing CL from 3 to 16 decreased the CFU counts significantly (*P*<.05). Note the log scale for the Y-axis. (*Adapted from* Zhang K, Cheng L, Weir MD, et al. Effects of quaternary ammonium chain length on the antibacterial and remineralizing effects of a calcium phosphate nanocomposite. Int J Oral Sci 2016;8(1):50; with permission.)

nanocomposite containing the antibacterial monomer with CL16 seemed to be promising to obtain the double benefits of being antibacterial and having remineralization capabilities to combat caries.

To further increase the antibacterial potency, an antibacterial monomer dimethyla-minododecyl methacrylate (DMADDM) was combined with nanoparticles of silver (NAg) in an experimental bonding agent containing NACP.[69] Due to the small size of NACP and NAg, these nanoparticles readily flowed into dentinal tubules to form resin tags (**Fig. 4**A–C),[69] which could potentially kill residual bacteria in the tubules and remineralize the remnants of caries-damaged tissues in the prepared tooth cavity.[64,69,70] The strong antibacterial activity was maintained during 6 months of water-aging, with no decrease in the killing potency at 6 months, compared with that at 1 day.[69] During the 6 months of water-aging, a commercial bonding agent control lost 35% of the dentin bond strength (see **Fig. 4**D).[69] However, the new antibacterial bonding agents showed no loss in dentin bond strength over 6 months, likely due to the antienzyme properties and the inhibition of matrix metalloproteinases, thereby protecting the hybrid layer via the antibacterial monomer.[71–74] Therefore, the new

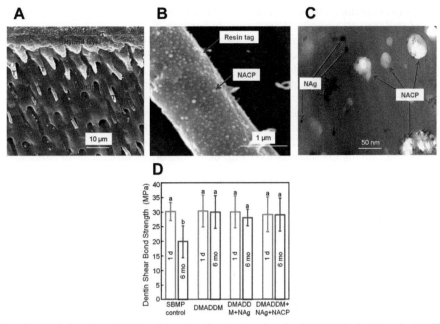

Fig. 4. Dentin bonding. (*A*) SEM of dentin-adhesive interface for DMADDM plus NAg plus NACP group (T, resin tag). (*B*) Higher magnification SEM of a resin tag showing NACP in tubules. (*C*) Higher magnification TEM indicating NAg and NACP in resin tag. (*D*) Dentin shear bond strengths (mean ± SD; n = 10). Dissimilar letters indicate significantly different values (*P*<.05). There was a 35% loss in bond strength for commercial group in water-aging for 6 months. There was no bond strength loss for groups containing DMADDM, NAg, and NACP. (*From* Zhang K, Cheng L, Wu EJ, et al. Effect of water-aging on dentin bond strength and anti-biofilm activity of bonding agent containing new monomer dimethylaminododecyl methacrylate. J Dent 2013;41(6):508; with permission.)

antibacterial bonding agent shows promise to inhibit biofilms and caries at the margins, with the potential to provide a stronger and longer-lasting bonded interface, in addition to the potential remineralization effect from NACP.

PROTEIN REPELLENT AND ANTIBACTERIAL COMPOSITES, ADHESIVES, AND CEMENTS

A dental resin, when placed in the oral environment in the presence of normal salivary flow, is quickly coated with a pellicle that is comprised of a layer of selectively adsorbed salivary proteins.[75] Early colonizing oral bacteria, such as mutans streptococci, adhere to resin and tooth surfaces via this layer, and this is the initial step in biofilm formation.[76] Therefore, it would be highly desirable to develop a new composite that can repel proteins, thereby hindering bacterial attachment. To this end, poly(ethylene glycol) and 2 pyridinium group-containing methacrylate monomers were immobilized to silicon wafer surfaces to achieve protein-repellent activity.[77] Hydrophilic surfaces are usually more resistant to protein adsorption and bacterial adhesion than hydrophobic surfaces. 2-methacryloyloxyethyl phosphorylcholine (MPC) is a methacrylate with a phospholipid polar group in the side chain, and is among the most common biocompatible and hydrophilic biomedical polymers.[78] MPC shows excellent resistance to protein adsorption and bacterial adhesion, and has been used in artificial blood vessels, artificial hip joints, and microfluidic devices.[78–82] The

MPC polymer coating renders the surfaces extremely hydrophilic, prevents the adhesion of proteins, and inhibits the adhesion of bacteria.[78–80]

Recently, MPC was incorporated into an experimental dental composite to render it protein-repellent.[83] Incorporation of 3% MPC and 1.5% dimethylaminohexadecyl methacrylate (DMAHDM) into the composite achieved protein-repellent and antibacterial capabilities without compromising the mechanical properties. The composite showed protein adsorption that was only one-tenth that of a commercial composite (**Fig. 5**A).[83] Lactic acid production by biofilms formed on the material was also greatly reduced (see **Fig. 5**B). The biofilm CFU on the composite with 3% MPC plus 1.5% DMAHDM was more than 3 orders of magnitude lower than that of the commercial control (see **Fig. 5**C). Further, incorporation of MPC and

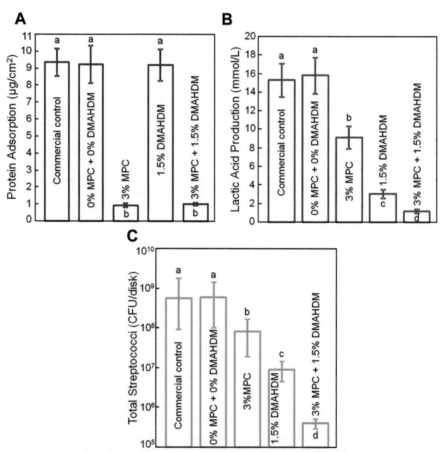

Fig. 5. Protein-repellent. (*A*) Bovine serum albumin adsorption onto composite surface. The composite with 3% MPC and the composite with 3% MPC plus 1.5% DMAHDM both had protein adsorption about 1/10 that of commercial composite. In each plot, dissimilar letters indicate significantly different values (*P*<.05). (*B*) Lactic acid production by biofilms was greatly reduced via MPC and DMAHDM. (*C*) Biofilm total streptococci CFU on composite with 3% MPC plus 1.5% DMAHDM was more than 3 orders of magnitude lower than commercial control. (*Adapted from* Zhang N, Ma J, Melo MA, et al. Protein-repellent and antibacterial dental composite to inhibit biofilms and caries. J Dent 2015;43(2):229–31; with permission.)

DMAHDM achieved biofilm reduction efficacy that was much greater than that using MPC or DMAHDM alone.[83] The reason for the synergistic effect obtained when using MPC and DMAHDM together is likely that the salivary protein coating on resin surfaces in vivo could reduce the contact-inhibition efficacy of DMAHDM. Hence, due to the protein-repellent function of MPC, the resin surface had adsorbed much less protein and, therefore, was more exposed to direct contact against bacteria and their biofilms, thereby increasing the contact-inhibition efficacy of DMAHDM. Therefore, using MPC plus DMAHDM together may have wide applicability to other dental materials.

In addition to restorative composites, a bonding agent incorporating combined MPC and DMAHDM has also been tested.[84] Adding 7.5% MPC and 5% DMAHDM into the primer and adhesive did not adversely affect the dentin shear bond strength, whereas the protein adsorption was nearly 20-fold less than that of a control. Biofilm CFU on the resin with 7.5% MPC plus 5% DMAHDM was 4 orders of magnitude less than that of the control.[84] Consistent with the results obtained for the composite,[83] the use of double agents (protein-repellent MPC plus antibacterial DMAHDM) synergistically in the dental adhesive achieved much stronger inhibition of biofilms than using each agent alone.

The protein-repellent method was further applied to developing a bioactive orthodontic cement.[85] Orthodontic treatments often cause white spot lesions in enamel due to biofilm accumulation and acid production.[86] Resin-modified glass ionomer cements (RMGIs) possess fluoride release and clinically acceptable enamel bond strength, and have been used as orthodontic cements.[87] However, white spot lesions around orthodontic brackets are still common, which jeopardizes the health and esthetics of the teeth. This indicates that fluoride ions alone cannot prevent enamel demineralization.[86] In a recent study, 4 bioactive agents (MPC, DMAHDM, NAg, and NACP) were incorporated into an RMGI.[85] The incorporation of MPC into RMGI reduced the protein adsorption by an order of magnitude. Via DMAHDM and NAg, the biofilm CFU was reduced by 3 orders of magnitude. This method seemed to be promising to yield a protein-repellent, antibacterial, and remineralizing orthodontic cement.[85] The combined use of 4 bioactive agents (MPC, DMAHDM, NAg, and NACP) may lead to the prevention of enamel white spot lesions, as well as caries-inhibition effects in other dental materials systems, which warrants further in vitro and in vivo investigations.

BIOCOMPATIBILITY OF ANTIBACTERIAL AND REMINERALIZING RESINS

For novel bioactive materials to be used in tooth restorations in patients, investigations are needed to ensure that the new materials are noncytotoxic and compatible with the dentin-pulp complex. Several studies have investigated the biocompatibility of antibacterial monomers and resins.[88–91] MDPB was shown to have a relatively low level of toxicity to human pulpal cells, with a cytotoxicity similar to the dimethacrylate monomer, TEGDMA, which has long been used in dentistry.[88] Another study showed that MDPB incorporation into a primer did not cause an increase in toxicity to pulpal cells.[89] Another study compared the cytotoxicity of MDPB with BisGMA, and showed that the inhibitory effects of MDPB on the proliferation and mineralization of odontoblast-like MDPC-23 rodent-derived cells were lower than BisGMA, indicating that MDPB was less cytotoxic than BisGMA.[90] In addition, an in vivo study investigated MDPB-containing primer in tooth cavities in dogs.[92] The results showed that restorations with experimental primer containing MDPB caused little or no pulpal inflammation in vivo.[92]

These results are consistent with a report on DMADDM that had a median lethal concentration of between 20 to 40 µg/mL, about 20-fold higher than that of a BisGMA control, indicating that DMADDM had a much lower cytotoxicity than BisGMA.[91] Another study tested the in vitro cytotoxicity of a series of QAMs including DMAHDM against human gingival fibroblasts and odontoblast-like MDPC-23 cells.[67] The results showed that increasing monomer concentration increased the cytotoxicity, and increasing the CL also increased the cytotoxicity. However, all the tested antibacterial monomers had less cytotoxicity than BisGMA, and similar cytotoxicity to those of 2-hydroxyethyl methacrylate (HEMA) and TEGDMA.[67] Furthermore, the testing using eluents from the polymerized resin specimens containing QAMs also showed that the fibroblast and odontoblast cytotoxicity was similar to commercial dental resin controls (without QAMs).[67]

Most studies evaluating the biocompatibility of antibacterial dental monomers have been conducted in vitro. However, several animal studies have also been performed, using models with monkeys,[93] dogs,[94] ferrets,[95] and rats.[96] Ethical and cost considerations make rodent models more preferable. A study showed that, after pulp-capping, the rat molar pulp healing was histologically similar to that in humans and other animal species.[96] Several studies used rats with maxillary molar models to examine class I[96] and class V restorations.[97] A recent study investigated antibacterial and remineralizing restorations containing DMADDM and NACP in a rat tooth cavity model.[98] NACP and DMADDM were incorporated into a composite and an adhesive. Four types of restorations were tested:

1. Control composite and control adhesive
2. Control composite plus DMADDM, and control adhesive plus DMADDM
3. Control composite plus NACP, and control adhesive plus NACP
4. Control composite plus DMADDM plus NACP, control adhesive plus DMADDM plus NACP.[98]

Occlusal deep cavities were prepared in the first molars of rats and restored with one of the 4 groups (**Fig. 6**A, B). The NACP group and DMADDM plus NACP group showed less inflammatory response in the pulp, with more tertiary dentin formation, than the control (see **Figs. 6**C, D). At 30 days, the NACP group and DMADDM plus NACP group had tertiary dentin thickness (TDT) that was 4 to 6 times that of the control (see **Fig. 6**E).[98] Groups with or without DMADDM had similar pulpal responses and tertiary TDT, indicating that DMADDM had no significant effect on pulpal inflammation and TDT. All the samples containing NACP, whether with or without DMADDM, yielded milder pulpal inflammation and much greater TDT, indicating that the presence of NACP was beneficial to the pulp, likely due to Ca and P ion release.[98] Therefore, the combined use of NACP and DMADDM in composites and adhesives are promising as a new therapeutic restorative system with the potential to not only combat oral pathogens and cariogenic biofilm acids but also facilitate the healing of the dentin-pulp complex.[98]

Regarding future work, although current restorative materials are relatively inert and replace the missing tooth structures, it would be highly desirable for future restorative materials to not only replace the missing tooth volume but also be bioactive and possess beneficial therapeutic properties. The development of new bioactive restorative materials, including remineralizing and antibacterial characteristics, although still in a relatively early stage, has achieved significant progress. Nonetheless, further studies are needed to improve and optimize the new bioactive materials, and investigate their antibacterial and remineralization efficacy in human in situ or in vivo models under clinically relevant conditions. More studies are also needed to thoroughly understand the remineralizing and antibacterial mechanisms and systematically establish the structure-property-clinical performance relationships for the new class of bioactive restorative materials.

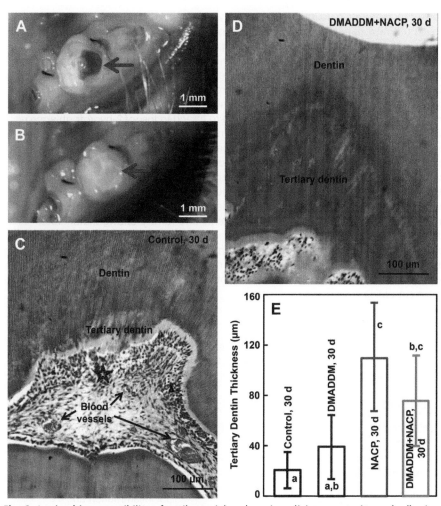

Fig. 6. In vivo biocompatibility of antibacterial and remineralizing composite and adhesive. (*A*) Rat tooth model (*arrow*), in which the right and left molars were used. (*B*) Occlusal cavity (*arrow*) was restored with bonding agent and composite. (*C*) Hematoxylin-eosin stain (H&E) at 30 days for control. Star indicates inflammatory cells and blood vessels by arrows. Control group exhibited slight inflammation. (*D*) H&E at 30 days for DMADDM plus NACP. NACP group and DMADDM plus NACP group showed normal pulp without inflammatory response, along with greater tertiary dentin thicknesses. (*E*) Tertiary dentin thickness data. Different letters indicate significantly different values (*P*<.05) . ([*A, B, E*] *Adapted from* Li F, Wang P, Weir MD, et al. Evaluation of antibacterial and remineralizing nanocomposite and adhesive in rat tooth cavity model. Acta Biomater 2014;10(6):2806–11, with permission; and [*C, D*] *From* Li F, Wang P, Weir MD, et al. Evaluation of antibacterial and remineralizing nanocomposite and adhesive in rat tooth cavity model. Acta Biomater 2014;10(6):2810, with permission.)

SUMMARY

Currently available dental composites and bonding agents are typically bioinert and replace the missing volume of the tooth but lack bioactivity to interact with either oral bacteria or pulp cells, despite biofilm acids and recurrent caries being a major cause of restoration failures. Several key approaches are being investigated to develop a new generation of bioactive dental composites and bonding agents with therapeutic functions. One approach incorporates NACP into composites and adhesives to remineralize existing lesions and inhibit future caries from occurring. A second approach develops antibacterial composites and bonding agents by copolymerizing QAMs in resins, to suppress biofilm growth and acid production. A third approach imparts a protein-repellent capability to resins, to repel proteins from the surface, thereby making it more difficult for bacteria to attach to the surface. A forth approach combines multiple bioactive agents for synergistic effects. For example, the use of both protein-repellent and antibacterial agents has been shown to result in a much greater reduction in biofilm growth than using a single agent alone. Furthermore, combining NACP with protein-repellent and antibacterial agents could yield a resin with not only much less biofilm plaque buildup and acid production but also with remineralization and acid-neutralizing capabilities. In vitro cell studies and in vivo animal models have indicated that these antibacterial and remineralizing materials not only possess cytotoxicity similar to, or less than, existing dental monomers and resins but also induce milder pulpal inflammation and facilitate the healing of the dentin-pulp complex. This new class of bioactive materials with remineralizing and antibacterial properties is promising to reverse tooth decay, regain lost minerals, and inhibit recurrent caries.

ACKNOWLEDGMENTS

We thank Drs Lei Cheng, Mary Anne S. Melo, Satoshi Imazato, Jack Ferracane, Ashraf F. Fouad, Joseph M. Antonucci, Nancy J. Lin, Sheng Lin-Gibson, Laurence C. Chow, Xianju Xie, Ling Zhang, Fang Li, and Lin Wang for discussions and experimental help.

REFERENCES

1. Bayne SC, Thompson JY, Swift EJ, et al. A characterization of first-generation flowable composites. J Am Dent Assoc 1998;129:567–77.
2. Watts DC, Marouf AS, Al-Hindi AM. Photo-polymerization shrinkage-stress kinetics in resin-composites: methods development. Dent Mater 2003;19:1–11.
3. Drummond JL. Degradation, fatigue, and failure of resin dental composite materials. J Dent Res 2008;87:710–9.
4. Lynch CD. Successful posterior composites. London: Quintessence Publishing Co.; 2008.
5. Ferracane JL. Resin composite - state of the art. Dent Mater 2011;27:29–38.
6. Demarco FF, Correa MB, Cenci MS, et al. Longevity of posterior composite restorations: not only a matter of materials. Dent Mater 2012;28:87–101.
7. Ferracane JL, Hilton TJ. Polymerization stress–is it clinically meaningful? Dent Mater 2016;32:1–10.
8. Xu X, Burgess JO. Compressive strength, fluoride release and recharge of fluoride-releasing materials. Biomaterials 2003;24:2451–61.
9. Samuel SP, Li S, Mukherjee I, et al. Mechanical properties of experimental dental composites containing a combination of mesoporous and nonporous spherical silica as fillers. Dent Mater 2009;25:296–301.
10. Milward PJ, Adusei GO, Lynch CD. Improving some selected properties of dental polyacid-modified composite resins. Dent Mater 2011;27:997–1002.
11. Hosoya Y, Shiraishi T, Odatsu T, et al. Effects of polishing on surface roughness, gloss, and color of resin composites. J Oral Sci 2011;53:283–91.

12. Wei YJ, Silikas N, Zhang ZT, et al. Hygroscopic dimensional changes of self-adhering and new resin-matrix composites during water sorption/desorption cycles. Dent Mater 2011;27:259–66.
13. Ferracane JL, Giannobile WV. Novel biomaterials and technologies for the dental, oral, and craniofacial structures. J Dent Res 2014;93:1185–6.
14. Stansbury JW, Idacavage MJ. 3D printing with polymers: challenges among expanding options and opportunities. Dent Mater 2016;32:54–64.
15. Deligeorgi V, Mjor IA, Wilson NH. An overview of reasons for the placement and replacement of restorations. Prim Dent Care 2001;8:5–11.
16. National Institute of Dental and Craniofacial Research (NIDCR) announcement # 13-DE-102, Dental Resin Composites and Caries, March 5, 2009.
17. Pallesen U, van Dijken JW, Halken J, et al. A prospective 8-year follow-up of posterior resin composite restorations in permanent teeth of children and adolescents in Public Dental Health Service: reasons for replacement. Clin Oral Investig 2014;18:819–27.
18. Bernardo M, Luis H, Martin MD, et al. Survival and reasons for failure of amalgam versus composite posterior restorations placed in a randomized clinical trial. J Am Dent Assoc 2007;138:775–83.
19. Bourbia M, Ma D, Cvitkovitch DG, et al. Cariogenic bacteria degrade dental resin composites and adhesives. J Dent Res 2013;92:989–94.
20. Svanberg M, Major IA, Ørstavik D. Mutans streptococci in plaque from margins of amalgam, composite and glass ionomer restorations. J Dent Res 1990;69:861–4.
21. Beyth N, Bahir R, Matalon S, et al. Streptococcus mutans biofilm changes surface-topography of resin composites. Dent Mater 2008;24:732–6.
22. Khalichi P, Singh J, Cvitkovitch DG, et al. The influence of triethylene glycol derived from dental composite resins on the regulation of Streptococcus mutans gene expression. Biomaterials 2009;30:452–9.
23. Breschi L, Mazzoni A, Ruggeri A, et al. Dental adhesion review: aging and stability of the bonded interface. Dent Mater 2008;24:90–101.
24. Spencer P, Ye Q, Park JG, et al. Adhesive/dentin interface: the weak link in the composite restoration. Ann Biomed Eng 2010;38:1989–2003.
25. Khvostenko D, Salehi S, Naleway SE, et al. Cyclic mechanical loading promotes bacterial penetration along composite restoration marginal gaps. Dent Mater 2015;31:702–10.
26. Skrtic D, Antonucci JM, Eanes ED, et al. Physiological evaluation of bioactive polymeric composites based on hybrid amorphous calcium phosphates. J Biomed Mater Res 2000;53B:381–91.
27. Dickens SH, Flaim GM, Takagi S. Mechanical properties and biochemical activity of remineralizing resin-based Ca-PO$_4$ cements. Dent Mater 2003;19:558–66.
28. Langhorst SE, O'Donnell JNR, Skrtic D. In vitro remineralization of enamel by polymeric amorphous calcium phosphate composite: quantitative microradiographic study. Dent Mater 2009;25:884–91.
29. Xu HHK, Sun L, Weir MD, et al. Nano dicalcium phosphate anhydrous-whisker composites with high strength and Ca and PO$_4$ release. J Dent Res 2006;85:722–7.
30. Xu HHK, Weir MD, Sun L, et al. Strong nanocomposites with Ca, PO$_4$ and F release for caries inhibition. J Dent Res 2010;89:19–28.
31. Yang B, Flaim G, Dickens SH. Remineralization of human natural caries and artificial caries-like lesions with an experimental whisker-reinforced ART composite. Acta Biomater 2011;7:2303–9.

32. Marovic D, Tarle Z, Hiller KA, et al. Reinforcement of experimental composite materials based on amorphous calcium phosphate with inert fillers. Dent Mater 2014;30:1052–60.
33. Weir MD, Chow LC, Xu HHK. Remineralization of demineralized enamel via calcium phosphate nanocomposite. J Dent Res 2012;91:979–84.
34. Melo MA, Weir MD, Rodrigues LK, et al. Novel calcium phosphate nanocomposite with caries-inhibition in a human in situ model. Dent Mater 2013;29:231–40.
35. Melo MA, Cheng L, Zhang K, et al. Novel dental adhesives containing nanoparticles of silver and amorphous calcium phosphate. Dent Mater 2013;29:199–210.
36. Moreau JL, Sun L, Chow LC, et al. Mechanical and acid neutralizing properties and inhibition of bacterial growth of amorphous calcium phosphate dental nanocomposite. J Biomed Mater Res B Appl Biomater 2011;98:80–8.
37. Melo MA, Orrego S, Weir MD, et al. Designing multiagent dental materials for enhanced resistance to biofilm damage at the bonded interface. ACS Appl Mater Interfaces 2016;8(18):11779–87.
38. Salehi S, Davis HB, Ferracane JL, et al. Sol-gel-derived bioactive glasses demonstrate antimicrobial effects on common oral bacteria. Am J Dent 2015;28:111–5.
39. Khvostenko D, Hilton TJ, Ferracane JL, et al. Bioactive glass fillers reduce bacterial penetration into marginal gaps for composite restorations. Dent Mater 2016;32:73–81.
40. Zhang L, Weir MD, Chow LC, et al. Novel rechargeable calcium phosphate dental nanocomposite. Dent Mater 2016;32:285–93.
41. Zhang L, Weir MD, Hack G, et al. Rechargeable dental adhesive with calcium phosphate nanoparticles for long-term ion release to inhibit caries. J Dent 2015;43:1587–95.
42. ten Cate JM. Biofilms, a new approach to the microbiology of dental plaque. Odontology 2006;94:1–9.
43. Totiam P, Gonzalez-Cabezas C, Fontana MR, et al. A new in vitro model to study the relationship of gap size and secondary caries. Caries Res 2007;41:467–73.
44. Imazato S, Ehara A, Torii M, et al. Antibacterial activity of dentine primer containing MDPB after curing. J Dent 1998;26:267–71.
45. Imazato S. Bio-active restorative materials with antibacterial effects: new dimension of innovation in restorative dentistry. Dent Mater J 2009;28:11–9.
46. Antonucci JM, Zeiger DN, Tang K, et al. Synthesis and characterization of dimethacrylates containing quaternary ammonium functionalities for dental applications. Dent Mater 2012;28:219–28.
47. Weng Y, Howard L, Guo X, et al. A novel antibacterial resin composite for improved dental restoratives. J Mater Sci Mater Med 2012;23:1553–61.
48. Xu X, Wang Y, Liao S, et al. Synthesis and characterization of antibacterial dental monomers and composites. J Biomed Mater Res B Appl Biomater 2012;100:1151–62.
49. Imazato S, Ma S, Chen JH, et al. Therapeutic polymers for dental adhesives: loading resins with bio-active components. Dent Mater 2014;30:97–104.
50. Imazato S, Kinomoto Y, Tarumi H, et al. Antibacterial activity and bonding characteristics of an adhesive resin containing antibacterial monomer MDPB. Dent Mater 2003;19:313–9.
51. Imazato S, Kuramoto A, Takahashi Y, et al. In vitro antibacterial effects of the dentin primer of Clearfil Protect Bond. Dent Mater 2006;22:527–32.
52. Li F, Chen J, Chai Z, et al. Effects of a dental adhesive incorporating antibacterial monomer on the growth, adherence and membrane integrity of Streptococcus mutans. J Dent 2009;37:289–96.

53. Beyth N, Yudovin-Farber I, Bahir R, et al. Antibacterial activity of dental composites containing quaternary ammonium polyethylenimine nanoparticles against *Streptococcus mutans*. Biomaterials 2006;27:3995–4002.
54. Xie D, Weng Y, Guo X, et al. Preparation and evaluation of a novel glass-ionomer cement with antibacterial functions. Dent Mater 2011;27:487–96.
55. Cheng L, Weir MD, Xu HHK, et al. Antibacterial amorphous calcium phosphate nanocomposites with a quaternary ammonium dimethacrylate and silver nanoparticles. Dent Mater 2012;28:561–72.
56. Cheng L, Zhang K, Melo MA, et al. Anti-biofilm dentin primer with quaternary ammonium and silver nanoparticles. Dent Mater 2012;91:598–604.
57. Zhang K, Melo MA, Cheng L, et al. Effect of quaternary ammonium and silver nanoparticle-containing adhesives on dentin bond strength and dental plaque microcosm biofilms. Dent Mater 2012;28:842–52.
58. Pashley DH, Tay FR, Breschi L, et al. State of the art etch-and-rinse adhesives. Dent Mater 2011;27:1–16.
59. Spencer P, Wang Y. Adhesive phase separation at the dentin interface under wet bonding conditions. J Biomed Mater Res 2002;62:447–56.
60. Ikemura K, Tay FR, Endo T, et al. A review of chemical-approach and ultramorphological studies on the development of fluoride-releasing dental adhesives comprising new pre-reacted glass ionomer (PRG) fillers. Dent Mater J 2008;27:315–29.
61. Ritter AV, Swift EJ Jr, Heymann HO, et al. An eight-year clinical evaluation of filled and unfilled one-bottle dental adhesives. J Am Dent Assoc 2009;140:28–37.
62. Van Meerbeek B, Yoshihara K, Yoshida Y, et al. State of the art of self-etch adhesives. Dent Mater 2011;27:17–28.
63. Blum IR, Hafiana K, Curtis A, et al. The effect of surface conditioning on the bond strength of resin composite to amalgam. J Dent 2012;40:15–21.
64. Imazato S, Tay FR, Kaneshiro AV, et al. An in vivo evaluation of bonding ability of comprehensive antibacterial adhesive system incorporating MDPB. Dent Mater 2007;23:170–6.
65. Hiraishi N, Yiu CK, King NM, et al. Effect of chlorhexidine incorporation into a self-etching primer on dentine bond strength of a luting cement. J Dent 2010;38:496–502.
66. Simoncic B, Tomcis B. Structures of novel antimicrobial agents for textiles - a review. Textile Res J 2010;80:1721–37.
67. Li F, Weir MD, Xu HK. Effects of quaternary ammonium chain length on antibacterial bonding agents. J Dent Res 2013;92:932–8.
68. Zhang K, Cheng L, Weir MD, et al. Effects of quaternary ammonium chain length on the antibacterial and remineralizing effects of a calcium phosphate nanocomposite. Int J Oral Sci 2016;8:45–53.
69. Zhang K, Cheng L, Wu EJ, et al. Effect of water-aging on dentin bond strength and anti-biofilm activity of bonding agent containing antibacterial monomer dimethylaminododecyl methacrylate. J Dent 2013;41:504–13.
70. Cheng L, Zhang K, Weir MD, et al. Effects of antibacterial primers with quaternary ammonium and nano-silver on *S. mutans* impregnated in human dentin blocks. Dent Mater 2013;29:462–72.
71. Donmez N, Belli S, Pashley DH, et al. Ultrastructural correlates of in vivo/in vitro bond degradation in self-etch adhesives. J Dent Res 2005;84:355–9.
72. Breschi L, Mazzoni A, Nato F, et al. Chlorhexidine stabilizes the adhesive interface: a 2-year in vitro study. Dent Mater 2010;26:320–5.

73. Tezvergil-Mutluay A, Agee KA, Uchiyama T, et al. The inhibitory effects of quaternary ammonium methacrylates on soluble and matrix-bound MMPs. J Dent Res 2011;90:535–40.
74. Li F, Majd H, Weir MD, et al. Inhibition of matrix metalloproteinase activity in human dentin via novel antibacterial monomer. Dent Mater 2015;31:284–92.
75. Lendenmann U, Grogan J, Oppenheim FG. Saliva and dental pellicle – a review. Adv Dent Res 2000;14:22–8.
76. Donlan RM, Costerton JW. Biofilms: survival mechanisms of clinically relevant microorganisms. Clin Microbiol Rev 2002;15:167–93.
77. Müller R, Eidt A, Hiller KA, et al. Influences of protein films on antibacterial or bacteria-repellent surface coatings in a model system using silicon wafers. Biomaterials 2009;30:4921–9.
78. Ishihara K, Nomura H, Mihara T, et al. Why do phospholipid polymers reduce protein adsorption? J Biomed Mater Res 1998;39:323–30.
79. Lewis AL. Phosphorylcholine-based polymers and their use in the prevention of biofouling. Colloids Surf B Biointerfaces 2000;18:261–75.
80. Sibarani J, Takai M, Ishihara K. Surface modification on microfluidic devices with 2-methacryloyloxyethyl phosphorylcholine polymers for reducing unfavorable protein adsorption. Colloids Surf B Biointerfaces 2007;54:88–93.
81. Kuiper KK, Nordrehaug JE. Early mobilization after protamine reversal of heparin following implantation of phosphorylcholine-coated stents in totally occluded coronary arteries. Am J Cardiol 2000;85:698–702.
82. Lewis AL, Tolhurst LA, Stratford PW. Analysis of a phosphorylcholine-based polymer coating on a coronary stent pre-and post-implantation. Biomaterials 2002;23: 1697–706.
83. Zhang N, Ma J, Melo MA, et al. Protein-repellent and antibacterial dental composite to inhibit biofilms and caries. J Dent 2015;43:225–34.
84. Zhang N, Weir MD, Bai YX, et al. Development of novel dental adhesive with double benefits of protein-repellent and antibacterial capabilities. Dent Mater 2015; 31:845–54.
85. Zhang N, Weir MD, Chen C, et al. Orthodontic cement with protein-repellent and antibacterial properties and the release of calcium and phosphate ions. J Dent 2016. http://dx.doi.org/10.1016/j.jdent.2016.05.001.
86. Chapman JA, Roberts WE, Eckert GJ, et al. Risk factors for incidence and severity of white spot lesions during treatment with fixed orthodontic appliances. Am J Orthod Dentofacial Orthop 2010;138:188–94.
87. Rogers S, Chadwick B, Treasure E. Fluoride-containing orthodontic adhesives and decalcification in patients with fixed appliances: a systematic review. Am J Orthod Dentofacial Orthop 2010;138:390.e1-8.
88. Imazato S, Ebi N, Tarumi H, et al. Bactericidal activity and cytotoxicity of antibacterial monomer MDPB. Biomaterials 1999;20:899–903.
89. Imazato S, Tarumi H, Ebi N, et al. Cytotoxic effects of composite restorations employing self-etching primers or experimental antibacterial primers. J Dent 2000; 28:61–7.
90. Nishida M, Imazato S, Takahashi Y, et al. The influence of the antibacterial monomer 12-methacryloyloxydodecylpyridinium bromide on the proliferation, differentiation and mineralization of odontoblast-like cells. Biomaterials 2010;31:1518–32.
91. Li F, Weir MD, Fouad AF, et al. Time-kill behaviour against eight bacterial species and cytotoxicity of antibacterial monomers. J Dent 2013;41:881–91.
92. Imazato S, Kaneko T, Takahashi Y, et al. In vivo antibacterial effects of dentin primer incorporating MDPB. Oper Dent 2004;29-4:369–75.

93. Cox CF, White KC, Ramus DL, et al. Reparative dentin: factors affecting its deposition. Quintessence Int 1992;23:257–70.
94. Tziafas D, Alvanou A, Papadimitriou S, et al. Effects of recombinant basic fibroblast growth factor, insulin-like growth factor-II and transforming growth factor-beta 1 on dog dental pulp cells in vivo. Arch Oral Biol 1998;43:431–44.
95. Smith AJ, Tobias RS, Plant CG, et al. In vivo morphogenetic activity of dentine matrix proteins. J Biol Buccale 1990;18:123–9.
96. Dammaschke T. Rat molar teeth as a study model for direct pulp capping research in dentistry. Lab Anim 2010;44:1–6.
97. Kawagishi E, Nakakura-Ohshima K, Nomura S, et al. Pulpal responses to cavity preparation in aged rat molars. Cell Tissue Res 2006;326:111–22.
98. Li F, Wang P, Weir MD, et al. Evaluation of novel antibacterial and remineralizing nanocomposite and adhesive in rat tooth cavity model. Acta Biomater 2014;10: 2804–13.

Advanced Scaffolds for Dental Pulp and Periodontal Regeneration

Marco C. Bottino, DDS, PhD[a],*, Divya Pankajakshan, PhD[a],
Jacques E. Nör, DDS, PhD[b]

KEYWORDS

- Biomaterials • 3D printing • Dental pulp • Pulpitis • Periodontitis • Scaffolds
- Regenerative endodontics • Guided tissue regeneration

KEY POINTS

- No current therapy exists that promotes regeneration of the pulp-dentin complex in cases of pulp necrosis.
- Antibiotic pastes used to eradicate root canal infection have been shown to negatively affect stem cell survival.
- Three-dimensional easy-to-fit antibiotic-eluting nanofibers, combined with injectable scaffolds, enriched or not with stem cells and/or growth factors, may lead to an increased likelihood of achieving predictable dental pulp regeneration in humans.
- Periodontitis is an aggressive disease that impairs the integrity of tooth-supporting structures and may lead to tooth loss.
- The latest advances related to membranes' biomodification to endow needed functionalities (eg, antimicrobial capacity) and technologies (additive manufacturing) to engineer patient-specific membranes/constructs to amplify both hard and soft tissue periodontal regeneration are presented.

INTRODUCTION

Caries and periodontitis are major disorders affecting teeth and their ancillary structures and, if not properly managed, may lead to tooth loss.[1,2] Recent estimates from the National Health and Nutrition Examination Survey show that, in the United States, nearly 8% of adults (aged 20–64 years) and 17% of seniors (aged ≥65 years) have periodontitis, whereas caries affects 37% of children (aged 2–8 years) in their

[a] Department of Cariology, Restorative Sciences and Endodontics, University of Michigan School of Dentistry, Ann Arbor, MI 48109, USA; [b] Department of Biomedical and Applied Sciences, Indiana, University School of Dentistry, Indianapolis, IN 46202, USA
* Corresponding author. 1011 N. University, Ann Arbor, MI 48109.
E-mail address: mbottino@umich.edu

Dent Clin N Am 61 (2017) 689–711
http://dx.doi.org/10.1016/j.cden.2017.06.009
0011-8532/17/© 2017 Elsevier Inc. All rights reserved.

deciduous teeth and 58% of adolescents (aged 12–19 years) in their permanent dentition. From these statistics, it becomes immediately clear that these two conditions remain a significant public health problem and require better strategies for disease prevention and clinical management.

A challenging problem for endodontists and pediatric dentists is the clinical management of immature (open apex) permanent teeth with necrotic pulp resulting from trauma or bacterial infection.[3] Over the years, the therapy of choice has followed the principles of apexification; that is, disinfection treatment with calcium hydroxide followed by root canal sealing with gutta-percha. However, the last decade has brought forward new prospects regarding dental pulp regeneration, thanks to evoked bleeding (EB), an approach that has been found to induce dentinal wall thickening and root end closure.[3–6] Nonetheless, despite the aforementioned clinical and histologic observations, the regenerative outcome of this patient-dependent and unpredictable therapy remains elusive.[6–11] Several aspects, including but not limited to the use of very cytotoxic antibiotic pastes, have been thought to account for the unsystematic success.[4] To circumvent the characteristic toxicity associated with commonly used antibiotic pastes and sodium hypochlorite, a more biocompatible strategy has recently been developed by our laboratory. A series of studies[3,12–20] have stressed the practicality and translational prospects of three-dimensional (3D) easy-to-fit antibiotic-eluting nanofibers as a localized, intracanal drug delivery strategy that, combined with injectable scaffolds, enriched or not with stem cells and/or growth factors (GFs), may lead to an increased likelihood of achieving predictable dental pulp regeneration in humans.

Considered to be one of the most aggressive chronic inflammatory oral diseases, periodontitis affects the integrity of both soft and hard tissue, and, in severe cases of tissue destruction, can result in tooth loss.[21] Originally, the principles of guided tissue regeneration have been followed to restore the architecture and functionality of the periodontal system. In essence, an occlusive biocompatible polymer-based membrane is used as a barrier to prevent epithelial and connective tissue migration into the regenerating site. In this way, slower migrating progenitor cells, located in the remaining periodontal ligament (PDL), are able to recolonize the root area and differentiate into new periodontal tissues.[22] Based on varying levels of clinical success with this approach, the last decade has witnessed significant advancement toward the generation of membranes with therapeutic properties. The work reported in the literature has included not only antimicrobials and inorganic particles (eg, calcium phosphates) but also biomolecules (eg, GFs) in the fabrication of membranes with therapeutic functions.[21,23] More recently, the combination of known materials and biomolecules with advanced technologies,[24–31] particularly 3D printing, has permitted translation of the first patient-specific scaffold modified with recombinant human platelet-derived growth factor-BB (rhPDGF-BB) for treating large periodontal defects.[26]

This 2-part review offers an update on progress related to advanced biomaterials for dental pulp and periodontal regeneration. To provide a better understanding of the regenerative strategies described herein, a concise but informative summary on dental stem cells is presented. The first part provides a short background on the EB strategy, the significance of a biocompatible disinfection, and major highlights on the use of scaffolds, stem cells, and GFs in dental pulp regeneration. The second part highlights the newest advances regarding the development of membranes with therapeutic properties and technologies, such as additive manufacturing, to engineer patient-specific membranes/scaffolds to amplify hard and soft tissue periodontal regeneration.

DENTAL STEM CELLS
Dental Stem Cells in Deciduous and Adult Teeth

Dental stem cells are considered a population of mesenchymal stem cells (MSCs), according to the minimal criteria defined by the International Society for Stem Cell Research.[32,33] Apart from showing plastic adherence and multilineage differentiation, dental stem cells show positive expression of specific surface antigen markers (eg, CD44, CD73, CD105).[33]

In 2000, Gronthos and colleagues[34] reported seminal work on the isolation and characterization of an MSC-like heterogeneous population of stem cells from the dental pulp tissue of human third molars, calling them postnatal dental pulp stem cells (DPSCs). The notable regenerative potential of DPSCs based on their differentiation into odontoblasts, osteoblasts, adipocytes, and neurons has been shown.[35–37] A few years later, a subpopulation of DPSCs that express certain hematopoietic lineage markers were similarly isolated from the pulp of exfoliated deciduous teeth (stem cells from human exfoliated deciduous teeth [SHED]).[38] The advantages of SHED, compared with DPSCs, are their higher proliferation rate and enhanced differentiation potential; for example, into odontoblasts and endothelial-like cells when implanted in vivo using a tooth slice/scaffold model.[38–40] The mechanistic pathways involved in the endothelial differentiation of SHED[41] and DPSCs[42] have recently been unveiled by our group.

Stem cells from the apical papilla (SCAP) were identified by Sonoyama and colleagues[43,44] as an embryonic-like soft tissue located at the apex of growing tooth roots. Apical papilla is speculated to be a source of so-called primary odontoblasts that synthesize primary tubular dentin, as opposed to the so-called replacement odontoblasts that form reparative dentin. A key benefit related to SCAPs pertains to the apical location, which supports tissue survival during pulp necrosis.[45] Specifically, SCAP coexpresses STRO-1+ with a range of osteogenic/dentinogenic markers and neural markers.[44] From a proliferation standpoint, SCAP shows a higher rate than DPSC and expresses, similarly to DPSCs, typical dentinogenic markers (eg, dentin sialophosphoprotein [DSPP]) on induction.[46]

Stem Cells in Periodontal Tissues and Dental Follicles

The PDL, a specialized connective tissue that links the radicular surface to the alveolar bone, was found to harbor a unique population of stem cells, ie, periodontal ligament stem cells (PDLSCs).[47] These cells express not only MSC markers but also tendon-specific markers. PDLSCs isolated from periodontal granulation tissue improved new bone formation when transplanted in calvarial defects in mice.[47] Another important stem cell niche is the dental follicle, a loose connective tissue surrounding the developing tooth, which later develops into the periodontium.[48] The dental follicle harbors dental follicle precursor cells (DFSCs). DFSCs can be maintained and expanded in cell culture, show a higher proliferation capacity compared with DPSCs, and have been found to be precursors of periodontal tissues cells (ie, fibroblasts in the PDL, alveolar bone cells, and cementoblasts).[48,49]

Several other candidate dental-derived stem cells for oral/craniofacial tissue regeneration isolated from salivary glands, oral mucosa, gingiva, and periosteum have been identified. However, their differentiation ability and in vivo regenerative potential remains unclear.[50] In summary, the multipotency, increased proliferation rates, and ease of accessibility make dental stem cells an attractive source for tissue regeneration. Next, selected studies involving the use of dental stem cells and advanced scaffolds for dental pulp and periodontal regeneration are discussed.

ADVANCED BIOMATERIALS FOR DENTAL PULP REGENERATION
Pulpal Disease

Root canal therapy involving chemomechanical debridement and sealing of the canal system with an inert rubber-like material remains the standard of care for necrotic mature teeth with closed apices.[51] However, immature permanent teeth have a wide-open root apex and thin root dentinal walls, making it virtually impossible to obtain an apical seal using the customary method.[3–5] Therefore, new clinical therapies (eg, EB) for dental pulp regeneration have been explored, particularly because apexification supports only apical closure and does not promote root maturation,[52,53] thus increasing the chance of root fracture on secondary trauma.[54,55]

Evoked Bleeding: The First Step Toward Dental Pulp Regeneration

In the early 1990s, tissue engineering emerged as a field tasked to provide a clinically translatable platform for tissue/organ regeneration.[56] Three major elements form the basis for tissue engineering, namely stem cells, bioactive signaling molecules, and scaffolds. Scaffolds, in turn, can have unique structural, chemical, mechanical, and biophysical properties. These properties have been explored individually and in tandem to ensure controllable tissue regeneration.

In recent years, the development of new clinical therapies for dental pulp regeneration, such as the EB method, have offered promise for improving treatment outcomes. In EB, succeeding proper root canal disinfection, the laceration of periapical tissue is deliberately performed to evoke bleeding and form a fibrin-based scaffold to interact with endogenous stem cells and GFs. The EB method has preferably used a triple-antimicrobial (ciprofloxacin [CIP], metronidazole [MET], and minocycline [MINO]) or double-antimicrobial (MINO free) component in a very concentrated antibiotic paste to accomplish disinfection. However, the specific therapeutic dose of the antibiotic mixtures that promotes maximum antimicrobial action, while reducing toxicity to the host tissues and residing cells, is not currently known. Regardless of the promising results achieved by EB when treating immature permanent teeth with necrotic pulp,[57] only 1 case report shows pulp-like tissue formation.[58] Most histologic findings have acknowledged the invagination of periapical tissue containing bonelike hard tissue and cementumlike tissue that has led to further root canal wall thickening.[59,60] Although the EB strategy has been proposed to treat immature teeth, a recent study also showed the influx of undifferentiated MSCs from the apical region into the pulpal space of mature teeth with apical lesions.[61]

Antibiotic-Eluting Polymer Nanofibers for Intracanal Drug Delivery

A significant amount of data has indicated that antibiotic pastes and chemical irrigants can affect the survival ability and function of dental stem cells.[3–5] In light of this, a biocompatible nanofiber–based intracanal drug delivery system has been proposed as a means to create a bacteria-free environment favorable to tissue regeneration.[3,12–20] In brief, a polymer solution loaded with the chosen antibiotics at the desired concentration needs to be prepared.[3,12,21] Following that, by adjusting electrospinning parameters (eg, flow rate, field strength), antibiotic-eluting nanofibers are obtained. The use of these therapeutic nanofibers processed as a three-dimensional (3D) tubular construct[3,17,62] that can be easily fitted into the root canal system of necrotic teeth (**Fig. 1**) holds great clinical potential, because it guarantees the release of antibiotics onto the dentinal walls where microbial biofilm has been found to be present.[3,12,14–16,18–20,62] As an example, triple (MET, CIP, and MINO) antibiotic–eluting nanofibers were developed and tested for antimicrobial efficacy

☐ **Synthesis**

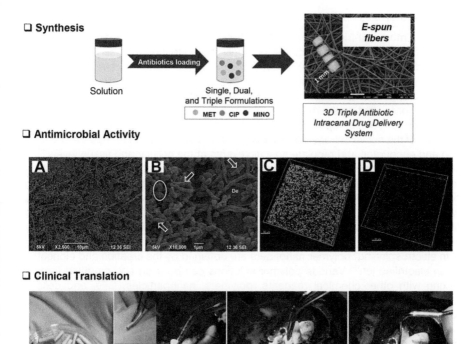

Fig. 1. Synthesis of triple antibiotic–eluting nanofibers. Polymer solubilization in hexafluoro-2-propanol. Single, dual, or triple antibiotic incorporation (MET, CIP, and MINO) into the solution before electrospinning. Representative scanning electron micrograph (SEM) of triple antibiotic–containing nanofibers and 3D constructs (in *yellow*, superimposed on the SEM image). Antimicrobial activity of triple antibiotic nanofibers against a 7-day dual-species (*Actinomyces naeslundii* and *Enterococcus faecalis*) biofilm formed on dentin specimens. (*A*) Lower-magnification SEM image showing a homogeneous distribution of the 2 bacterial cells. (*B*) Higher-magnification SEM image revealing the rod-shaped *A naeslundii* (arrows) and cocci-shaped *E faecalis* (circle) bacterial cells over the dentin (De) surface. Confocal laser scanning micrographs of (*C*) 7-day dual-species biofilm growth on dentin (live bacteria = *green*) and (*D*) Confocal image showing the elimination of most of the bacteria (dead bacteria = *red*) by the formulated triple antibiotic nanofibers. Scale bars = 30 μm. Clinical translation: placement of 3D tubular triple antibiotic–eluting construct into the root canal of a periapical lesion dog model, to act as a localized intracanal drug delivery system. (*Adapted from* Pankajakshan D, Albuquerque MT, Evans JD, et al. Triple antibiotic polymer nanofibers for intracanal drug delivery: effects on dual species biofilm and cell function. J Endod 2016;42(10):1492; with permission.)

against a dual-species bacterial biofilm.[20] Infected dentin exposed to the triple antibiotic–eluting nanofibers revealed significant bacterial death based on confocal laser scanning microscopy data (see **Fig. 1**). Numerous studies[3,12–16,18–20] have been published and provided critical information to test the clinical efficacy of 3D tubular antibiotic-eluting nanofibers using animal models of periapical disease (see **Fig. 1**).

Advanced Scaffolds and Regenerative Strategies

Besides a more cell-friendly disinfection strategy, several developments in tissue engineering and regenerative medicine, primarily related to the synthesis scaffolds, have provided the foundational knowledge for reliable and predictable regeneration of the pulp-dentin complex. According to the American Society for Testing Materials (ASTM; designation F2150), a scaffold is defined as "the support, delivery vehicle, or matrix for facilitating the migration, binding, or transport of cells or bioactive molecules used to replace, repair, or regenerate tissues." It should precisely replicate the features of the native extracellular matrix (ECM) at the nanoscale to regulate cell function and encourage and regulate specific events at the cellular and tissue levels.[63–65] Moreover, scaffolds should be synthesized from biocompatible and biodegradable materials to avoid immune responses. A myriad of polymers, both synthetic (eg, poly[lactic] acid [PLA]) and natural (eg, collagen), have been used in gas foaming, as well as salt leaching techniques, to obtain macroporous scaffolds. Meanwhile, nanofibrous scaffolds have been processed via electrospinning, self-assembly, and phase separation.[63,66,67]

In electrospinning, polymer nanofibers are obtained by the creation and elongation of an electrified jet.[68] Various polymer solutions can be used and modified through mixing with other chemical reagents, polymers, nanoparticles, GFs, and cells to generate unique nanofibers.[68] Meanwhile, molecular self-assembly has been used to fabricate nanofibrous scaffolds through spontaneous molecular arrangement via noncovalent interactions.[63] This technique allows recapitulation of collagen's supramolecule formation and enhances cell adhesion.[63] Moreover, these unique nanofibers present major clinical advantages because they are assembled in solution and result in gels that are biocompatible and can be used for stem cell transplant.[66,67,69–71] However, this technique has limitations in terms of controlling pore size/shape within the scaffold and in producing suitable mechanical properties.[63,70] Accordingly, an alternative method, commonly referred to as thermally induced phase separation, has been incorporated in the fabrication of macropore/micropore networks within 3D nanofibrous scaffolds.[63] Taken together, recent advances in biomaterials have allowed researchers to obtain scaffolds that can be easily injected in the desired site to aid in stem cell transplant or to serve as delivery vehicles for bioactive factors. The latest developments include the testing of innovative scaffolds/stem cell constructs in conjunction with therapeutic agents, and these are presented next as evidence of the translational potential of tissue engineering in regenerative endodontics.

A well-known approach, the tooth slice/scaffold model, which uses immunodeficient mice and tooth fragments/segments,[40] has provided key insight into the use of injectable scaffolds and stem cells toward dental pulp regeneration (**Fig. 2**). Puramatrix, a self-assembling peptide hydrogel[71] mixed with SHED, generated a pulp-like tissue with odontoblasts capable of producing new tubular dentin. Moreover, the engineered pulp (see **Fig. 2**) showed similar cellularity and vascularization compared with human pulps.[67]

Over the past decade, multidomain peptides (MDPs) consisting of short sequences of amino acids that self-assemble to form fibers in aqueous solution, have been the focus of Professors D'Souza and Hartgerink's groups.[66,72] MDPs with the cell adhesion motif arginine-glycine-aspartic acid (RGD), matrix metalloproteinase (MMP)–cleavable site, and heparin-binding domains allowed GF conjugation and assisted in its slow release. On injection into dentin cylinders and subsequent implantation in immunocompromised mice for 5 weeks, the scaffold was entirely degraded and replaced by collagenous ECM. Vascularized soft connective tissue resembling dental pulp could be visualized and the cells at the cell-dentin interface appeared in intimate association with the dentin wall.[66]

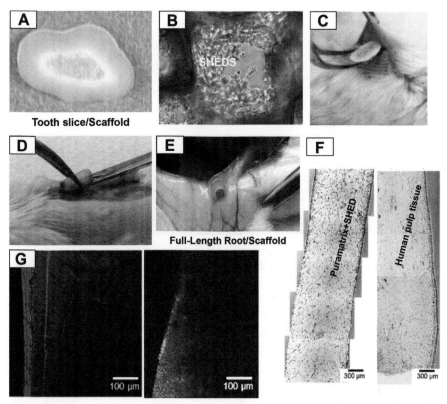

Fig. 2. The tooth slice and full-length root/scaffold models. (*A*) Tooth slice provided from the cervical third of a human third molar with a highly porous PLLA (Poly[lactic acid]) scaffold placed within the pulp chamber. (*B*) SHED proliferation into the tooth slice/scaffold. (*C*) Insertion of a tooth slice and scaffold containing SHED into the subcutaneous space of the dorsum of an immunodeficient mouse. (*D*) Subcutaneous transplant of a human full-length root injected with hydrogel-based nanofibrous scaffolds containing SHEDs. (*E*) The engineered pulp-like tissue and human pulp tissue (control) in the root canal. (*F*) Layer of dentin formation after pulp tissue induction in PuraMatrix plus SHEDs. (*G*) Dentin slice with no SHEDs. (*From* Albuquerque MT, Valera MC, Nakashima M, et al. Tissue-engineering-based strategies for regenerative endodontics. J Dent Res 2014;93(12):1227; with permission.)

A well-known hydrogel (ie, gelatin methacrylate [GelMA]) was recently investigated for the first time for dental pulp regeneration.[73] GelMA is composed of denatured collagen and retains RGD adhesive domains and MMP-sensitive sites to enhance cell binding and matrix degradation. Furthermore, it is suitable for cell encapsulation and easily tunable by varying the concentrations of GelMA and photoinitiators. Professor Yelick's group showed the formation of patent blood vessels filled with host blood cells following subcutaneous implantation of in vitro cultured human umbilical vein endothelial cells (HUVECs)/DPSCs/GelMA injected into the tooth.[73]

Biodegradable polymer microspheres have been used as cell carriers for the regeneration and repair of irregularly shaped tissue defects because of their suitability for injection, controllable biodegradability, and the capacity for drug incorporation and release.[74] In this way, nanostructured, self-assembling microspheres were used (**Fig. 3**A, B) to deliver DPSCs into the pulpal space.[75,76] The investigators reported

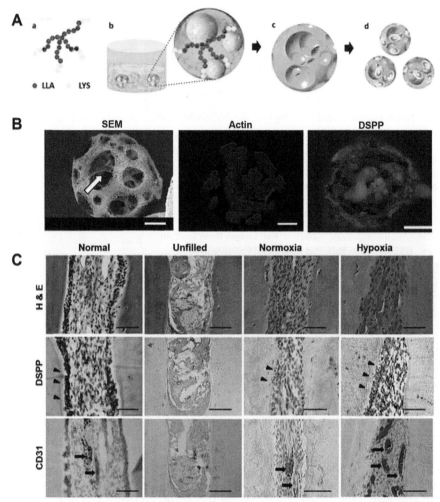

Fig. 3. (*A*) The fabrication of nanofibrous spongy microspheres (NF-SMS) for stem cell delivery through injection. (*a*) SS-PLLA-b-PLYS (star-shaped poly[L-lactic acid]-block-polylysine [PLLA-b-PLYS] copolymer). (*b*) Emulsions self-assembled from SS-PLLA-b-PLYS, with 1 polymer solution droplet containing multiple glycerol domains. (*c*) NF-SMS were obtained after phase separation and freeze drying. (*d*) The porous structure of NF-SMS allows efficient cell loading and delivery through injection. (*B*) Interactions of human dental pulp stem cells (hDPSCs) with the microspheres. SEM image of hDPSCs seeded on a nanofibrous spongy microsphere (NF-SMS) for 24 hours showing the attachment of cells on both the surface and interior (*arrow*) of the spheres, with abundant cellular processes. Laser scanning confocal light microscope image of DPSCs seeded on NF-SMS for 24 hours, showing cells attached on the surface and inner pores of NF-SMS. DSPP immunofluorescence staining of hDPSCs on NF-SMS after odontogenic induction for 4 weeks. Blue indicates nuclei; green indicates DSPP; red indicates F-actin. (*C*) Pulp tissue regeneration enhanced by hypoxia-primed hDPSCs/NF-SMS in maxillary first molar of immunodeficient rats. From left to right, the first column is the normal pulp, the second column is the unfilled pulp canal group, the third column is the normoxia group, and the last column is the hypoxia group. Hematoxylin-eosin (H&E) staining showed that no pulp-like tissue was formed in the unfilled group, whereas neo pulp-like tissue formed in the normoxia and hypoxia groups. DSPP

on the synthesis of a novel, star-shaped block copolymer, poly(L-lactic acid)-block-poly-(L-lysine), capable of self-assembling into nanofibrous spongy microspheres (NF-SMS). The NF-SMS supported DPSC proliferation and showed DSPP expression in vitro.[75,76] DPSCs in NF-SMS, when exposed to hypoxic conditions, showed increased vascular endothelial growth factor (VEGF) expression. Following 4 weeks' implantation in an in situ pulp regeneration model, the cells in the hypoxia-primed group showed columnar odontoblastic cell arrangement at the dentin-pulp interface, similar to that of native teeth. Hypoxia-primed human dental pulp stem cells (hDPSCs)/NF-SMS effectively regenerated pulp-like tissue with higher vascularity compared with the normoxia conditions (see **Fig. 3**C).[75]

Nanostructured microspheres have also been investigated for GF delivery. A recent study elegantly described a strategy to allow dual drug delivery.[77] A microsphere platform was used to concurrently release fluocinolone acetonide (FA) to suppress inflammation and bone morphogenetic protein (BMP) 2 to enhance odontogenic differentiation of DPSCs. A constant linear release of FA and a rapid BMP-2 release was observed in in vitro systems that reduced inflammation on DPSCs and enhanced differentiation.[77]

Cell-Free Approaches for Dental Pulp Regeneration

The identification of biomolecules, including but not limited to GFs and matrix molecules sequestered within dentin and dental pulp, affords a unique opportunity to make these signaling cues available in the regenerative process after a biocompatible disinfection approach. It has been suggested that the release of these biomolecules by certain irrigants and medicaments can potentially circumvent the use of nonhuman exogenous biomolecules and avoid their short half-lives.[78] Meanwhile, the use of exogenous bioactive molecules that can be adsorbed, tethered, or encapsulated into scaffolds to attract stem/progenitor cells adjacent to the root apices of endodontically treated teeth has shown great clinical prospects. Professor Mao's group reported[79] on the regeneration of dental-pulp–like tissue based solely on the intracanal delivery of fibroblast growth factor 2 (FGF2) and/or VEGF without stem cell transplant. A recellularized and revascularized connective tissue integrated with the native dentinal wall in root canals was observed following in vivo implantation of endodontically treated human teeth in mouse dorsum for 3 weeks. In addition, combined delivery of a cocktail of GFs (FGF2, VEGF, and PDGF) with a basal set of nerve GF and BMP-7 led to the formation of tissues with patent vessels and new dentin regeneration.[79]

Clinical Translation

Over the past 5 years, unprecedented preclinical (animal model) demonstration[80–82] of pulp regeneration by CD31⁻ side population (SP) cells and CD105⁺ cells has suggested that clinically effective human pulp regeneration is closer than it has ever been. Remarkably, this specific subfraction of DPSCs revealed higher angiogenic

---

immunohistochemistry staining was positive in the hypoxia group and the normal pulp group at the dentin-pulp interface (*black triangles*). CD31 staining showed more blood vessels in the hypoxia group than in the normoxia group (*black arrows*). ([A, B] *Adapted from* Kuang R, Zhang Z, Jin X, et al. Nanofibrous spongy microspheres enhance odontogenic differentiation of human dental pulp stem cells. Adv Healthc Mater 2015;4(13):1993–2000, with permission; and [C] *From* Kuang R, Zhang Z, Jin X, et al. Nanofibrous spongy microspheres for the delivery of hypoxia-primed human dental pulp stem cells to regenerate vascularized dental pulp. Acta Biomater 2016;33:232, with permission.)

and neurogenic potential than bone marrow–derived or adipose-derived MSCs.[80–82] Evidence for complete pulp regeneration with adequate vasculature and innervation (**Fig. 4**A–C) into the pulpectomized root canals of dogs after autologous transplant of CD31⁻ (SP) cells or CD105⁺ cells associated with stromal cell–derived factor-1 (SDF-1) and a collagen scaffold has been shown.[80–82] Moreover, new dentin formation along the dentinal wall was observed (see **Fig. 4**D).

To expedite the clinical translation of the aforementioned approach in humans, it is key to obtain clinical-grade stem cells based on good-manufacturing-practice conditions. A safe technique that isolates DPSC subsets has recently been devised by using an optimized granulocyte colony–stimulating factor (G-CSF)–induced mobilization.[83] The mobilized DPSCs (MDPSCs) showed stem cell properties, including high proliferation rate, migratory activity, and expression of multiple trophic factors.[83] Preclinical efficacy and safety tests were performed in dogs using clinical-grade G-CSF and collagen with MDPSCs, which resulted in complete pulp regeneration (see **Fig. 4**E) with coronal dentin formation in the pulpectomized root canal and reduced number of inflammatory cells, decrease in cell death, and the major increase in neurite outgrowth.[84] These preclinical results of efficacy and safety of stem cell transplant led to the initiation of a clinical trial with the consent of the Japanese Ministry of Health, Labor and Welfare.[85]

ADVANCED BIOMATERIALS FOR PERIODONTAL REGENERATION
Periodontal Disease

Periodontitis, a chronic inflammatory disease, occurs when bacteria-stimulated inflammation or infection of the gingival tissue progressively destroys the periodontium.[21] Tissue integrity is compromised by the loss of soft tissue attachment to the root surface, which results in periodontal pocket formation and subsequent loss of the alveolar bone, ultimately resulting in tooth loss.[21] According to Eke and colleagues,[86] the prevalence of varying degrees of periodontitis in the US adult population has been estimated to be nearly 47%.

Traditional Membranes for Periodontal Regeneration

Periodontal regeneration is attributed to a complete recovery of both architecture and function, manifested as alveolar bone regeneration and new connective attachment through collagen fibers functionally oriented on the newly regenerated cementum.[21,87,88] As stated earlier, the use of synthetic or tissue-derived (collagen) membranes as barriers for guided tissue/bone regeneration procedures with or without calcium phosphate bone graft materials has been the treatment of choice.[21] According to their degradation behavior, membrane materials can be grouped into 2 classes: nonresorbable and resorbable.[21] Ideally, these membranes need to have biocompatibility to allow host integration without eliciting inflammatory responses, and a proper degradation profile that not only matches that of the new tissue formation but more importantly allows sufficient maturation of the tissue before the membrane starts to degrade.[21,25] Also, these membranes need to possess sufficient initial strength to allow clinical handling and placement.[21]

One of the major drawbacks of nonresorbable membranes (polytetrafluoroethylene) is the necessity for a secondary surgery for removal.[21] Resorbable membranes were developed to eliminate the pain and discomfort, as well as the financial burden, associated with a second surgery.[89–92] Most resorbable synthetic membranes are based on polyesters and/or their copolymers.[91–101] Collagen membranes derived from the ECM of human skin and other sources have become important alternatives to their

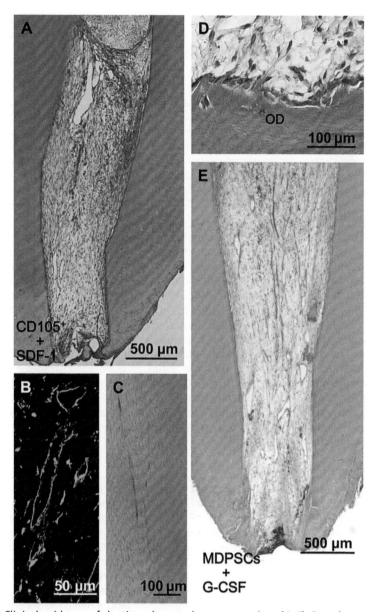

Fig. 4. Clinical evidence of dentin-pulp complex regeneration. (*A–E*) Complete regeneration of pulp tissue after autologous transplant of CD105+ cells with stromal cell–derived factor-1 (SDF-1) in the pulpectomized root canal in dogs. (*B*) Immunostaining with BS-1 lectin. (*C*) Immunostaining with PGP (protein gene product) 9.5. (*D*) Odontoblastic cell lining to newly formed osteodentin/tubular dentin (OD), along with the dentinal wall. (*E*) Complete regeneration of pulp tissue after autologous transplant of mobilized dental pulp stem cells (MDPSCs) with granulocyte colony–stimulating factor (G-CSF) in the pulpectomized root canal in dogs. (*From* Albuquerque MT, Valera MC, Nakashima M, et al. Tissue-engineering-based strategies for regenerative endodontics. J Dent Res 2014;93(12):1228; with permission.)

synthetic counterparts, because of their excellent cell affinity and biocompatibility.[89,102,103] Regrettably, type-I collagen has many limitations, such as low strength and fast degradation, that support the need for an improved material.[21]

Membranes with therapeutic properties

Numerous attempts, with varying degrees of clinical success, have been made to develop a membrane with the right combination of mechanical, degradation, and biological characteristics required for guided tissue regeneration.[21,23] Although progress has been made, these requirements are only being approached in recent published work. Advances related to membranes' biomodification to endow needed functionalities (eg, antimicrobial, antiinflammatory, cell differentiation capacities) and technologies (eg, additive manufacturing) to engineer patient-specific membranes and constructs to amplify both hard and soft tissue periodontal regeneration are presented next.

Antimicrobial

Infection is the foremost reason for clinical failure of periodontal regeneration. Therefore, it is extremely important to control and/or eradicate bacterial contamination of the periodontal defect.[104,105] A wide range of antimicrobials, including but not limited to tetracycline hydrochloride, MET, and amoxicillin, have been incorporated into polymer membranes.[106–108] Furtos and colleagues[109] reported on the synthesis of nanocomposite polycaprolactone (PCL)-based membranes modified with amoxicillin and nanohydroxyapatite to provide antimicrobial and osteoconductive properties, respectively. Based on the well-known side effects, such as bacterial strain resistance, associated with the overuse of antibiotics, alternative agents, such as zinc oxide (ZnO) nanoparticles, have been proposed by our group.[110] Successful synthesis of PCL-based nanofibrous membranes using ZnO has recently been reported (**Fig. 5**).[110] The antimicrobial action of cytocompatible ZnO-modified membranes was tested against *Porphyromonas gingivalis* and *Fusobacterium nucleatum*. All membranes containing different concentrations of ZnO showed significant antimicrobial action against the periodontopathogens tested.[110]

Calcium Phosphates and Bioactive Glass

A naturally occurring mineral form of calcium phosphate, hydroxyapatite (HAp), constitutes up to 70% of the dry weight of bone.[111] Scaffold processing techniques, such as coelectrospinning of HAp nanoparticles,[112–118] have been used to produce composite membranes with improved strength and bioactivity.[119,120] A recent study combined electrospinning with melt plotting to generate a hierarchical PCL/β-tricalcium phosphate (TCP) scaffold embedded with collagen nanofibers.[121] Scanning electron micrographs of the constructs revealed uniform distribution of β-TCP particles in PCL struts and well-layered collagen nanofibers between composite struts. The combination of collagen nanofibers and β-TCP was found to provide synergistic effects related to cell activity.[121]

Over the past decade, bioglass, another material with demonstrated properties related to bone formation, osteogenic differentiation, and activation of gene expression, has been used to modify periodontal membranes. For example, El-Fiqi and colleagues[122] synthesized via electrospinning PCL-gelatin nanofibrous membranes modified with mesoporous bioglass (mBG) nanoparticles to provide the long-term delivery of dexamethasone. PDLSCs showed increased proliferation and differentiation on these membranes. The mBG/PCL-gelatin membranes revealed excellent strength, elasticity, and hydrophilicity, compared with their mBG-free counterparts. Dexamethasone was released in a linear fashion up to 28 days after a rapid initial burst (~30%) within the first 24 hours.[122]

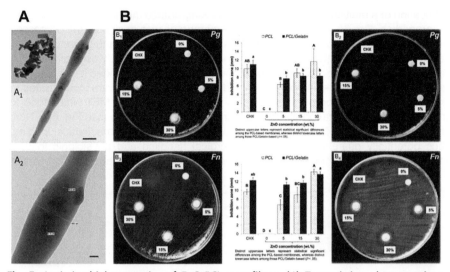

Fig. 5. Antimicrobial properties of ZnO-PCL nanofibers. (*A*) Transmission electron micrographs (TEMs) of PCL nanofibers incorporated with ZnO nanoparticles. (*A₁, A₂*) TEMs showing ZnO nanoparticles within the neat PCL fibers at different magnifications. (*A₁*, inset) TEM shoing the overall morphology and size distribution of the ZnO nanoparticles. (*B*) Representative agar plates and data of the antibacterial activity obtained with the positive control (chlorhexidine [CHX]) and the PCL-based and PCL/gelatin (GEL)-based membranes containing different concentrations of ZnO. (*B₁, B₂*) The results compared with *Porphyromonas gingivalis* (*Pg*) and *Fusobacterium nucleatum* (*Fn*) (*B₃, B₄*). (*Adapted from* Münchow EA, Albuquerque MTP, Zero B, et al. Development and characterization of novel ZnO-loaded electrospun membranes for periodontal regeneration. Dent Mater 2015;31(9):1038–51; with permission.)

Growth Factors

The local delivery of GFs (eg, BMP-2) has shown enhanced periodontal healing and regeneration by modulating the cellular activity and providing stimuli to cells to differentiate and synthesize the ECM to develop new tissues.[21] The potent stimulatory effects of PDGF-BB, a commercially available molecule for periodontal regeneration, as a chemoattractant and mitogen, along with its ability to promote angiogenesis, were reported by Phipps and colleagues.[123] PDGF-BB was physically adsorbed to blended (PCL–collagen I) nanofibers embedded with HAp nanoparticles. A sustained release of PDGF-BB was seen for 8 weeks in addition to enhanced MSC chemotaxis.[123]

A recent strategy to promote bone regeneration relates to endogenous stem/progenitor cell recruitment/homing to the injury site by increasing local concentrations of cytokines and chemokines at the injured site. SDF-1α is key in MSC homing and localization within the bone marrow. Ji and colleagues[124] reported on the synthesis of SDF-1α modified polymer membranes. The membranes were able to amplify chemotactic migration of MSCs. In vivo, after 8 weeks, SDF-1α–loaded membranes led to a 6-fold increase in bone formation compared with SDF-1α–free counterparts.

Multilayered membranes and multiphasic patient-specific scaffolds

It has become evident that a multiphasic periodontal membrane/scaffold using a tissue-specific structure with compositional and structural variation to recapitulate the structural organization or cellular and biochemical composition of native tissues is critical for periodontal regeneration. With this in mind, our group reported on the fabrication of a multilayered, tissue-specific biodegradable membrane with therapeutic properties (**Fig. 6**A, B).[125] The innovative membrane was designed and processed via sequential electrostatic spinning to present a core layer (CL) and 2 functional surface layers (SLs) that interface with hard and soft tissues. The CL was engineered by spinning a poly(DL-lactide-co-ε-caprolactone) (PLCL) layer surrounded by 2 composite layers consisting of a gelatin/polymer blend. HAp nanoparticles were incorporated to enhance bone formation on the SL facing the bone defect and MET was added to inhibit bacterial colonization on the SL facing the epithelial tissue (see **Fig. 6**B). Note that no delamination of the layered structure was observed on mechanical loading, thus potentially guaranteeing adequate surgical handling and physiologic loading in vivo.[125] Taken together, this study showed that sequential electrospinning can be

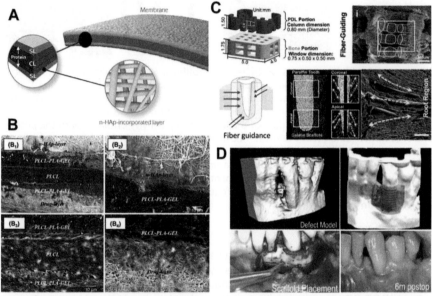

Fig. 6. Multilayered/multiphasic scaffolds for periodontal regeneration. (*A*) The multilayered periodontal membrane processed via multilayered electrospinning showing the details of the core layer (CL) and the functional surface layers (SL). (*B*) Cross-sectional SEM micrographs of the multilayered membrane. (*B₁*) General view of the functionally graded membrane, (*B₂*) interface between the n-HAp–containing layer and the poly(DL-lactide-co-ε-caprolactone) (PLCL)/PLA/ GEL, (*B₃*) CL structure, and (*B₄*) interface between the MET-loaded layer and the PLCL/PLA/GEL. (*C*) Design of a customized scaffold using 3D printing. Scaffold design consists of a PDL portion and a bone portion. This design was further modified to improve the fiber-guiding potential as well as the direction of the PDL to mimic the topography of the different kinds of fibers in the PDL (*first row*). Digitalized cross-sectional view of a 3D-reconstructed image. Longitudinal cross-sectional image showing pore morphologies at coronal and apical portions. Scanning electron microscopy image showing longitudinal pores produced by a freeze-casting method. (*D*) 3D printing using PCL was made to fit the periosseous defect based on the patient's cone beam computed tomography scan. 6m postop, 6 months postoperative. ([*A, B*] *Adapted from* Bottino MC, Thomas V, Janowski GM. A novel spatially designed and functionally graded electrospun membrane for periodontal regeneration. Acta Biomater 2011;7(1):216–24, with permission; and [*C, D*] *From* Larsson L, Decker AM, Nibali L, et al. Regenerative medicine for periodontal and peri-implant diseases. J Dent Res 2016;95(3):262, with permission.)

used to fabricate tissue-specific multilayered membranes with desired physicochemical, mechanical, and biological cues that could ultimately lead to enhanced periodontal regeneration.[125]

More recently, advances in tissue engineering and scaffold synthesis have permitted the development of mechanically competent, tissue-specific, and multiphasic 3D scaffolds for periodontal regeneration, all of which have been addressed in exceptional review articles.[24–31,126] Ivanovski and colleagues[25] provided a comprehensive perspective regarding the association between scaffolds with cells and/or GFs to engineer 3D structures capable of influencing a spatiotemporal wound-healing cascade to encourage predictable regeneration. Notably, the ability to form highly complex 3D multiphasic scaffolds with tissue compartmentalization properties to encourage (1) bone and periodontal attachment formation and integration, (2) promotion of cementum formation onto the root surface, and (3) the establishment of suitably oriented PDL fibers that attach to regenerated bone and cementum have significantly advanced periodontal tissue engineering. The design and fabrication of multiphasic scaffolds need to mimic the anatomy of the defect, which, in turn, will permit cell delivery and neovascularization, an also provide space for new tissue formation. Moreover, these constructs must also follow the general principles of the scaffolds' design, namely (1) biocompatibility and degradability with a tunable degradation rate to complement cell and tissue growth and proper maturation; (2) a highly porous 3D framework with surface properties that enhance cell attachment, migration, proliferation, and differentiation; and (3) an open interconnected structure that allows the flow transport of nutrients and metabolic waste.[24,25]

Remarkably, Giannobile's group recently reported on the clinical findings of a 3D-printed, bioresorbable (PCL), patient-specific scaffold and signaling growth factor to treat a large periodontal osseous defect caused by generalized aggressive periodontitis (see **Fig. 6C, D**).[26] Specifically, selective laser sintering was used to print an HAp-containing PCL-based scaffold according to the anatomic configuration of the defect, as revealed by the patient's cone beam computed tomography. The design consisted of perforations for fixation, an internal port for delivery of recombinant human PDGF-BB (rhPDGF-BB), and pegs oriented perpendicular to the root for PDL formation.[27] The adaptation ratio based on the methodology for PDL fiber guidance was defined based on micro-CT information. Before implantation, the scaffold was immersed in rhPDGF-BB, filled with autologous blood, and stabilized over the defect with resorbable pins. No clinical signs of chronic inflammation or rejection associated with the presence of the scaffold were seen during the first year. In vitro studies showed a burst release of rhPDGF-BB within 180 minutes. The scaffold remained covered for 12 months, revealing a 3-mm gain of clinical attachment and partial root coverage. However, scaffold exposure was noticed after 1 year (13 months) and, although palliative strategies were performed to save the treatment, the implanted material was removed (~76% of the molecular weight) for analyses. Although the success of this clinical study was modest, given that complete regeneration of the periodontium was not observed, it provided key information to drive the field forward, particularly regarding the aspects associated with scaffold design and fabrication.

SUMMARY

The unprecedented histologic findings reported by Nygaard-Ostby and Hjortdal,[127] and Ostby,[128] who showed that periapical tissue laceration may lead to vascularized tissue formation within the root canal system and root maturation, have laid the groundwork for dental pulp tissue engineering. Over the past decade, in spite of significant advancement and amendments of the EB technique, thanks to accumulating evidence regarding key aspects deemed to negatively affect clinical outcome (eg, cytotoxic antibiotic pastes and sodium hypochlorite irrigation), only 1 report has shown pulp-like tissue formation. As a result, numerous research groups have been working intensively on tissue engineering–based strategies for regenerative endodontics. A variety of scaffolds, associated or not with stem cells and GFs, have been explored. Based on current knowledge, a key aspect for clinical success is the development of a biocompatible disinfection approach. Our group has focused on the design and synthesis of 3D patient-specific cytocompatible antibiotic–containing nanofibers for intracanal drug delivery. In vivo preclinical (animal) studies are currently being conducted to validate these results. Nonetheless, the development of a regenerative strategy using advanced scaffolds, loaded or not with stem cells and/or GFs to stimulate pulp and dentin regeneration after attaining a bacteria-free niche, is warranted to establish novel therapeutics to treat teeth with necrotic pulp.

Regarding periodontal tissue engineering, regenerative strategies with membranes associated or not with grafting materials have been used with distinct levels of clinical success. With the aging population, it is crucial to find a tissue-engineering/regenerative medicine approach that allows for the fabrication of scaffolds that can ultimately guide reliable and predictable regeneration of multiple periodontal tissues. Current evidence, including the results of the first 3D-printed patient-specific scaffold, suggests that both biologically modified and multilayered tissue-specific scaffolds should be used. Although that case report was considered unsuccessful in the long term, several issues were raised and will help move the field forward. For example, it is well known that vascularization of the scaffold/cell construct is an essential step in tissue healing, because this process provides the nutrients and oxygen needed for bone cells to survive, and facilitates removal of cell waste products. Therefore, a more open and interconnected porous structure might amplify bone regeneration and vascularization. In addition, the compartmentalized delivery of biologics to the PDL-forming region of the scaffold, along with osteogenic molecules (eg, BMPs) to the bone region, may further facilitate tissue growth and remodeling.

ACKNOWLEDGMENTS

M.C. Bottino thanks former students/postdoctoral researchers from the Indiana University School of Dentistry (IUSD), Drs Maria T. P. de Albuquerque, Eliseu A. Münchow, and Krzysztof Kamocki, for their contributions to electrospun nanofibers research. The authors apologize for not citing all relevant references because of space limitations. M.C. Bottino acknowledges funding from the National Institutes of Health (NIH)/National Institute of Dental and Craniofacial Research (NIDCR) (grant DE023552). J.E. Nör acknowledges NIH/NIDCR grant R01DE21410.

REFERENCES

1. Caton J, Bostanci N, Remboutsika E, et al. Future dentistry: cell therapy meets tooth and periodontal repair and regeneration. J Cell Mol Med 2011;15(5): 1054–65.
2. Mitsiadis TA, Orsini G, Jimenez-Rojo L. Stem cell-based approaches in dentistry. Eur Cell Mater 2015;30:248–57.
3. Albuquerque MT, Valera MC, Nakashima M, et al. Tissue-engineering-based strategies for regenerative endodontics. J Dent Res 2014;93(12):1222–31.
4. Diogenes AR, Ruparel NB, Teixeira FB, et al. Translational science in disinfection for regenerative endodontics. J Endod 2014;40(4 Suppl):S52–7.

5. Galler KM. Clinical procedures for revitalization: current knowledge and considerations. Int Endod J 2016;49(10):926–36.

6. Diogenes A, Henry MA, Teixeira FB, et al. An update on clinical regenerative endodontics. Endod Top 2013;28(1):2–23.

7. Banchs F, Trope M. Revascularization of immature permanent teeth with apical periodontitis: new treatment protocol? J Endod 2004;30(4):196–200.

8. Bose R, Nummikoski P, Hargreaves K. A retrospective evaluation of radiographic outcomes in immature teeth with necrotic root canal systems treated with regenerative endodontic procedures. J Endod 2009;35(10):1343–9.

9. Cehreli ZC, Isbitiren B, Sara S, et al. Regenerative endodontic treatment (revascularization) of immature necrotic molars medicated with calcium hydroxide: a case series. J Endod 2011;37(9):1327–30.

10. Iwaya SI, Ikawa M, Kubota M. Revascularization of an immature permanent tooth with apical periodontitis and sinus tract. Dent Traumatol 2001;17(4):185–7.

11. Petrino JA, Boda KK, Shambarger S, et al. Challenges in regenerative endodontics: a case series. J Endod 2010;36(3):536–41.

12. Bottino MC, Kamocki K, Yassen GH, et al. Bioactive nanofibrous scaffolds for regenerative endodontics. J Dent Res 2013;92(11):963–9.

13. Bottino MC, Arthur RA, Waeiss RA, et al. Biodegradable nanofibrous drug delivery systems: effects of metronidazole and ciprofloxacin on periodontopathogens and commensal oral bacteria. Clin Oral Investig 2014;18(9):2151–8.

14. Palasuk J, Kamocki K, Hippenmeyer L, et al. Bimix antimicrobial scaffolds for regenerative endodontics. J Endod 2014;40(11):1879–84.

15. Albuquerque MT, Ryan SJ, Munchow EA, et al. Antimicrobial effects of novel triple antibiotic paste-mimic scaffolds on *Actinomyces naeslundii* biofilm. J Endod 2015;41(8):1337–43.

16. Albuquerque MT, Valera MC, Moreira CS, et al. Effects of ciprofloxacin-containing scaffolds on *Enterococcus faecalis* biofilms. J Endod 2015;41(5):710–4.

17. Bottino MC, Yassen GH, Platt JA, et al. A novel three-dimensional scaffold for regenerative endodontics: materials and biological characterizations. J Tissue Eng Regen Med 2015;9(11):E116–23.

18. Kamocki K, Nor JE, Bottino MC. Effects of ciprofloxacin-containing antimicrobial scaffolds on dental pulp stem cell viability – In vitro studies. Arch Oral Biol 2015;60(8):1131–7.

19. Kamocki K, Nor JE, Bottino MC. Dental pulp stem cell responses to novel antibiotic-containing scaffolds for regenerative endodontics. Int Endod J 2015;48(12):1147–56.

20. Pankajakshan D, Albuquerque MT, Evans JD, et al. Triple antibiotic polymer nanofibers for intracanal drug delivery: effects on dual species biofilm and cell function. J Endod 2016;42(10):1490–5.

21. Bottino MC, Thomas V, Schmidt G, et al. Recent advances in the development of GTR/GBR membranes for periodontal regeneration–a materials perspective. Dent Mater 2012;28(7):703–21.

22. Karring T, Warrer K. Development of the principle of guided tissue regeneration. Alpha Omegan 1992;85(4):19–24.

23. Larsson L, Decker AM, Nibali L, et al. Regenerative medicine for periodontal and peri-implant diseases. J Dental Res 2016;95(3):255–66.

24. Carter S-SD, Costa PF, Vaquette C, et al. Additive biomanufacturing: an advanced approach for periodontal tissue regeneration. Ann Biomed Eng 2017;45(1):12–22.

25. Ivanovski S, Vaquette C, Gronthos S, et al. Multiphasic scaffolds for periodontal tissue engineering. J Dental Res 2014;93(12):1212–21.
26. Rasperini G, Pilipchuk SP, Flanagan CL, et al. 3D-printed bioresorbable scaffold for periodontal repair. J Dent Res 2015;94(9 Suppl):153S–7S.
27. Park CH, Rios HF, Jin Q, et al. Tissue engineering bone-ligament complexes using fiber-guiding scaffolds. Biomaterials 2012;33(1):137–45.
28. Pilipchuk SP, Monje A, Jiao Y, et al. Integration of 3D printed and micropatterned polycaprolactone scaffolds for guidance of oriented collagenous tissue formation in vivo. Adv Healthc Mater 2016;5(6):676–87.
29. Park CH, Rios HF, Jin Q, et al. Biomimetic hybrid scaffolds for engineering human tooth-ligament interfaces. Biomaterials 2010;31(23):5945–52.
30. Park CH, Kim KH, Rios HF, et al. Spatiotemporally controlled microchannels of periodontal mimic scaffolds. J Dent Res 2014;93(12):1304–12.
31. Park CH, Rios HF, Taut AD, et al. Image-based, fiber guiding scaffolds: a platform for regenerating tissue interfaces. Tissue Eng Part C Methods 2014; 20(7):533–42.
32. Dominici M, Le Blanc K, Mueller I, et al. Minimal criteria for defining multipotent mesenchymal stromal cells. The International Society for Cellular Therapy position statement. Cytotherapy 2006;8(4):315–7.
33. Gronthos S, Brahim J, Li W, et al. Stem cell properties of human dental pulp stem cells. J Dent Res 2002;81(8):531–5.
34. Gronthos S, Mankani M, Brahim J, et al. Postnatal human dental pulp stem cells (DPSCs) in vitro and in vivo. Proc Natl Acad Sci U S A 2000;97(25):13625–30.
35. Arthur A, Rychkov G, Shi S, et al. Adult human dental pulp stem cells differentiate toward functionally active neurons under appropriate environmental cues. Stem Cells 2008;26(7):1787–95.
36. Iohara K, Zheng L, Ito M, et al. Side population cells isolated from porcine dental pulp tissue with self-renewal and multipotency for dentinogenesis, chondrogenesis, adipogenesis, and neurogenesis. Stem Cells 2006;24(11):2493–503.
37. Jo YY, Lee HJ, Kook SY, et al. Isolation and characterization of postnatal stem cells from human dental tissues. Tissue Eng 2007;13(4):767–73.
38. Miura M, Gronthos S, Zhao M, et al. SHED: stem cells from human exfoliated deciduous teeth. Proc Natl Acad Sci U S A 2003;100(10):5807–12.
39. Cordeiro MM, Dong Z, Kaneko T, et al. Dental pulp tissue engineering with stem cells from exfoliated deciduous teeth. J Endod 2008;34(8):962–9.
40. Sakai VT, Zhang Z, Dong Z, et al. SHED differentiate into functional odontoblasts and endothelium. J Dent Res 2010;89(8):791–6.
41. Bento LW, Zhang Z, Imai A, et al. Endothelial differentiation of SHED requires MEK1/ERK signaling. J Dent Res 2013;92(1):51–7.
42. Zhang N, Chen B, Wang W, et al. Isolation, characterization and multi-lineage differentiation of stem cells from human exfoliated deciduous teeth. Mol Med Rep 2016;14(1):95–102.
43. Sonoyama W, Liu Y, Fang D, et al. Mesenchymal stem cell-mediated functional tooth regeneration in swine. PLoS One 2006;1:e79.
44. Sonoyama W, Liu Y, Yamaza T, et al. Characterization of the apical papilla and its residing stem cells from human immature permanent teeth: a pilot study. J Endod 2008;34(2):166–71.
45. Huang GT, Sonoyama W, Liu Y, et al. The hidden treasure in apical papilla: the potential role in pulp/dentin regeneration and bioroot engineering. J Endod 2008;34(6):645–51.

46. Huang GT, Yamaza T, Shea LD, et al. Stem/progenitor cell-mediated de novo regeneration of dental pulp with newly deposited continuous layer of dentin in an in vivo model. Tissue Eng Part A 2010;16(2):605–15.
47. Seo BM, Miura M, Gronthos S, et al. Investigation of multipotent postnatal stem cells from human periodontal ligament. Lancet 2004;364(9429):149–55.
48. Shoi K, Aoki K, Ohya K, et al. Characterization of pulp and follicle stem cells from impacted supernumerary maxillary incisors. Pediatr Dent 2014;36(3): 79–84.
49. Guo W, Gong K, Shi H, et al. Dental follicle cells and treated dentin matrix scaffold for tissue engineering the tooth root. Biomaterials 2012;33(5):1291–302.
50. Bakopoulou A, About I. Stem cells of dental origin: current research trends and key milestones towards clinical application. Stem Cells Int 2016;2016:4209891.
51. Huang GT. Dental pulp and dentin tissue engineering and regeneration: advancement and challenge. Front Biosci (Elite Ed) 2011;3:788–800.
52. Jeeruphan T, Jantarat J, Yanpiset K, et al. Mahidol study 1: comparison of radiographic and survival outcomes of immature teeth treated with either regenerative endodontic or apexification methods: a retrospective study. J Endod 2012;38(10):1330–6.
53. Wang X, Thibodeau B, Trope M, et al. Histologic characterization of regenerated tissues in canal space after the revitalization/revascularization procedure of immature dog teeth with apical periodontitis. J Endod 2010;36(1):56–63.
54. Andreasen JO, Farik B, Munksgaard EC. Long-term calcium hydroxide as a root canal dressing may increase risk of root fracture. Dent Traumatol 2002;18(3): 134–7.
55. Cvek M. Prognosis of luxated non-vital maxillary incisors treated with calcium hydroxide and filled with gutta-percha. A retrospective clinical study. Endod Dent Traumatol 1992;8(2):45–55.
56. Langer R, Vacanti JP. Tissue engineering. Science 1993;260(5110):920–6.
57. Conde MCM, Chisini LA, Sarkis-Onofre R, et al. A scoping review of root canal revascularization: relevant aspects for clinical success and tissue formation. Int Endod J 2016. [Epub ahead of print].
58. Shimizu E, Jong G, Partridge N, et al. Histologic observation of a human immature permanent tooth with irreversible pulpitis after revascularization/regeneration procedure. J Endod 2012;38(9):1293–7.
59. Martin G, Ricucci D, Gibbs JL, et al. Histological findings of revascularized/revitalized immature permanent molar with apical periodontitis using platelet-rich plasma. J Endod 2013;39(1):138–44.
60. Becerra P, Ricucci D, Loghin S, et al. Histologic study of a human immature permanent premolar with chronic apical abscess after revascularization/revitalization. J Endod 2014;40(1):133–9.
61. Chrepa V, Henry MA, Daniel BJ, et al. Delivery of apical mesenchymal stem cells into root canals of mature teeth. J Dental Res 2015;94(12):1653–9.
62. Porter ML, Munchow EA, Albuquerque MT, et al. Effects of novel 3-dimensional antibiotic-containing electrospun scaffolds on dentin discoloration. J Endod 2016;42(1):106–12.
63. Gupte MJ, Ma PX. Nanofibrous scaffolds for dental and craniofacial applications. J Dent Res 2012;91(3):227–34.
64. Huang GT. Pulp and dentin tissue engineering and regeneration: current progress. Regen Med 2009;4(5):697–707.

65. Li WJ, Tuli R, Okafor C, et al. A three-dimensional nanofibrous scaffold for cartilage tissue engineering using human mesenchymal stem cells. Biomaterials 2005;26(6):599–609.

66. Galler KM, Hartgerink JD, Cavender AC, et al. A customized self-assembling peptide hydrogel for dental pulp tissue engineering. Tissue Eng Part A 2012; 18(1–2):176–84.

67. Rosa V, Zhang Z, Grande RH, et al. Dental pulp tissue engineering in full-length human root canals. J Dent Res 2013;92(11):970–5.

68. Reneker DH, Yarin AL. Electrospinning jets and polymer nanofibers. Polymer 2008;49(10):2387–425.

69. Ishimatsu H, Kitamura C, Morotomi T, et al. Formation of dentinal bridge on surface of regenerated dental pulp in dentin defects by controlled release of fibroblast growth factor-2 from gelatin hydrogels. J Endod 2009;35(6):858–65.

70. Zhang H, Liu S, Zhou Y, et al. Natural mineralized scaffolds promote the dentinogenic potential of dental pulp stem cells via the mitogen-activated protein kinase signaling pathway. Tissue Eng Part A 2012;18(7–8):677–91.

71. Cavalcanti BN, Zeitlin BD, Nor JE. A hydrogel scaffold that maintains viability and supports differentiation of dental pulp stem cells. Dent Mater 2013;29(1): 97–102.

72. Moore AN, Perez SC, Hartgerink JD, et al. Ex vivo modeling of multidomain peptide hydrogels with intact dental pulp. J Dent Res 2015;94(12):1773–81.

73. Khayat A, Monteiro N, Smith EE, et al. GelMA-encapsulated hDPSCs and HUVECs for dental pulp regeneration. J Dental Res 2017;96(2):192–9.

74. Zhang Z, Eyster TW, Ma PX. Nanostructured injectable cell microcarriers for tissue regeneration. Nanomedicine (Lond) 2016;11(12):1611–28.

75. Kuang R, Zhang Z, Jin X, et al. Nanofibrous spongy microspheres for the delivery of hypoxia-primed human dental pulp stem cells to regenerate vascularized dental pulp. Acta Biomater 2016;33:225–34.

76. Kuang R, Zhang Z, Jin X, et al. Nanofibrous spongy microspheres enhance odontogenic differentiation of human dental pulp stem cells. Adv Healthc Mater 2015;4(13):1993–2000.

77. Niu X, Liu Z, Hu J, et al. Microspheres assembled from chitosan-graft-poly(lactic acid) micelle-like core-shell nanospheres for distinctly controlled release of hydrophobic and hydrophilic biomolecules. Macromol Biosci 2016;16(7):1039–47.

78. Smith AJ, Duncan HF, Diogenes A, et al. Exploiting the bioactive properties of the dentin-pulp complex in regenerative endodontics. J Endod 2016;42(1): 47–56.

79. Kim JY, Xin X, Moioli EK, et al. Regeneration of dental-pulp-like tissue by chemotaxis-induced cell homing. Tissue Eng Part A 2010;16(10):3023–31.

80. Ishizaka R, Iohara K, Murakami M, et al. Regeneration of dental pulp following pulpectomy by fractionated stem/progenitor cells from bone marrow and adipose tissue. Biomaterials 2012;33(7):2109–18.

81. Nakashima M, Iohara K. Regeneration of dental pulp by stem cells. Adv Dent Res 2011;23(3):313–9.

82. Iohara K, Imabayashi K, Ishizaka R, et al. Complete pulp regeneration after pulpectomy by transplantation of CD105+ stem cells with stromal cell-derived factor-1. Tissue Eng Part A 2011;17(15–16):1911–20.

83. Murakami M, Horibe H, Iohara K, et al. The use of granulocyte-colony stimulating factor induced mobilization for isolation of dental pulp stem cells with high regenerative potential. Biomaterials 2013;34(36):9036–47.

84. Iohara K, Murakami M, Takeuchi N, et al. A novel combinatorial therapy with pulp stem cells and granulocyte colony-stimulating factor for total pulp regeneration. Stem Cells Transl Med 2013;2(7):521–33.

85. Nakashima M, Iohara K, Murakami M, et al. Pulp regeneration by transplantation of dental pulp stem cells in pulpitis: a pilot clinical study. Stem Cell Res Ther 2017;8(1):61.

86. Eke PI, Dye BA, Wei L, et al. Prevalence of periodontitis in adults in the United States: 2009 and 2010. J Dent Res 2012;91(10):914–20.

87. Chen FM, Jin Y. Periodontal tissue engineering and regeneration: current approaches and expanding opportunities. Tissue Eng Part B Rev 2010;16(2): 219–55.

88. Chen FM, Zhang J, Zhang M, et al. A review on endogenous regenerative technology in periodontal regenerative medicine. Biomaterials 2010;31(31): 7892–927.

89. Behring J, Junker R, Walboomers XF, et al. Toward guided tissue and bone regeneration: morphology, attachment, proliferation, and migration of cells cultured on collagen barrier membranes. A systematic review. Odontology 2008;96(1):1–11.

90. Kasaj A, Reichert C, Gotz H, et al. In vitro evaluation of various bioabsorbable and nonresorbable barrier membranes for guided tissue regeneration. Head Face Med 2008;4:22.

91. Sculean A, Nikolidakis D, Schwarz F. Regeneration of periodontal tissues: combinations of barrier membranes and grafting materials - biological foundation and preclinical evidence: a systematic review. J Clin Periodontol 2008;35: 106–16.

92. Gentile P, Chiono V, Tonda-Turo C, et al. Polymeric membranes for guided bone regeneration. Biotechnol J 2011;6(10):1187–97.

93. Geurs NC, Korostoff JM, Vassilopoulos PJ, et al. Clinical and histologic assessment of lateral alveolar ridge augmentation using a synthetic long-term bioabsorbable membrane and an allograft. J Periodontol 2008;79(7):1133–40.

94. Gielkens PFM, Schortinghuis J, de Jong JR, et al. The influence of barrier membranes on autologous bone grafts. J Dental Res 2008;87(11):1048–52.

95. Jovanovic SA, Nevins M. Bone formation utilizing titanium-reinforced barrier membranes. Int J Periodontics Restorative Dent 1995;15(1):56–69.

96. Milella E, Barra G, Ramires PA, et al. Poly(L-lactide)acid/alginate composite membranes for guided tissue regeneration. J Biomed Mater Res 2001;57(2): 248–57.

97. Coonts BA, Whitman SL, O'Donnell M, et al. Biodegradation and biocompatibility of a guided tissue regeneration barrier membrane formed from a liquid polymer material. J Biomed Mater Res 1998;42(2):303–11.

98. Hou LT, Yan JJ, Tsai AYM, et al. Polymer-assisted regeneration therapy with Atrisorb® barriers in human periodontal intrabony defects. J Clin Periodontol 2004;31(1):68–74.

99. Donos N, Kostopoulos L, Karring T. Alveolar ridge augmentation using a resorbable copolymer membrane and autogenous bone grafts - an experimental study in the rat. Clin Oral Implants Res 2002;13(2):203–13.

100. Klinge U, Klosterhalfen B, Muller M, et al. Foreign body reaction to meshes used for the repair of abdominal wall hernias. Eur J Surg 1999;165(7):665–73.

101. Laurell L, Gottlow J. Guided tissue regeneration update. Int Dent J 1998;48(4): 386–98.

102. Santos A, Goumenos G, Pascual A. Management of gingival recession by the use of an acellular dermal graft material: a 12-case series. J Periodontol 2005;76(11):1982–90.

103. Felipe M, Andrade PF, Grisi MFM, et al. Comparison of two surgical procedures for use of the acellular dermal matrix graft in the treatment of gingival recession: a randomized controlled clinical study. J Periodontol 2007;78(7):1209–17.

104. Haffajee AD, Socransky SS. Microbial etiological agents of destructive periodontal diseases. Periodontol 2000 1994;5:78–111.

105. Slots J, MacDonald ES, Nowzari H. Infectious aspects of periodontal regeneration. Periodontol 2000 1999;19:164–72.

106. Kenawy ER, Bowlin GL, Mansfield K, et al. Release of tetracycline hydrochloride from electrospun poly(ethylene-co-vinylacetate), poly(lactic acid), and a blend. J Control Release 2002;81(1–2):57–64.

107. He CL, Huang ZM, Han XJ. Fabrication of drug-loaded electrospun aligned fibrous threads for suture applications. J Biomed Mater Res A 2009;89A(1):80–95.

108. Zamani M, Morshed M, Varshosaz J, et al. Controlled release of metronidazole benzoate from poly epsilon-caprolactone electrospun nanofibers for periodontal diseases. Eur J Pharm Biopharm 2010;75(2):179–85.

109. Furtos G, Rivero G, Rapuntean S, et al. Amoxicillin-loaded electrospun nanocomposite membranes for dental applications. J Biomed Mater Res B Appl Biomater 2017;105(5):966–76.

110. Munchow EA, Albuquerque MT, Zero B, et al. Development and characterization of novel ZnO-loaded electrospun membranes for periodontal regeneration. Dent Mater 2015;31(9):1038–51.

111. Rai JJ, Kalantharakath T. Biomimetic ceramics for periodontal regeneration in infrabony defects: a systematic review. J Int Soc Prev Community Dent 2014;4(Suppl 2):S78–92.

112. Bishop A, Balazsi C, Yang JHC, et al. Biopolymer-hydroxyapatite by electrospinning. Polym Adv Technol 2006;17(11–12):902–6.

113. Thomas V, Dean DR, Vohra YK. Nanostructured biomaterials for regenerative medicine. Curr Nanosci 2006;2(3):155–77.

114. Deng XL, Sui G, Zhao ML, et al. Poly(L-lactic acid)/hydroxyapatite hybrid nanofibrous scaffolds prepared by electrospinning. J Biomater Sci Polym Ed 2007;18(1):117–30.

115. Thomas V, Dean DR, Jose MV, et al. Nanostructured biocomposite scaffolds based on collagen coelectrospun with nanohydroxyapatite. Biomacromolecules 2007;8(2):631–7.

116. Erisken C, Kalyon DM, Wang HJ. Functionally graded electrospun polycaprolactone and beta-tricalcium phosphate nanocomposites for tissue engineering applications. Biomaterials 2008;29(30):4065–73.

117. Jose MV, Thomas V, Johnson KT, et al. Aligned PLGA/HA nanofibrous nanocomposite scaffolds for bone tissue engineering. Acta Biomater 2009;5(1):305–15.

118. Jose MV, Thomas V, Xu YY, et al. Aligned bioactive multi-component nanofibrous nanocomposite scaffolds for bone tissue engineering. Macromol Biosci 2010;10(4):433–44.

119. Wu XN, Miao LY, Yao YF, et al. Electrospun fibrous scaffolds combined with nanoscale hydroxyapatite induce osteogenic differentiation of human periodontal ligament cells. Int J Nanomedicine 2014;9:4135–43.

120. Ribeiro N, Sousa SR, van Blitterswijk CA, et al. A biocomposite of collagen nano-fibers and nanohydroxyapatite for bone regeneration. Biofabrication 2014;6(3): 035015.
121. Yeo M, Lee H, Kim G. Three-dimensional hierarchical composite scaffolds consisting of polycaprolactone, beta-tricalcium phosphate, and collagen nanofibers: fabrication, physical properties, and in vitro cell activity for bone tissue regeneration. Biomacromolecules 2011;12(2):502–10.
122. El-Fiqi A, Kim JH, Kim HW. Osteoinductive fibrous scaffolds of biopolymer/mesoporous bioactive glass nanocarriers with excellent bioactivity and long-term delivery of osteogenic drug. ACS Appl Mater Interfaces 2015;7(2):1140–52.
123. Phipps MC, Xu Y, Bellis SL. Delivery of platelet-derived growth factor as a chemotactic factor for mesenchymal stem cells by bone-mimetic electrospun scaffolds. PLoS One 2012;7(7):e40831.
124. Ji W, Yang F, Ma J, et al. Incorporation of stromal cell-derived factor-1alpha in PCL/gelatin electrospun membranes for guided bone regeneration. Biomaterials 2013;34(3):735–45.
125. Bottino MC, Thomas V, Janowski GM. A novel spatially designed and functionally graded electrospun membrane for periodontal regeneration. Acta Biomater 2011;7(1):216–24.
126. Obregon F, Vaquette C, Ivanovski S, et al. Three-dimensional bioprinting for regenerative dentistry and craniofacial tissue engineering. J Dental Res 2015; 94(9_suppl):143S–52S.
127. Nygaard-Ostby B, Hjortdal O. Tissue formation in the root canal following pulp removal. Scand J Dent Res 1971;79(5):333–49.
128. Ostby BN. The role of the blood clot in endodontic therapy. An experimental histologic study. Acta Odontol Scand 1961;19:324–53.

An Overview of Dental Adhesive Systems and the Dynamic Tooth–Adhesive Interface

Ana Bedran-Russo, DDS, MS, PhD[a,]*,
Ariene A. Leme-Kraus, DDS, MS, PhD[b],
Cristina M.P. Vidal, DDS, MS, PhD[c], Erica C. Teixeira, DDS, MS, PhD[c]

KEYWORDS

• Dental adhesives • Dentin • Enamel • Bond strength • Biodegradation • Technology

KEY POINTS

- There are 2 adhesive strategies of contemporary dental adhesive systems to bond to enamel and dentin. Strategies can be accomplished in 1 to 3 steps.
- Resin acidity and hydrophilicity increase the susceptibility for degradation of the adhesive interface; altered forms of enamel and dentin can negatively affect bonding to enamel and dentin.
- Adhesive interfaces are susceptible to biodegradation.
- Degradation includes interaction with the dental biofilm, active bacterial enzymes, and activation of endogenous enzymes.
- Some restorative strategies that might influence the long-term outcome of the dynamic tooth adhesive–interface are summarized.

Adhesion has revolutionized contemporary restorative dentistry with 3 ground-breaking research advances:

1. Dental surfaces modification by acid etching,
2. The development of methacrylate-based resin composite chemistry, and
3. The development of hydrophilic resin chemistry.

Disclosure Statement: The authors have nothing to disclose.
[a] Department of Restorative Dentistry, University of Illinois at Chicago College of Dentistry, 801 South Paulina Street, Room 531, Chicago, IL 60612, USA; [b] Department of Restorative Dentistry, University of Illinois at Chicago College of Dentistry, 801 South Paulina Street, Chicago, IL 60612, USA; [c] Department of Operative Dentistry, The University of Iowa College of Dentistry and Dental Clinics, 801 Newton Road, Iowa City, IA 52242, USA
* Corresponding author.
E-mail address: bedran@uic.edu

Dent Clin N Am 61 (2017) 713–731
http://dx.doi.org/10.1016/j.cden.2017.06.001
dental.theclinics.com

Adhesive restorative dentistry affects virtually every dental practice because it is integral to many procedures, including dental sealant placement, bonding of orthodontic brackets, direct composites restorations, intraradicular posts cementation, cementation of inlay or onlay tooth-colored restorations, full-coverage all-ceramic crowns, bonded bridges, and root canal obturation. This review focuses on dental restorative applications of dental adhesives.

CLASSIFICATION OF CONTEMPORARY DENTAL ADHESIVE SYSTEMS

Dental adhesives are often commercially categorized into generations reflecting the handling technique or advances in formulations rather than new adhesion concepts or mechanisms. A close look into the chemistry of dental adhesives and their mechanism of adhesion to dentin yield 2 major adhesive concepts:

1. Reliance on the complete removal of the smear layer (ie, the layer of debris formed after cavity preparation) and superficial demineralization of dentin and enamel, and
2. Partial superficial dissolution and incorporation of the smear layer into the adhesive interface.

Both concepts promote adhesion by micromechanical retention to the underlying dental tissues. However, an additional chemical bond to the substrate is present, particularly in the latter concept.

Multiple or single steps are commercially available within the 2 major categories of systems, being referred to as etch and rinse and self-etch (**Fig. 1**). Etch-and-rinse systems (also known as total etch) require separate acid etching and rinsing steps followed by the application of the primer and adhesive in 2 separate or one combined step (see **Fig. 1**). Self-etch systems do not require a separate etching step; rather, acidic primers are used to promote partial dissolution of the smear layer and infiltration of primers by an etching or primer step followed by an adhesive application (2-step systems) or through a single formulation with an adhesive resin (all-in-one system; see **Fig. 1**). More recently, the term universal systems has been used to define dental adhesive systems that can be applied either in etch-and-rinse or self-etch modes (see **Fig. 1**).

THE CHEMISTRY OF DENTAL ADHESIVES SYSTEMS

Overall, adhesion is attainable when the following are present: clean dental surfaces, good surface wettability, diffusion of the adhesive resin monomers within enamel and

Contemporary Dental Adhesive Systems					Characteristics			Longevity
System Mode	Delivery	Adhesion Steps			Acidity	Hydrophilicity	Bond Stability[b]	
		Etching	Primer	Adhesive				
Etch-and-rinse	3-step				+	+	+ + + +	Stability
	2-step				+ +	+ +	+ + +	Degree of Conversion / Solvent Evaporation
Self-etch	2-step				+ + +	+ +	+ + + +	Acidity / Hydrophilicity
	1-step				+ + + +	+ + +	+	Degradation
Universal	1 or 2 steps[a]				+ + +	+ +	+ (+) +	

Fig. 1. Current contemporary dental adhesives systems and characteristics affecting the long-term stability of dentin–resin interfaces. Symbol (+) indicates scale ranging from lowest (+) to highest (++++). [a] The adhesive system support optional pre-etching of enamel or dentin (2- step) or self-etching mode (1-step). [b] Depicts relative values of dentin bond strength, note that average bond strengths can greatly vary among brands, studies and application modes (for universal systems). Degree of conversion = polymerization rates of adhesive.

dentin, and adequate resin polymerization. The adhesive systems consist of a blend of methacrylate-based resin monomers with either 2 (cross-linking monomers) or 1 (functional monomers) polymerizable ends, organic solvents, a photoinitiator system, and often nanofillers (**Fig. 2**).[1] The chemistry of dental adhesive resins must fulfill the requirements for adhesion to different dental substrates: enamel, dentin, and cementum. Functional hydrophilic resin monomers facilitate resin infiltration within the demineralized and moist dentin surface whereas hydrophobic cross-linking resin monomers provide the mechanical strength, stability and compatibility between the adhesive system and the bulk restorative resin or resin cement.[2]

Resin monomers with 2 or more polymerizable groups are necessary to form a highly cross-linked network to provide the strength and stability of the adhesive layer.[1,2] Examples of cross-linking monomers with a more hydrophobic nature are bisphenol A-glycidyl methacrylate, triethylene glycol dymethacrylate (TEGDMA), urethane dimethacrylate, and ethoxylated bisphenol-A dimethacrylate. The difference in molecular weight among the resin monomers is important, because low-molecular-weight monomers dissolve the high-molecular-weight monomers, improving the wettability of the resin blend.

Functional monomers usually have 1 functional group (eg, hydroxyl groups) and a single polymerizable group to form linear polymer chains (see **Fig. 2**). One example is hydroxyethyl methacrylate (HEMA), a hydrophilic monomer that facilitates resin

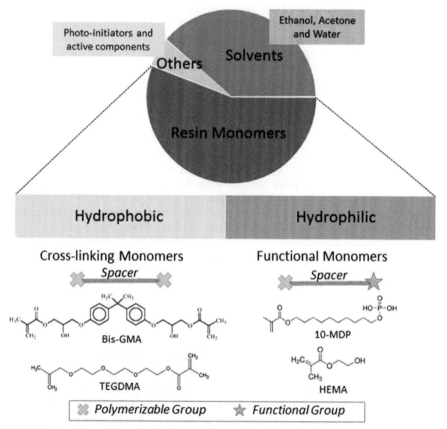

Fig. 2. Composition of dental adhesives and examples of cross-linking and functional monomers used in contemporary adhesive systems.

diffusion within the moist collagen network and is commonly present in contemporary adhesive systems. The importance of HEMA to adhesion in a wet environment is due to its amphiphilic nature, in addition to its low molecular weight that makes HEMA a suitable solvent for high-molecular-weight monomers. As a disadvantage, the incorporation of HEMA to adhesive–resin blends have made dental adhesives too hydrophilic and thus more susceptible to hydrolysis.[3]

In self-etch adhesive systems, the functional groups in the resin monomers are usually acidic, and are also important for etching the enamel and dentin surfaces. Examples of acidic functional resin monomers are 4-methacryloyloxyethyl trimellitate anhydride, 10-methacryloyloxydecyl dihydrogenphosphate (10-MDP), and 2-(methacryloyloxyethyl)phenyl hydrogenphosphate. The functional groups with self-etching ability are either carboxyl or phosphate, and they can also establish ionic bonds with calcium from hydroxyapatite. Overall, 10-MDP is the most popular and highly stable acidic monomer; its stability is attributed to the long carbonyl chain (spacer) between the functional and the polymerizable groups in the monomer structure (see **Fig. 2**). Additionally, the phosphate functional group is capable of forming strong ionic bonds with hydroxyapatite, owing to the low solubility of the resulting calcium salts.[4,5]

Solvents such as ethanol, acetone, and water are added to the adhesive blends to lower viscosity and promote resin infiltration.[1] Solvents are also essential for the effective "wet-bonding" technique of etch-and-rinse systems and dental surface etching by acidic primers in self-etching systems. In etch-and-rinse systems, ethanol plays key roles during the infiltration of the resin monomers within the wet collagen network and further helps in the evaporation of excess water by forming water–ethanol aggregates.[1,6] Remaining solvent within the adhesive layers may impair adhesive polymerization, lowering the mechanical properties and resulting in increased degradation over time.[7,8] Therefore, thorough and careful air drying of the adhesive, exceeding the time recommended by most manufacturers, is necessary to remove excess solvent before the light curing of the adhesive.

Another component that plays significant roles in both the attainment of bond strength and forming a stable adhesive interface is the photoinitiator system. The traditionally used photoinitiator system camphorquinone-amine possesses hydrophobic characteristics and, therefore, may be subjected to phase separation resulting in poor polymerization of the more hydrophilic portion of the adhesive systems.[9,10] Research toward the use of alternative photoinitiator systems have introduced diphenyl(2,4,6-trimethylbenzoyl)phosphine oxide and others like 2-hydroxy-3-(3,4 dimethyl-9-oxo-9H-thioxanthen-2-yloxy)-N,N,N-trimethyl-1-propanaminium chloride (QTX).[10–12] Specifically, the use of QTX has been explored because, as a water-soluble photoinitiator, it may improve the polymerization of the more hydrophilic components of the adhesive resin blends.[10,13]

Active ingredients may also be added to the adhesive resin chemistry for specific functions, such as methacryloyloxydodecylpyridinium bromide in the adhesive resin and benzalkonium chloride in the etching component to impart antibacterial activity.[1] Although the contribution of these specific ingredients have been demonstrated in in vitro studies, more studies are necessary to confirm their clinical efficiency.[14]

Finally, the compatibility and ratio of the various components of adhesive systems is essential to maximize performance. The one-step self-etch systems are chemically more unstable owing to an imbalance between the adhesive blends. The chemistry incompatibility leads to phase separation of the adhesive components, resulting in a porous and poorly polymerized adhesive layer.[9] The sealing ability of these systems is also compromised because of the high amount of hydrophilic monomers that entrap water within the bonding layer and thus can accelerate the degradation of the adhesive interface.

ADHESIVE BONDING MECHANISMS TO ENAMEL AND DENTIN
Bonding to Enamel

Enamel is the hardest tissue in the human body. It is composed of 96 wt. % mineral, 1 wt. % organic matrix, and 3 wt. % water. Hydroxyapatite crystals are orderly deposited to form highly complex enamel prisms. The enamel prisms run almost perpendicularly from the dentin–enamel junction to the outer enamel surface. An acid-resistant aprismatic enamel surface provides additional protection against enamel dissolution in the oral environment.

Adhesion of methacrylate-based resins to enamel is highly predictable and achievable in most adhesive restorative procedures. The micromechanical bonding mechanism is provided by formation of resin tags and microtags on the superficially demineralized enamel (**Fig. 3**). Phosphoric acid is the acid conditioner of choice for dental tissues. Phosphoric acid increases the surface area, surface energy, and wettability of enamel, which are key physical properties for the infiltration of resin and the formation of resin tags after light curing. Although the bond strength values to enamel are not as high as those to dentin, the bond strength is highly stable because of the nature of the enamel (high inorganic phase and minimal water content). It is unquestionable that pre-etching of the enamel provides the highest enamel bond strength for all contemporary dental adhesives, including self-etching systems.[15]

Bonding to Dentin

Dentin is the bulk tissue of the tooth and thus plays a key role in the clinical outcomes of adhesive restorations. Dentin is highly mineralized, but with lower mineral content

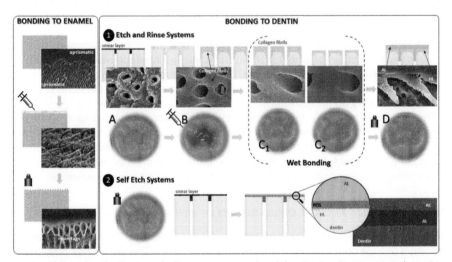

Fig. 3. Mechanism of adhesion of adhesives to enamel and dentin. Bonding to enamel requires superficial demineralization for the formation of resin tags and microtags. Bonding to dentin: (1) (*A*) smear layer on dentin tubules and intratubular and intertubular dentin. (*B*) Etch-and-rinse systems use a separate step of etching, resulting in removal of smear layer and exposure of collagen after superficial mineral removal. (*C1, C2*) The importance of surface moisture to maintain the collagen interfibrillar spaces for the infiltration of resin monomers. (*D*) Formation of the hybrid layer. (2) The smear layer is incorporated into the adhesive interface; the hybrid layer is thinner and irregular. Chemical bonding is achievable with certain adhesives brands (*green stars*).

(70 wt. % mineral) and much higher organic composition (20 wt. % organic phase) and water than enamel. The morphology of dentin is highly intricate. Dentin tubules, extending from the pulp complex to the dentin–enamel junction or cementum, are surrounded by a highly mineralized intratubular dentin that is bordered by less mineralized intertubular dentin (see **Fig. 3**). The intertubular dentin is rich in type I collagen fibrils and noncollagenous molecules, both of which are essential components of the dentin–adhesive interface.

There are significant variations in the biochemistry, morphology, and mechanical properties of the different types of dentin, dentin of different ages, within different dentin depths, and between crown and root dentin. Hence, dentin is a dynamic tissue and becomes modified over time owing to physiologic or pathologic conditions. The composition and morphology provides the necessary elasticity and toughness to support the enamel and protect the pulp tissue over a lifespan.

The high fluid content (10 wt. %) in the form of bound and unbound water and the extracellular protein content makes the mechanism of enamel adhesion unachievable in dentin. The dentin is highly hydrophilic and thus not well-suited for the infiltration of hydrophobic resin monomers. As with enamel, surface etching of dentin increases the bond strength owing to the removal of the smear layer (see **Fig. 3**). However, acceptable dentin–resin adhesion is only feasible with the hydrophilic and amphiphilic resin chemistry. Hydrophilic resin monomers can infiltrate the demineralized dentin surface rich in type I collagen fibrils, encapsulating the exposed dentin matrix and forming the so-called hybrid layer.[16] The hybridization of dentin surfaces is the primary mechanism of micromechanical retention of etch-and-rinse adhesive systems. To achieve good adhesion, a wet surface is necessary to maintain the interfibrillar spaces of the exposed collagen network for the infiltration of resin monomers into the demineralized dentin. Thus, the clinician must leave the cavity preparation visually wet, but without excessive water pooling, and immediately place the adhesive systems (see **Fig. 3**). Although this bonding to moist dentin is technique sensitive, it remains the most predictable adhesion mechanism for dentin.

Self-etch adhesive systems can still form hybrid layers, but the incorporation and/or partial demineralization of smear layer at the adhesive interface results in a thin and irregularly formed hybrid layer (see **Fig. 3**). Evidence of chemical bonding between certain acidic primers, such as 10-MDP functional monomer and the mineral phase of dentin, provides additional retention.

There is large variability in the adhesion of self-etching systems to enamel and dentin, reflecting the high variability in performance of various commercially available systems. The clinical performance of self-etching systems continues to improve, particularly with the technique of selective etching of enamel, where phosphoric acid etching of enamel only is performed before using the self-etch adhesive.

THE ORAL BIOFILM AND THE DEGRADATION OF DENTAL ADHESIVE INTERFACES

Microorganisms present in the oral cavity adhere to tooth surfaces (dental plaque), forming a diverse community that functions as a biofilm.[17] The biofilm has physiologic roles; however, changes in the microflora phenotype and genotype can favor the establishment of an acidogenic stage, resulting in the demineralization of enamel and dentin.[18] Biofilms form and interact differently with the various microenvironments in the oral cavity and such interaction is driven by modifications in dental plaque ecology, restorative material, chemistry and surface characteristics.

Oral biofilm formation is greater on resin composites than sound enamel and other restorative materials such as amalgam, glass ionomer cements, and ceramics.[19,20]

The more extensive biofilm formation and acid production on resin composites is a result of increased growth of microorganisms, mainly owing to genetic modifications of bacteria virulence induced by resin components.[21–23] Indeed, different monomers can increase the activity of a variety of cariogenic bacteria species. For example, TEGDMA stimulates growth of *Streptococcus sobrinus* and *Lactobacillus acidophilus*, which have high cariogenic potential for the development of primary and secondary caries, respectively.[24] The cariogenic effect is triggered by high amounts of TEGDMA monomer released from the resin composite matrix owing to increased hydrophilicity and greater unpolymerized content in the material.

Moreover, oral bacteria can induce the biodegradation of resin-based materials by esterase activity, resulting in the release of hydrolyzed byproducts from monomers. For example, triethylene glycol is released from TEGDMA, which stimulates the growth of microorganisms, especially at lower pH levels.[25] In particular for adhesive systems, the esterase activity of cariogenic bacteria can degrade cured resins, especially self-etching systems that present a more hydrophilic chemical composition.[26] However, phosphate derivatives of methacrylates present in those adhesives (such as 10-MDP) can release acidic polymers that actually inhibit bacterial growth owing to a very low pH.[27] Thus, the hydrophilicity of the adhesive system as well as its pH can influence bacterial growth.

Of great importance is that biofilm formation on resin composite is influenced by factors that can be controlled by the clinician, such as the quality of the light curing and finishing procedures.[28] Short light curing times may result in a lesser degree of conversion of monomer to polymer, leaving more residual unpolymerized monomers in the materials and enhancing *Streptococcus mutans* colonization.[29] Also, *S mutans* colonization is lower on polished resin surfaces[30] or nanofilled resin composite.[28] Resin composite surfaces with deep and large depressions or exposure of resin matrix are more prone to biofilm formation,[31] because these features promote a niche for bacteria to better resist shear forces and removal.

DEGRADATION OF DENTAL ADHESIVE INTERFACES: BIOLOGICAL CONSIDERATIONS

The main clinical shortcomings of resin composite restorations are marginal degradation, fracture, debonding, and secondary caries.[32–35] Although the proper handling of materials will maximize their performance, intrinsic (chemistry, bonding mechanism, biology) and extrinsic (oral environment) factors will affect the longevity of adhesive restorations. The mechanisms of degradation of the dental adhesive interfaces are complex, primarily driven by breakdown of the adhesive system, and the underlying dental tissue, potentially mediated by biological or environmental responses. Such mechanisms are described below and are summarized in **Table 1**.

The Stability of Dental Resin Chemistry

The resin chemistry of adhesive systems dramatically influences their stability in the oral environment. The major biological concern is the release of free monomers and/or products from the resin matrix either during the polymerization reaction or over time owing to biodegradation and erosion.[36] Unreacted monomers can diffuse and leach out of the resin matrix,[37] potentially causing cytotoxic reactions in the pulp.[38] This is a concern, particularly in deep cavities owing to increased permeability as a result of the reduced thickness of remaining dentin.[39] Commonly used monomers, such as bisphenol A-glycidyl methacrylate, urethane dimethacrylate, TEGDMA, and HEMA, present cytotoxic potential.[40] Newly developed adhesive formulations, such as the universal systems, have shown favorable results in reducing in vitro

Table 1
Summary of the contributors and the mechanism of the degradation of adhesive interfaces

Structure/Material		Characteristic/ Mechanism	Result	Contribution to Failure
Dental resins	Resin composite	Rough surface Leached/ unreacted resins	Favors biofilm formation and growth Favors acidogenic biofilm	Resin degradation by esterases Secondary caries Increases interfacial
	Adhesive system	Unreacted/ leached resins	Increase water/ saliva sorption Hydrolysis of resin Reach pulp tissue	porosity Pulp response Susceptibility to degradation
		Incomplete monomer infiltration	Exposed dentin organic matrix	Enzymes degrade anchoring collagen
		Etching technique/pH	Activation of endogenous proteases[a]	Loss of interfacial bonding/seal
Dental tissues	Latent endogenous proteases[a]	Latent enzymes activate at low pH	Degradation of dentin matrix	Increases interfacial porosities
	Inherent moisture	Water trapped at the adhesive interface	Hydrolysis of resin	Loss of interfacial bonding or seal
Oral environment	Bacterial esterases Salivary esterases	Enzymatic activity Enzymatic activity	Resin polymer degradation and release of monomers and byproducts	Enzymes degrade anchoring collagen Increases interfacial
	Biofilm	Leached or unreacted resins	Favors biofilm formation and growth Favors acidogenic biofilm	porosities Loss of interfacial bonding/seal Secondary caries

[a] Endogenous proteases are matrix metalloproteinases and cysteines cathepsins in dentin.

cytotoxicity.[41] Clinicians should be careful when light curing resin composite and adhesive systems to ensure that the distance between the light curing unit tip and the resin surface is as short as possible and that enough energy is delivered directly to the material to optimize the degree of conversion and reduce cytotoxic effects.

The breakdown and release of unbound monomers from the resin matrix can also take place by enzymatic catalysis,[36] along with pH changes and oxidation, leading to the degradation of resin-based materials.[42] In fact, the hydrolysis of monomers is aggravated by water sorption through nanoporosities within the hybrid layer that accelerates the degradation of the adhesive resin and results in areas of unprotected collagen fibrils and a weaker dentin–resin bond.[43]

The main enzymes involved in the degradation of resin-based materials are believed to be salivary esterases.[44] Esterases are released by salivary glands, gingival crevicular fluid, and oral microorganisms.[42] Esterases can hydrolytically degrade condensation bonds in resin monomers, such as esters and urethanes. Hydrolysis depends on water sorption, which is more likely to occur in adhesive systems composed of hydrophilic and acidic resin monomers acting as semipermeable membranes that allow water movement through the interface, regardless of the etch-and-rinse or self-etch strategy.[3,45,46]

Hence, esterases can act synergistically to promote resin composite biodegradation.[47,48] Therefore, resin composite degradation by esterases are dependent on adhesive or resin monomer formulation and the individual's salivary composition.

The Breakdown of Dentin: Host Response Mechanism

The degradation of the extracellular matrix exposed by the partial demineralization and incomplete infiltration of resin monomers can destabilize the underlying dentin and the hybrid layer. The presence of denuded collagen fibrils is more common in etch-and-rinse systems, owing to discrepancies in depth of acid etching and resin infiltration. For self-etching systems, the dentin matrix can be exposed after hydrolytic degradation of resin monomers.[49] Because collagen breakdown has been shown to take place even in the absence of bacteria, a host response mechanism was proposed to explain such degradation, previously attributed to water hydrolysis, saliva, and/or bacteria.[50]

Matrix metalloproteases (MMPs) were the first enzymes linked to a host triggered degradation of collagen by the cleavage of the extracellular matrix components within the dentin–resin interface.[51] Members of this family of zinc- and calcium-dependent endopeptidases were further identified in dentin,[52–54] whereas a wider gene expression profile for many different MMPs was reported in pulp tissue and odontoblasts.[55] MMPs are synthesized as inactive zymogens that remain trapped within the mineralized dentin and are activated by other proteases or by an acidic environment. However, it is in neutral pH that MMP reach the highest activity.

Cysteine cathepsins (CCs) are another family of host enzymes found in dentin and capable of degrading extracellular matrix components.[56] In contrast with MMPs, CCs are active at slightly acidic pH and most are unstable at neutral pH.[57] Although the role of CCs in the dentin organic matrix degradation was explored mainly in caries disease, a synergy between these 2 families of enzymes was proposed to explain collagen degradation at the adhesive interfaces.[58,59]

The ability of MMPs to contribute to the degradation of the dentin matrix and the hybrid layer was confirmed in vitro and in vivo by the investigation of protease inhibitors as part of the bonding protocol.[60–64] The low pH of phosphoric acid etching and acidic primers can activate MMPs and CCs, whereas the latter can release even more active enzymes, enhancing the proteolytic potency of MMPs.[58] In fact, both etch-and-rinse and self-etch strategies can activate endogenous enzymes.[65–67] When the pH is neutral, MMPs cleave exposed collagen fibrils that anchor the restoration to dentin, resulting in decreased bond strength and increased permeability at the dentin–adhesive interface.

Interestingly, a combined effect of endogenous MMPs and esterases from saliva was reported recently to promote adhesive interface degradation, especially when using an etch-and-rinse adhesive system.[68] Such findings confirm that a complex mechanism is involved in the degradation of hybrid layers. Future research should clarify such interactions to develop novel biomaterials that can inhibit different pathways of degradation.

CLINICAL CONSIDERATIONS WHEN USING CONTEMPORARY ADHESIVE SYSTEMS

The first step in ensuring that the adhesive system placement steps will go smoothly is to review handling instructions. Manufacturers provide easy to follow instructions to maximize the bonding technique steps and indications (ie, direct vs indirect restorations) of individual products. In general, when performing a dental adhesive procedure, the clinician must be aware that bonding to enamel is more predictable than that of dentin or cementum owing to the composition differences among these substrates. Thus, restorations with margins in enamel yield better outcomes.[69,70]

Contamination by saliva and blood during restorative procedure decreases the bond strength[71,72] and must be avoided. If accidental contamination occurs, there are experimentally tested strategies to minimize the negative effects of contamination, including re-etching the surface, rinsing and drying the contaminated surface, and the application of additional coats of adhesive.

Table 2 provides a few strategies and their purpose reported in the literature that might influence the long-term outcome of the dynamic tooth–adhesive interface. Additional considerations are described to maximize performance of adhesive systems.

Table 2
Strategies to optimize bonding and potentially the long-term outcomes of adhesive restorations

Strategy	Purpose	Technique
Field control[73,74]	Prevent contamination of prepared tooth structure (ie, with saliva, blood)	Optimal use of rubber dam isolation
Enamel grinding[73,75]	Expose enamel rods, increase bond effectiveness and durability	Bevel cavosurface of cavity preparation using fine diamond or hand instruments
Selective etching[76]	Improve bond strength and reduce microleakage	Apply phosphoric acid to enamel and rinse before using self-etch system
Wet bonding technique	Prepare dentin for hybridization	Remove excess of water from acid-etched dentin with sponges; apply primer on moist dentin
Dentin desensitizer[77,78]	Occlude dentinal tubules to reduce permeability and sensitivity	Additional step before primer application
Matrix metalloproteinase inhibitors[60,63]	Inhibit activation of endogenous enzymes responsible for the degradation of collagen fibrils	Extra step used as an additional primer of dentin (ie, 2% chlorhexidine) or within exiting primer
Enhanced solvent evaporation[7]	Remove interfacial water	Critical air drying of primer or adhesive layer before light curing
Hydrophobic coating[79]	Reduce water sorption and stabilize hybrid layer over time	Multiple layers of a hydrophobic resin layer might be applied
Dentin impregnation[80]	Enhance dentin impregnation of resin monomer into tubules	Increased application time of adhesive resin with vigorous brushing technique
Extended polymerization[81]	Improve polymerization (degree of conversion) and reduce permeability	Curing times used beyond manufacturer recommendation (ie, from 20 s to 40 s, to 60 s)
Wet ethanol bonding[82,83]	Permits the use of hydrophobic resins that absorb little water	Rub of ethanol in dentin before primer application (ie, 100% for 1 min); protocol is not completely established for clinical user

Substrate

Adhesive systems are formulated to bond to sound tooth structure. However, dental restorative procedures are often carried out on altered forms of enamel and dentin. There are significant compositional and morphologic differences between the dental substrate that impairs adhesion. It is well-known that bonding is higher in superficial dentin than deep dentin because of the increased number of tubules in the latter.[84] Furthermore, tubular fluid percolating from the pulp to the dentin surface can be detrimental to the bonding of certain adhesive systems.[77,85]

In enamel, dental fluorosis decreases the bond strength of etch-and-rinse and self-etching systems.[86] Thus, etching enamel for additional time is recommended. Amelogenesis imperfecta impairs bond strength to enamel, regardless of the adhesive strategy, possibly owing to a very mild etching of the enamel surface.[87] Similarly, bond strength is lower in tetracycline-stained teeth.[88]

Carious dentin is another commonly altered substrate that clinicians manage daily. Studies have shown that dentin with caries has lower hardness and produces lower bond strength owing to the low mineralization and collagen disorganization.[89] With new techniques involving minimally invasive dentistry and selective caries removal, the clinician will often need to bond to these less than ideal substrates when using resin-based materials. However, if the restoration margin is in sound dentin and/or enamel the outcome might not be affected. Therefore, it is crucial for optimization of bonding procedures to have a safe bonding zone containing sound dentin.

Restoration of noncarious cervical lesions are also a challenge, because sclerotic dentin is generally hypermineralized with the presence of intratubular mineral deposits. It has been recommended for noncarious cervical lesion surfaces to be gently mechanically roughened and surface etched with phosphoric acid for additional time (up to 30 seconds) to increase adhesion of selective materials.[90,91] Dentin desensitizers have been suggested to decrease the permeability of the substrate and reduce sensitivity, especially when using the etch-and-rinse approach (see **Table 2**). Desensitizers that do not precipitate at the surface of the tooth do not affect the bond strength of most contemporary systems.[78,92] In addition, the proximity of these lesions to the gingival tissue make class V preparations a challenge for the use of dentin bonding agents. A metaanalysis has shown that field isolation and type of adhesive system are factors that affect the clinical performance of these restorations.[73,74]

In addition, in vitro studies have shown that even the wetness of the acid-etched dentin from the bonding protocol can affect the performance of adhesive systems, and it can be material dependent.[93,94] Therefore, the conditioning of the dentin substrate is important consideration before the application of the primer or adhesive layer (see **Table 2**).

Material

According to most clinical studies, 3-step etch-and-rinse systems and 2-step self-etch systems have shown better performance than other systems with a reduced numbers of steps.[73,95] Self-etch systems are appealing products in clinical practice because of their reduced number of steps and anecdotal evidence of a low incidence of postoperative sensitivity.[96] In addition, they are less sensitive to the application technique as indicated by low variation in bond strength results.[85,97] However, studies have reported poorer clinical outcomes for all-in-one systems. Furthermore, acid etching with phosphoric acid, which has a much lower pH than the acids used in most self-etching systems, remains the most adequate strategy to achieve high bond strength to enamel.[70,76] Even with self-etching systems, selective etching and enamel grinding are indicated for a variety of clinical procedures, for example, class IV preparations.

With the etch-and-rinse approach, studies have investigated extensively the importance of the hybrid layer and the effective infiltration by resin monomers. The degradation of exposed collagen fibrils is known to be a problem for the tooth–resin interface. A few clinical strategies to overcome this problem are shown in **Table 2**, such as the use of MMPs inhibitors, as mentioned.[61,64]

Compatibility to Luting Cements

The material dependence of the self-etch adhesive systems regarding performance and clinical indications was made clear once these systems began to be used with autocured and dual-cured composites to bond indirect restoration and core buildup restorations on damaged teeth.[98–100] Light-cured resins with the adjunct of an adhesive system are used to bond porcelain or resin composite veneers. On the other hand, bonding all-ceramic restorations onto teeth with short clinical crowns benefit from the advantages of adhesive cementation and a dual-cured cement is usually indicated. The acidic monomers present in self-etch systems might affect the polymerization of dual-cured and self-cured resins.[100] The practitioner must investigate the manufacturers' recommendations before using multiple different systems. Lately, there is a trend to use self-adhesive luting resins, which might change the clinical vulnerability of using incompatible systems.

Preventive and Therapeutic Sealants

Resin-based sealants, used to seal incipient lesions in permanent tooth surfaces, has been shown to be an effective method for preventing and arresting caries. In this procedure, the enamel is etched and a sealant material is applied to fissures and pits acting as a protective layer against plaque retention. A recent clinical article showed that the use of an adhesive system (etch and rinse and self-etch) before placement of sealant (bonded sealant) produced higher retention rates over a 2-year follow-up period than that of the conventional technique, where only acid etching was performed before resin sealant application (no separate adhesive system). The same was not observed with a self-etch system without etching the enamel surface.[101] Additional clinical trials are necessary to investigate the performance of other contemporary adhesive systems for fissure sealing.

THE FUTURE FOR ADHESIVE SYSTEMS: TECHNOLOGICAL AND FUNDAMENTAL TRENDS

Adhesive dentistry continuously evolves fundamentally and technologically. Incremental advances in response to limitations in physical and chemical properties and handling are common and easier to implement than wholesale changes from the development of totally new materials. Innovative strategies for new materials have been aided by the identification of the effects of key biological and environmental factors. Below are examples of new concepts that may drive the development of novel dental adhesives to be implemented in clinical use.

Chemistry of Adhesive Systems

Current efforts are directed toward the modification of the chemistry of traditional monomers and the development of new monomers and resin composite formulations to enhance the chemical stability of resin-based restorations.[102,103] New resin chemistry free of ester bonds, such as ether-based monomers[102] and methacrylamide-based monomers, show or promise resistance against esterase degradation. Thiolene chemistries are resistant to water degradation and have been explored for the optimization of the physical characteristics and the polymerization mechanism for clinical use.[104–106]

The incorporation of antimicrobials and enzymatic inhibitors has been widely explored and limitations include the lack of substantivity and sustained effects. More recently, the inclusion of bioactive glass fillers, as antimicrobial and remineralizing agents, to an experimental resin showed effectiveness in reducing biofilm formation and penetration within adhesive interfaces.[107] The incorporation of natural-derived plant compounds has also been shown to be an option for obtaining resins with antimicrobial properties.[108] Moreover, novel monomers containing amorphous calcium phosphate have shown the potential to prevent periodontitis-related bacteria and might have potential clinical use to restore class V cavities.[109]

Biologically Driven Strategies

Biologically inspired strategies have been of particular interest to solve the many limitations of dental adhesion. Many of these strategies mimic natural biological processes to develop novel biomaterials. This approach has been particularly used to stabilize and even reinforce the dental substrate in intimate contact with the adhesive interface. Biomimetic analogs, such as polyacrylic acid and sodium trimetaphosphate, have been elegantly shown to regulate mineral deposition in dentin and promote remineralization at the adhesive interface.[110,111]

Other biomimetic approaches use physiologic processes in dentin to mediate physicochemical modification of the dentin matrix using chemical agents. Experimental studies have explored multifunctional synthetic and natural chemical agents to reinforce and stabilize the dentin–adhesive interface. Plant-derived compounds have attracted particular attention owing to their potency, bioavailability, and potential biocompatibility. A range of biological responses are elicited, such as increased collagen cross-linking and inactivation of endogenous and exogenous proteases.[112] Such effects have been shown to increase the mechanical properties of both dentin[113] and the dentin–resin interface.[94] Enrichment of these bioactives has shown remarkably stable adhesion on wet surfaces,[114] as well as the ability to inhibit artificial secondary caries around dentin–resin margins.[115]

Catechol containing molecules are known to adhere to wet surfaces.[116,117] The synergistic role in adhesion of catecholamine functionalized monomers allied to the micromechanical interlocking of the polymerized resin with the dentin collagen network are promising for the future of adhesion to teeth.[118]

SUMMARY

Significant improvements to the chemistry and handling of adhesive systems have broadened the use of adhesive restorative dentistry. However, adhesive systems remain technique sensitive, and proper use of the material is the first step to achieving clinically acceptable bonds to enamel and dentin. Once in service, resin–tooth interfaces are highly susceptible to degradation in the oral environment. Bacteria, endogenous enzymes, and inherent resin chemistry limitations can further determine the longevity of dental restorations. The clinician must be aware of dental tissue variation and optimization strategies for individual decision making of the best adhesive system and bonding technique.

REFERENCES

1. Van Landuyt KL, Snauwaert J, De Munck J, et al. Systematic review of the chemical composition of contemporary dental adhesives. Biomaterials 2007;28(26): 3757–85.
2. Moszner N, Salz U, Zimmermann J. Chemical aspects of self-etching enamel-dentin adhesives: a systematic review. Dent Mater 2005;21(10):895–910.
3. Malacarne J, Carvalho RM, de Goes MF, et al. Water sorption/solubility of dental adhesive resins. Dent Mater 2006;22(10):973–80.
4. Yoshida Y, Nagakane K, Fukuda R, et al. Comparative study on adhesive performance of functional monomers. J Dent Res 2004;83(6):454–8.
5. Yoshihara K, Yoshida Y, Nagaoka N, et al. Adhesive interfacial interaction affected by different carbon-chain monomers. Dent Mater 2013;29(8):888–97.
6. Chiba A, Zhou J, Nakajima M, et al. The effects of ethanol on the size-exclusion characteristics of type I dentin collagen to adhesive resin monomers. Acta Biomater 2016;33:235–41.
7. Bail M, Malacarne-Zanon J, Silva SM, et al. Effect of air-drying on the solvent evaporation, degree of conversion and water sorption/solubility of dental adhesive models. J Mater Sci Mater Med 2012;23(3):629–38.
8. Ito S, Hashimoto M, Wadgaonkar B, et al. Effects of resin hydrophilicity on water sorption and changes in modulus of elasticity. Biomaterials 2005;26(33): 6449–59.
9. Abedin F, Ye Q, Good HJ, et al. Polymerization- and solvent-induced phase separation in hydrophilic-rich dentin adhesive mimic. Acta Biomater 2014;10(7): 3038–47.
10. Abedin F, Ye Q, Parthasarathy R, et al. Polymerization behavior of hydrophilic-rich phase of dentin adhesive. J Dent Res 2015;94(3):500–7.
11. Schneider LF, Cavalcante LM, Prahl SA, et al. Curing efficiency of dental resin composites formulated with camphorquinone or trimethylbenzoyl-diphenyl-phosphine oxide. Dent Mater 2012;28(4):392–7.
12. Dressano D, Palialol AR, Xavier TA, et al. Effect of diphenyliodonium hexafluorophosphate on the physical and chemical properties of ethanolic solvated resins containing camphorquinone and 1-phenyl-1,2-propanedione sensitizers as initiators. Dent Mater 2016;32(6):756–64.
13. Hayakawa T, Horie K. Effect of water-soluble photoinitiator on the adhesion between composite and tooth substrate. Dent Mater 1992;8(6):351–3.
14. Cocco AR, Rosa WL, Silva AF, et al. A systematic review about antibacterial monomers used in dental adhesive systems: current status and further prospects. Dent Mater 2015;31(11):1345–62.
15. Luhrs AK, Guhr S, Schilke R, et al. Shear bond strength of self-etch adhesives to enamel with additional phosphoric acid etching. Oper Dent 2008;33(2):155–62.
16. Nakabayashi N, Kojima K, Masuhara E. The promotion of adhesion by the infiltration of monomers into tooth substrates. J Biomed Mater Res 1982;16(3): 265–73.
17. Marsh PD. Dental plaque as a microbial biofilm. Caries Res 2004;38(3):204–11.
18. Takahashi N, Nyvad B. Caries ecology revisited: microbial dynamics and the caries process. Caries Res 2008;42(6):409–18.
19. Konishi N, Torii Y, Kurosaki A, et al. Confocal laser scanning microscopic analysis of early plaque formed on resin composite and human enamel. J Oral Rehabil 2003;30(8):790–5.

20. Rosentritt M, Hahnel S, Groger G, et al. Adhesion of Streptococcus mutans to various dental materials in a laminar flow chamber system. J Biomed Mater Res B Appl Biomater 2008;86(1):36–44.
21. Shemesh M, Tam A, Aharoni R, et al. Genetic adaptation of Streptococcus mutans during biofilm formation on different types of surfaces. BMC Microbiol 2010;10:51.
22. Khalichi P, Singh J, Cvitkovitch DG, et al. The influence of triethylene glycol derived from dental composite resins on the regulation of Streptococcus mutans gene expression. Biomaterials 2009;30(4):452–9.
23. Sadeghinejad L, Cvitkovitch DG, Siqueira WL, et al. Mechanistic, genomic and proteomic study on the effects of BisGMA-derived biodegradation product on cariogenic bacteria. Dent Mater 2017;33(2):175–90.
24. Hansel C, Leyhausen G, Mai UE, et al. Effects of various resin composite (co) monomers and extracts on two caries-associated micro-organisms in vitro. J Dent Res 1998;77(1):60–7.
25. Khalichi P, Cvitkovitch DG, Santerre JP. Effect of composite resin biodegradation products on oral streptococcal growth. Biomaterials 2004;25(24):5467–72.
26. Bourbia M, Ma D, Cvitkovitch DG, et al. Cariogenic bacteria degrade dental resin composites and adhesives. J Dent Res 2013;92(11):989–94.
27. Brambilla E, Ionescu A, Mazzoni A, et al. Hydrophilicity of dentin bonding systems influences in vitro Streptococcus mutans biofilm formation. Dent Mater 2014;30(8):926–35.
28. Pereira CA, Eskelson E, Cavalli V, et al. Streptococcus mutans biofilm adhesion on composite resin surfaces after different finishing and polishing techniques. Oper Dent 2011;36(3):311–7.
29. Brambilla E, Gagliani M, Ionescu A, et al. The influence of light-curing time on the bacterial colonization of resin composite surfaces. Dent Mater 2009;25(9):1067–72.
30. Ionescu A, Wutscher E, Brambilla E, et al. Influence of surface properties of resin-based composites on in vitro Streptococcus mutans biofilm development. Eur J Oral Sci 2012;120(5):458–65.
31. Park JW, Song CW, Jung JH, et al. The effects of surface roughness of composite resin on biofilm formation of Streptococcus mutans in the presence of saliva. Oper Dent 2012;37(5):532–9.
32. Morimoto S, Rebello de Sampaio FB, Braga MM, et al. Survival rate of resin and ceramic inlays, onlays, and overlays: a systematic review and meta-analysis. J Dent Res 2016;95(9):985–94.
33. Kopperud SE, Tveit AB, Gaarden T, et al. Longevity of posterior dental restorations and reasons for failure. Eur J Oral Sci 2012;120(6):539–48.
34. Astvaldsdottir A, Dagerhamn J, van Dijken JW, et al. Longevity of posterior resin composite restorations in adults - a systematic review. J Dent 2015;43(8):934–54.
35. Rho YJ, Namgung C, Jin BH, et al. Longevity of direct restorations in stress-bearing posterior cavities: a retrospective study. Oper Dent 2013;38(6):572–82.
36. Goldberg M. In vitro and in vivo studies on the toxicity of dental resin components: a review. Clin Oral Investig 2008;12(1):1–8.
37. Kwon HJ, Oh YJ, Jang JH, et al. The effect of polymerization conditions on the amounts of unreacted monomer and bisphenol A in dental composite resins. Dent Mater J 2015;34(3):327–35.
38. Chen RS, Liuiw CC, Tseng WY, et al. The effect of curing light intensity on the cytotoxicity of a dentin-bonding agent. Oper Dent 2001;26(5):505–10.

39. Galler K, Hiller KA, Ettl T, et al. Selective influence of dentin thickness upon cyto-toxicity of dentin contacting materials. J Endod 2005;31(5):396–9.
40. Urcan E, Scherthan H, Styllou M, et al. Induction of DNA double-strand breaks in primary gingival fibroblasts by exposure to dental resin composites. Biomaterials 2010;31(8):2010–4.
41. Elias ST, Santos AF, Garcia FC, et al. Cytotoxicity of universal, self-etching and etch-and-rinse adhesive systems according to the polymerization time. Braz Dent J 2015;26(2):160–8.
42. Santerre JP, Shajii L, Leung BW. Relation of dental composite formulations to their degradation and the release of hydrolyzed polymeric-resin-derived products. Crit Rev Oral Biol Med 2001;12(2):136–51.
43. Hashimoto M, Ohno H, Sano H, et al. In vitro degradation of resin-dentin bonds analyzed by microtensile bond test, scanning and transmission electron microscopy. Biomaterials 2003;24(21):3795–803.
44. Chauncey HH. Salivary enzymes. J Am Dent Assoc 1961;63(3):360–8.
45. Tay FR, Pashley DH, Suh BI, et al. Single-step adhesives are permeable membranes. J Dent 2002;30(7–8):371–82.
46. Tay FR, Pashley DH, Suh B, et al. Single-step, self-etch adhesives behave as permeable membranes after polymerization. Part I. Bond strength and morphologic evidence. Am J Dent 2004;17(4):271–8.
47. Finer Y, Santerre JP. Biodegradation of a dental composite by esterases: dependence on enzyme concentration and specificity. J Biomater Sci Polym Ed 2003; 14(8):837–49.
48. Finer Y, Jaffer F, Santerre JP. Mutual influence of cholesterol esterase and pseudocholinesterase on the biodegradation of dental composites. Biomaterials 2004;25(10):1787–93.
49. Hashimoto M. A review–micromorphological evidence of degradation in resin-dentin bonds and potential preventional solutions. J Biomed Mater Res B Appl Biomater 2010;92(1):268–80.
50. Pashley DH, Tay FR, Yiu C, et al. Collagen degradation by host-derived enzymes during aging. J Dent Res 2004;83(3):216–21.
51. Nagase H, Visse R, Murphy G. Structure and function of matrix metalloproteinases and TIMPs. Cardiovasc Res 2006;69(3):562–73.
52. Niu LN, Zhang L, Jiao K, et al. Localization of MMP-2, MMP-9, TIMP-1, and TIMP-2 in human coronal dentine. J Dent 2011;39(8):536–42.
53. Mazzoni A, Mannello F, Tay FR, et al. Zymographic analysis and characterization of MMP-2 and -9 forms in human sound dentin. J Dent Res 2007;86(5):436–40.
54. Sulkala M, Tervahartiala T, Sorsa T, et al. Matrix metalloproteinase-8 (MMP-8) is the major collagenase in human dentin. Arch Oral Biol 2007;52(2):121–7.
55. Palosaari H, Pennington CJ, Larmas M, et al. Expression profile of matrix metalloproteinases (MMPs) and tissue inhibitors of MMPs in mature human odontoblasts and pulp tissue. Eur J Oral Sci 2003;111(2):117–27.
56. Tersariol IL, Geraldeli S, Minciotti CL, et al. Cysteine cathepsins in human dentin-pulp complex. J Endod 2010;36(3):475–81.
57. Turk V, Stoka V, Vasiljeva O, et al. Cysteine cathepsins: from structure, function and regulation to new frontiers. Biochim Biophys Acta 2012;1824(1):68–88.
58. Tjaderhane L, Nascimento FD, Breschi L, et al. Optimizing dentin bond durability: control of collagen degradation by matrix metalloproteinases and cysteine cathepsins. Dent Mater 2013;29(1):116–35.
59. Nascimento FD, Minciotti CL, Geraldeli S, et al. Cysteine cathepsins in human carious dentin. J Dent Res 2011;90(4):506–11.

60. Breschi L, Mazzoni A, Nato F, et al. Chlorhexidine stabilizes the adhesive interface: a 2-year in vitro study. Dent Mater 2010;26(4):320–5.
61. Zhou J, Tan J, Yang X, et al. MMP-inhibitory effect of chlorhexidine applied in a self-etching adhesive. J Adhes Dent 2011;13(2):111–5.
62. Silva Sousa AB, Vidal CM, Leme-Kraus AA, et al. Experimental primers containing synthetic and natural compounds reduce enzymatic activity at the dentin-adhesive interface under cyclic loading. Dent Mater 2016;32(10):1248–55.
63. Carrilho MR, Geraldeli S, Tay F, et al. In vivo preservation of the hybrid layer by chlorhexidine. J Dent Res 2007;86(6):529–33.
64. Hebling J, Pashley DH, Tjaderhane L, et al. Chlorhexidine arrests subclinical degradation of dentin hybrid layers in vivo. J Dent Res 2005;84(8):741–6.
65. Nishitani Y, Yoshiyama M, Wadgaonkar B, et al. Activation of gelatinolytic/collagenolytic activity in dentin by self-etching adhesives. Eur J Oral Sci 2006;114(2):160–6.
66. Mazzoni A, Pashley DH, Nishitani Y, et al. Reactivation of inactivated endogenous proteolytic activities in phosphoric acid-etched dentine by etch-and-rinse adhesives. Biomaterials 2006;27(25):4470–6.
67. Mazzoni A, Scaffa P, Carrilho M, et al. Effects of etch-and-rinse and self-etch adhesives on dentin MMP-2 and MMP-9. J Dent Res 2013;92(1):82–6.
68. Serkies KB, Garcha R, Tam LE, et al. Matrix metalloproteinase inhibitor modulates esterase-catalyzed degradation of resin-dentin interfaces. Dent Mater 2016;32(12):1513–23.
69. Peumans M, Kanumilli P, De Munck J, et al. Clinical effectiveness of contemporary adhesives: a systematic review of current clinical trials. Dent Mater 2005;21(9):864–81.
70. Peumans M, De Munck J, Mine A, et al. Clinical effectiveness of contemporary adhesives for the restoration of non-carious cervical lesions. A systematic review. Dent Mater 2014;30(10):1089–103.
71. Cobanoglu N, Unlu N, Ozer FF, et al. Bond strength of self-etch adhesives after saliva contamination at different application steps. Oper Dent 2013;38(5):505–11.
72. Aboushelib MN. Clinical performance of self-etching adhesives with saliva contamination. J Adhes Dent 2011;13(5):489–93.
73. Mahn E, Rousson V, Heintze S. Meta-analysis of the influence of bonding parameters on the clinical outcome of tooth-colored cervical restorations. J Adhes Dent 2015;17(5):391–403.
74. Wang Y, Li C, Yuan H, et al. Rubber dam isolation for restorative treatment in dental patients. Cochrane Database Syst Rev 2016;(9):CD009858.
75. Perdigao J, Geraldeli S. Bonding characteristics of self-etching adhesives to intact versus prepared enamel. J Esthet Restor Dent 2003;15(1):32–41 [discussion: 42].
76. Szesz A, Parreiras S, Reis A, et al. Selective enamel etching in cervical lesions for self-etch adhesives: a systematic review and meta-analysis. J Dent 2016;53:1–11.
77. Perdigao J. Dentin bonding-variables related to the clinical situation and the substrate treatment. Dent Mater 2010;26(2):e24–37.
78. Lee J, Sabatini C. Glutaraldehyde collagen cross-linking stabilizes resin-dentin interfaces and reduces bond degradation. Eur J Oral Sci 2017;125(1):63–71.
79. Sadek FT, Pashley DH, Nishitani Y, et al. Application of hydrophobic resin adhesives to acid-etched dentin with an alternative wet bonding technique. J Biomed Mater Res A 2008;84(1):19–29.

80. Hashimoto M, Sano H, Yoshida E, et al. Effects of multiple adhesive coatings on dentin bonding. Oper Dent 2004;29(4):416–23.

81. Cadenaro M, Breschi L, Rueggeberg FA, et al. Effect of adhesive hydrophilicity and curing time on the permeability of resins bonded to water vs. ethanol-saturated acid-etched dentin. Dent Mater 2009;25(1):39–47.

82. Sadek FT, Braga RR, Muench A, et al. Ethanol wet-bonding challenges current anti-degradation strategy. J Dent Res 2010;89(12):1499–504.

83. Ayar MK. A review of ethanol wet-bonding: principles and techniques. Eur J Dent 2016;10(1):155–9.

84. Giannini M, Carvalho RM, Martins LR, et al. The influence of tubule density and area of solid dentin on bond strength of two adhesive systems to dentin. J Adhes Dent 2001;3(4):315–24.

85. Perdigao J. New developments in dental adhesion. Dent Clin North Am 2007; 51(2):333–57, viii.

86. Ertugrul F, Turkun M, Turkun LS, et al. Bond strength of different dentin bonding systems to fluorotic enamel. J Adhes Dent 2009;11(4):299–303.

87. Yaman BC, Ozer F, Cabukusta CS, et al. Microtensile bond strength to enamel affected by hypoplastic amelogenesis imperfecta. J Adhes Dent 2014;16(1): 7–14.

88. Liu HL, Liang KN, Cheng L, et al. The adhesive properties of two bonding systems to tetracycline stained dentin. Zhonghua Kou Qiang Yi Xue Za Zhi 2016; 51(1):42–5 [in Chinese].

89. Hosoya Y, Tay FR. Hardness, elasticity, and ultrastructure of bonded sound and caries-affected primary tooth dentin. J Biomed Mater Res B Appl Biomater 2007;81(1):135–41.

90. Luque-Martinez IV, Mena-Serrano A, Munoz MA, et al. Effect of bur roughness on bond to sclerotic dentin with self-etch adhesive systems. Oper Dent 2013; 38(1):39–47.

91. Tay FR, Pashley DH. Resin bonding to cervical sclerotic dentin: a review. J Dent 2004;32(3):173–96.

92. Pashley DH, Tay FR, Breschi L, et al. State of the art etch-and-rinse adhesives. Dent Mater 2011;27(1):1–16.

93. Tay FR, Gwinnett AJ, Pang KM, et al. Variability in microleakage observed in a total-etch wet-bonding technique under different handling conditions. J Dent Res 1995;74(5):1168–78.

94. Leme AA, Vidal CM, Hassan LS, et al. Potential role of surface wettability on the long-term stability of dentin bonds after surface biomodification. J Biomech 2015;48(10):2067–71.

95. van Dijken JW, Pallesen U. Long-term dentin retention of etch-and-rinse and self-etch adhesives and a resin-modified glass ionomer cement in non-carious cervical lesions. Dent Mater 2008;24(7):915–22.

96. Sancakli HS, Yildiz E, Bayrak I, et al. Effect of different adhesive strategies on the post-operative sensitivity of class I composite restorations. Eur J Dent 2014;8(1):15–22.

97. Cardoso MV, de Almeida Neves A, Mine A, et al. Current aspects on bonding effectiveness and stability in adhesive dentistry. Aust Dent J 2011; 56(Suppl 1):31–44.

98. Cheong C, King NM, Pashley DH, et al. Incompatibility of self-etch adhesives with chemical/dual-cured composites: two-step vs one-step systems. Oper Dent 2003;28(6):747–55.

99. Schittly E, Bouter D, Le Goff S, et al. Compatibility of five self-etching adhesive systems with two resin luting cements. J Adhes Dent 2010;12(2):137–42.
100. Tay FR, Pashley DH, Yiu CK, et al. Factors contributing to the incompatibility between simplified-step adhesives and chemically-cured or dual-cured composites. Part I. Single-step self-etching adhesive. J Adhes Dent 2003;5(1):27–40.
101. Erbas Unverdi G, Atac SA, Cehreli ZC. Effectiveness of pit and fissure sealants bonded with different adhesive systems: a prospective randomized controlled trial. Clin Oral Investig 2016. [Epub ahead of print].
102. Gonzalez-Bonet A, Kaufman G, Yang Y, et al. Preparation of dental resins resistant to enzymatic and hydrolytic degradation in oral environments. Biomacromolecules 2015;16(10):3381–8.
103. Cramer NB, Stansbury JW, Bowman CN. Recent advances and developments in composite dental restorative materials. J Dent Res 2011;90(4):402–16.
104. Boulden JE, Cramer NB, Schreck KM, et al. Thiol-ene-methacrylate composites as dental restorative materials. Dent Mater 2011;27(3):267–72.
105. Cramer NB, Couch CL, Schreck KM, et al. Properties of methacrylate-thiol-ene formulations as dental restorative materials. Dent Mater 2010;26(8):799–806.
106. Cramer NB, Couch CL, Schreck KM, et al. Investigation of thiol-ene and thiol-ene-methacrylate based resins as dental restorative materials. Dent Mater 2010;26(1):21–8.
107. Khvostenko D, Hilton TJ, Ferracane JL, et al. Bioactive glass fillers reduce bacterial penetration into marginal gaps for composite restorations. Dent Mater 2016;32(1):73–81.
108. Mankovskaia A, Levesque CM, Prakki A. Catechin-incorporated dental copolymers inhibit growth of streptococcus mutans. J Appl Oral Sci 2013;21(2):203–7.
109. Wang L, Melo MA, Weir MD, et al. Novel bioactive nanocomposite for Class-V restorations to inhibit periodontitis-related pathogens. Dent Mater 2016;32(12): e351–61.
110. Tay FR, Pashley DH. Biomimetic remineralization of resin-bonded acid-etched dentin. J Dent Res 2009;88(8):719–24.
111. Liu Y, Li N, Qi Y, et al. The use of sodium trimetaphosphate as a biomimetic analog of matrix phosphoproteins for remineralization of artificial caries-like dentin. Dent Mater 2011;27(5):465–77.
112. Vidal CM, Aguiar TR, Phansalkar R, et al. Galloyl moieties enhance the dentin biomodification potential of plant-derived catechins. Acta Biomater 2014; 10(7):3288–94.
113. Bedran-Russo AK, Pauli GF, Chen SN, et al. Dentin biomodification: strategies, renewable resources and clinical applications. Dent Mater 2014;30(1):62–76.
114. Leme-Kraus AA, Aydin B, Vidal CM, et al. Biostability of the proanthocyanidins-dentin complex and adhesion studies. J Dent Res 2017;96(4):406–12.
115. Kim GE, Leme-Kraus AA, Phansalkar R, et al. Effect of bioactive primers on bacterial-induced secondary caries at the tooth-resin interface. Oper Dent 2017;42(2):196–202.
116. Lee H, Dellatore SM, Miller WM, et al. Mussel-inspired surface chemistry for multifunctional coatings. Science 2007;318(5849):426–30.
117. Maier GP, Rapp MV, Waite JH, et al. BIOLOGICAL ADHESIVES. Adaptive synergy between catechol and lysine promotes wet adhesion by surface salt displacement. Science 2015;349(6248):628–32.
118. Lee SB, Gonzalez-Cabezas C, Kim KM, et al. Catechol-functionalized synthetic polymer as a dental adhesive to contaminated dentin surface for a composite restoration. Biomacromolecules 2015;16(8):2265–75.

Polymer-Based Direct Filling Materials

Carmem S. Pfeifer, DDS, PhD

KEYWORDS

- Dental composites • Polymerization • Clinical longevity • Caries

KEY POINTS

- Review of the literature on conventional materials and current drawbacks, including wear and polymerization stress.
- Summary of claims and properties of newer materials, and their relationship (or lack thereof) with the increase in clinical longevity in dental composite restorations.
- Evidence from the last 10 years on novel materials and techniques, such as bulk fill and self-adhesive composites.
- Analysis of clinical trials available using most current materials and techniques.
- Brief outlook to the future and latest research on materials intended to better withstand the environmental and bacterial challenges in the oral cavity.

INTRODUCTION

Since their introduction to the market more than 60 years ago, modern resin composite restorative materials have undergone substantial development and improvement. Even larger posterior restorations now show good clinical performance when built with current materials.[1–3] More and more, amalgams are falling out of favor for such applications for a number of different reasons, but are composite materials truly a complete substitute? Most of the developments throughout the history of composites have concentrated on the inorganic filler portion, and the advent of microhybrid and nanohybrid formulations has made it possible to obtain highly esthetic and wear-resistant restorations recommended for use as universal restoratives.

More recently, especially in the last 15 years or so, the technological advances have focused on the organic matrix, with a heavy emphasis on producing low shrinkage and low stress materials. The rationale is that polymerization shrinkage and the consequent stress that develops at the tooth–restoration interface produces gaps that, in turn, make the restoration more prone to recurrent decay.[4] This premise has been challenged in the past few years, especially because materials that have been shown

Division of Biomaterials and Biomechanics, Department of Restorative Dentistry, Oregon Health & Science University, 2730 Southwest Moody Avenue, Room 6N036, Portland, OR 97201, USA
E-mail address: pfeiferc@ohsu.edu

Dent Clin N Am 61 (2017) 733–750
http://dx.doi.org/10.1016/j.cden.2017.06.002
0011-8532/17/© 2017 Elsevier Inc. All rights reserved.

dental.theclinics.com

to present low shrinkage and stress in in vitro testing were not able to outperform so-called conventional materials in clinical trials.[5,6] More recent advances include bulk fill composites and materials claiming to be self-adhesive to the tooth, with the main goal of simplifying the technique-sensitive restorative procedure to avoid inherent operative errors. As it stands, composite restorations present an average lifespan of about 10 years or less, with the main reasons for failure being secondary caries and fracture.[7–11] Therefore, even with the tremendous advances made in the recent past, there remains room for improvement.

This article examines the scientific evidence available in the last 10 years to provide insight into novel techniques and materials available to the clinician. From the more than 3000 papers published on dental composites and related techniques in that period, this review focuses on novel materials or restorative protocols developed, and on how those have influenced clinical practice. The term "conventional composite" in this article refers to composite materials with regular consistency (not flowable or packable) and whose placement protocol recommends increments no thicker than 2 mm, preceded by the application of an adhesive system.

THE EVOLUTION OF FILLER SYSTEMS

Current commercially available composite materials can be classified according to their filler type (Table 1). Excellent, in-depth reviews focusing specifically on the filler technology can be found in the literature,[12–14] and a summary is provided here. Micro-fill composites contain colloidal silica particles with average size of 50 nm. To enhance filler loading levels, monomers are highly filled with colloidal silica and polymerized by heat. These prepolymerized composites are then ground to a relatively fine powder on order of 50 μm in size, and then redispersed in the final composite for a total filler content (including prepolymers) of about 70 wt%, according to the manufacturers (available from: http://www.ivoclarvivadent.com/en/products/restorative-materials/composites/heliomolar). These materials present excellent polishability,[15] but do not perform well in more mechanically challenging situations, so their main indication is for highly esthetic areas, and relatively small class III and class V restorations.[16] To try to overcome these challenges and expand the indications of esthetic direct restorations, the materials evolved into hybrids and midifills having glass fillers with variable sizes in combination with the 50-nm colloidal silica. This aimed to improve filler loading and, therefore, mechanical properties, while maintaining reasonable esthetic characteristics.[17] In fact, generally, midifills and hybrids have ranked among the materials with the greatest fracture toughness, flexural strength, and elastic modulus,[18] which makes them very good choices for midsize to larger posterior restorations.[19] However, loss of surface gloss and wear of the restorations remain a clinical concern, even within a relatively short time after restoration placement,[20–22] and especially in larger posterior preparations. Wear and esthetics were the main driving forces for the development of even smaller sized filler technologies, in an attempt to combine smooth, esthetic surfaces with longer lasting restorations, capable of withstanding occlusal challenges.

Microhybrid composites were then developed. Together with nanohybrid materials, they comprise the most abundant categories of composite currently on the market. These materials have also been extensively characterized in the literature, both in in vitro and in clinical studies.[23–28] They are considered to be universal composites, recommended for use in anterior and posterior restorations. In vitro studies comparing the mechanical properties of microhybrid and nanohybrid composites with those of

Table 1
Classification of conventional resin composite materials currently available on the market according to their filler type

Type of Composite	Comparative Filler Size and Distribution	Average Filler Size	Commercial Examples
Microfill		40–50 nm	Durafill VS (Heraeus Kulzer Inc), Renamel Microfill (Cosmedent, Inc), Matrixx Restoratives Anterior Microfill (Discus Dental), and EPIC-TMPT (Parkell, Inc), Heliomolar/Heliomolar HB (Ivoclar Vivadent) and Virtuoso Sculptable (Den-Mat)
Hybrid		10–50 μm + 40 nm	Herculite XRV (Sybron Dental Specialties Inc/Kerr Dental), Spectrum TPH (DENTSPLY Caulk), and Charisma (Heraeus Kulzer Inc).
Midifill		1–10 μm + 40 nm	Z100 (3M-ESPE), Clearfil Photo posterior (Kuraray America, Inc)
Minifill or microhybrid		0.6–1 μm + 40 nm	Filtek Z250 (3M ESPE), Synergy D6 (Coltène/Whaledent Inc), Gradia Direct (GC America), Point 4 (Kerr Dental), Renamel Universal Microhybrid (Cosmedent), Tetric Ceram (Ivoclar Vivadent, Inc), and Venus (Heraeus Kulzer Inc)
Nanohybrid		0.6–1 μm + 5–100 nm	Premise (Kerr Dental), Aelite Aesthetic Enamel (Bisco, Inc), Clearfil Majesty Esthetic (Kuraray America, Inc), Artiste (MANUF) and Z250 XT (3M-ESPE).

(continued on next page)

Table 1
(continued)

Type of Composite	Comparative Filler Size and Distribution	Average Filler Size	Commercial Examples
Nanofill		5–100 nm	Filtek Supreme Plus (3M-ESPE), Clearfil Majesty posterior (Kuraray America, Inc) and Estelite Sigma 1 (Tokuyama)

Modified from Ferracane JL. Resin composite–state of the art. Dent Mater 2011;27(1):32; with permission.

hybrids and midifills concluded that, as general categories, and because of the great variations among different commercial brands, there is no difference between microhybrid and nanohybrid materials.[29,30] However, in terms of polishability and long-term gloss retention, microhybrids and nanohybrids have demonstrated far superior performance both in in vitro[20,31] and in clinical studies[32] compared with their predecessors. In general, their clinical performance is excellent with some examples of up to a 10-year follow-up studies showing failure rates of less than 3%.[1,33,34] It is noteworthy that the differences between microhybrid and nanohybrid materials are in fact very subtle. Because of the size distribution of particles (see **Table 1**), the overall particle size is very similar for the 2 categories.

True nanofill composites contain filler particles with the smallest size available to date, ranging from 5 to 100 nm. These materials do not contain additional glass particles that exceed the nanoscale (ie, >100 nm). Their obvious advantage is the excellent esthetic made possible by the fact that the dentist can obtain highly polished surfaces, which can retain their gloss even after long-term use.[13] Different manufacturers rely on different strategies to decrease the filler size and still keep the overall filler loading high, such as the clustering of nanoparticles via water dispersion and spray drying (Filtek Supreme, 3M-ESPE, Maplewood, MN). Other nanohybrids have used different approaches to achieve low overall average particle size, but high filler fraction, such as the use of prepolymerized composite particles redispersed in the matrix (such as in Tetric Evo-Ceram, Ivoclar-Vivadent, Schaan, Liechtenstein), or the solvent-driven dispersion of particles in the matrix, followed by atomization and prepolymerization (CeramX, Dentsply-Sirona, York, PA). One study has indeed demonstrated color stability and gloss retention for several nanohybrid and nanofill materials after simulated clinical conditions.[21] A comprehensive literature review of in vitro studies, however, concluded that nanofill composites were no better than microhybrids in terms of surface smoothness and/ or gloss, before and after surface challenges.[13] Nanofills have also been demonstrated to behave very similarly in vitro to nanohybrid and microhybrids, both in terms of mechanical properties and depth of cure.[35,36] Clinical studies with follow-up times of up to 5 years have demonstrated an annual failure rate for nanofilled composites of less than 3%, deeming these materials clinically acceptable and within the range of survival of microhybrid and nanohybrid materials.[37–39]

NEWER MONOMERS AND LOW SHRINKAGE, LOW STRESS COMPOSITES

Although the evolution of fillers improved the wear and fracture characteristics of dental composites, most of the development in the organic matrix in the last 10 to 20 years has been dedicated to producing low-shrinking materials.[40] It has long been demonstrated that the composite polymerization shrinkage that takes place, when confined by the adhesion to the relatively rigid cavity walls, leads to stress development at the tooth–restoration interface.[41] This can have several deleterious effects on the restoration, such as debonding and formation of marginal gaps,[42] and induction of cracks near the margin[43] (**Fig. 1**). Other than being responsible for postoperative sensitivity, it is logical to assume that the formation of gaps facilitates bacterial recolonization and secondary decay, a long held assumption.[44] At least 1 study was able to successfully demonstrate the formation of biofilm at the bottom of an artificially created gap in a restoration subjected to cariogenic and mechanical challenges.[45] Another study demonstrated that the presence of adhesive in the gap significantly reduced the formation of carious lesions.[46,47]

With that in mind, manufacturers developed new products based on a few different shrinkage and/or stress reduction strategies. Some products rely on the use of monomers of higher molecular weight compared with the conventional bisphenol A (BPA) diglycidyl dimethacrylate/TEGDMA mixtures.[48] Larger monomers lead to less shrinkage because of the lower concentration of reactive functional groups ($C=C$) per unit volume. This is the same rationale for why the inclusion of prepolymerized additives reduce shrinkage and stress, as has been recently demonstrated with nanogels in experimental dental composites.[49] **Table 2** shows a comparison of molecular structures, molecular weights (sizes) and commercial brands for some of these new monomers. One other product is based on ring opening polymerization (Filtek LS, 3M-ESPE; see **Table 2**), with intrinsically lower shrinkage than conventional methacrylate polymerization.[50,51] In vitro studies comparing "low-shrinkage" products have shown that they indeed present lower volumetric shrinkage, but not all of them result in lower stress.[48,52,53] This is because the stress, apart from the shrinkage, also depends on the final degree of conversion and elastic modulus of the composite,[4] so comparisons among commercial brands is often difficult. In general terms, the stress increases for higher shrinkage, higher conversion, and higher stiffness materials.[4] When experimental materials are used, under controlled conditions (geometry, photoactivation protocol) and known composition, those relationships are usually straightforward. However, for commercial materials, it is impossible to control all the variables simultaneously, because of the differences in type and concentration of initiators, type

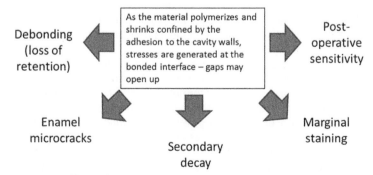

As the material polymerizes and shrinks confined by the adhesion to the cavity walls, stresses are generated at the bonded interface – gaps may open up

Debonding (loss of retention)

Post-operative sensitivity

Enamel microcracks

Secondary decay

Marginal staining

Fig. 1. Deleterious effects of polymerization stress at the bonded interface.

Table 2
Molecular structures of several examples of monomers used in modern dental composites

Monomer	Molecular Weight (g/Mol)	Commercial Example
BisGMA	512	Present in several brands in different
BisEMA	540	combinations—Filtek Supreme
UDMA	470	(3M-ESPE), Aelite (Bisco Dental Inc), Tetric
TEGDMA	286	Evo Ceram (Ivoclar-Vivadent), etc
DX-511 (DuPont monomer)	895	Venus Diamond (Heraeus-Kulzer)
Dimer-acid dimethacrylate	870	N'Durance (Septodont-Confidental)
TCD-urethane (tricyclodecane urethane)	510	Kalore (GC America)
Silorane	470	Filtek LS (3M-ESPE)

and concentrations of monomer species, filler type, and so on. For example, 1 study demonstrated that the ring opening–based material produced the lowest shrinkage while showing one of the highest elastic moduli among the materials tested, including the conventional control.[53] Interestingly, the stress values for that material were actually higher than the conventional control, likely owing to the high modulus, and despite the lower shrinkage. Other composites showed lower stress than the control in that study, with comparable modulus, which is an encouraging result.[53] This demonstrates the complexity of the polymerization stress issue in commercial materials, even in controlled, in vitro studies, where biological factors such as the biofilm and complex occlusal loading do not come into play.

Despite the encouraging in vitro evidence and despite the intuitive correlation between shrinkage or gap formation and secondary caries development, clinical studies have failed to demonstrate this effect, at least with the available "low-shrink" materials.[5,6,44,54] This is due to the biological factors mentioned (biofilm formation, dietary and hygiene habits of the patient, and unique occlusal loading situations). For example, in studies evaluating 1 low-shrinking composite and a conventional control, the incidence of restoration failure and recurrent decay was similar for either material.[5,6,55] The reason for the lack of correlation between marginal gaps and secondary decay stem from the fact that biofilm formation and caries development are multifactorial processes, and the presence of gaps alone do not guarantee that demineralization will take place. However, just because a direct correlation has not been found between improved clinical performance and the use of reduced stress materials, the presence of marginal gaps resulting from polymerization stress remains consequential. As mentioned, at least in vitro, the presence of caries-forming bacteria has been identified at the bottom of gaps at the margin of restorations subjected to cyclic loading.[45] There are no clinical or in vivo studies correlating gap formation and the development of secondary decay.

Still, the subject of polymerization stress continues to be investigated. More recently, materials capable of directly reducing stress have been introduced. Examples range from thiol-ene-methacrylate formulations[56,57] to covalent adaptable networks.[58] In the case of thiol-ene methacrylates, the presence of thiols leads to delay at the point in conversion when gelation and vitrification take place, that is, the point where the liquid resin polymerizes sufficiently to form a network with substantial rigidity.[59] By delaying gelation, the impact of stresses is reduced, because they do not reach a high level until the network is mostly formed, and therefore, the overall stress is drastically reduced.[59] There are currently no commercial materials based on this technology, although it has been licensed by dental companies. Another example of stress-reducing material is based on the covalent adaptable networks concept.[58] These monomers contain allyl disulfide functionalities in their backbone, capable of recycling crosslinks (ie, breaking them in response to internal stress and then reforming them) without decreasing the overall crosslinking density. The effect of this mechanism is that the network can adapt to dimensional changes and strain as it is forming, generating far less stress overall.[58] Its use for dental materials has been introduced with model molecules, later optimized for use in commercial materials. The only example of a commercial material containing this type of chemistry is Filtek Bulk Fill (3M-ESPE). This material has only been evaluated as part of bulk fill studies, where the main focus was not the stress development aspect, but the depth of cure and the influence of the placement technique.[60,61] However, in selected publications, this material showed less gap formation compared with that of a conventional composite of the same manufacturer when the material was placed in a single increment, presumably owing to the reduced polymerization stress.[62] Finally, other materials contain proprietary compounds ("stress modulators") that are, according to the manufacturer, capable of stress relaxation. This is the case for SDR Flow (Dentsply-Caulk). This material has indeed shown low stress values[63] and adequate depth of cure,[60] as will be discussed in the appropriate section.

Although the longevity of resin dental composites has been increasing, perhaps owing to better materials, but also owing to more acceptance and better training by practitioners, the current placement protocol is still considered time-consuming and technique sensitive compared with the placement of amalgam. Depending on the adhesive system selected, the number of application steps can vary from 1 (with universal, self-etching adhesives) to more than 3 (with etch-and-rinse, 3-component adhesives). In every step, there is a possibility for error, especially when bonding to dentin, where the moisture content of the substrate, if not controlled, can affect clinical longevity.[64–66] The other main sensitivity issue involves the depth of cure of current composites. In general, the recommendation for conventional materials is to use increments no thicker than 2 mm.[67] However, if the tip of the light source is not properly positioned, or for the material located at the bottom of a proximal box, there is the possibility for insufficient light to reach the full depth of even a 2-mm increment.[68] All of this has prompted manufacturers to develop materials that could be placed in 1 increment, and/or without the need for an adhesive step, as will be explored in the following sections.

BULK FILL MATERIALS

The rationale for the use of bulk fill materials is to streamline the restorative process in the operatory. However, the insertion of composites in a single increment has long been contraindicated for 2 main reasons. (1) Conventional materials need to be placed in increments no thicker than 2 mm to ensure proper monomer to polymer conversion at the bottom of the increment. This is even more critical at the bottom of, for example, a proximal box of a large class II restoration, where light access is often compromised.[69] (2) Especially for class I and class V restorations, the cavity configuration factor (C-factor, the ratio of surface area of bonded to nonbonded interfaces in a preparation) is high and this has been correlated, in general, with increase in stress.[70] This correlation is not without controversy; it is often seen as an oversimplification of the subject, because it overlooks the volume of the restoration[70] and the condition of the remaining tooth structure.[71–73] However, at least for conventional composites, because of the C-factor versus stress correlation, the use of incremental placement is still recommended to minimize the bonded surface on each increment, reducing the relative C-factor in each increment, and therefore, reducing overall stress.[60] This was indeed observed in several in vitro studies.[60,74] In one of them, the deflection of aluminum molds of various thicknesses was measured for conventional composites placed in a single or multiple increments, with the results showing that the single increment technique always resulted in greater wall deflection.[72] There is also some clinical evidence that incremental technique improves the outcomes of restorations of conventional dental composites.[2,75] In 1 clinical study, premolars scheduled for extraction for orthodontic reasons received standardized preparations and were restored with either a single or several increments. The results demonstrated a lower incidence of marginal gaps for restorations placed using the incremental technique.[75]

In recent years, manufacturers have introduced modifications in the materials to try to overcome the 2 main drawbacks mentioned and allow for bulk placement of restorations, including:

1. Use of flowable materials, with lower filler content;
2. Modifications to the filler type to improve light transmission in depth;
3. Use of more efficient initiators; and
4. Modifications to the monomer system to allow for stress relief during curing.

These strategies are summarized in **Fig. 2.**

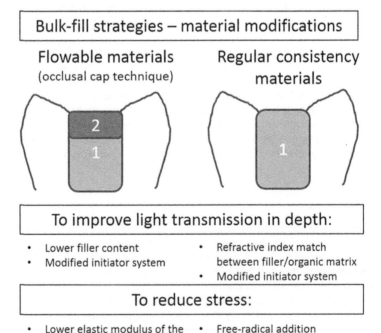

Fig. 2. Different strategies to build bulk fill restorations as a function of the materials used.

For the materials that use the flowable strategy, the rationale is that the lower filler content (in general) would decrease the light scattering through the material and provide a better degree of conversion in depth.[76–78] This is was shown to be generally true for blue wavelengths, but shorter wavelengths in the ultraviolet range were shown to be significantly limited in terms of penetration depth despite the increased translucency of the material.[79] However, because of the low resistance to wear expected with lower filler contents, the clinical placement technique calls for bulk fill of the cavity preparation with the flowable material, except for the last 2 mm of the occlusal surface, which needs to be filled with a conventional, highly filled material. In other words, the restoration still has a "cap" made of a hybrid or microhybrid regular consistency composite to ensure sufficient mechanical strength to withstand occlusal loading and reduce the amount of wear.[63,80] The degree of conversion of such flowable bulk fill materials at the bottom of 4-mm increments was indeed shown to be similar to that of the top in some studies.[81] One potential added advantage observed with this technique is that the composite adaptation to the cavity walls may improve,[60] as expected based on the low viscosity of the flowable materials. As for the polymerization stress, some studies actually found increased values with the use of bulk fill flowable composites compared with a conventional ones depending on the C-factor,[82] but because the degree of conversion was not measured in that study, it is not possible to determine whether greater conversion from the bulk fill materials, associated with the greater shrinkage obtained, played a role in determining the stress values. There is evidence, however, for increased gap formation at the base of such restorations owing to the greater shrinkage observed.[60,82] One other study used finite element analysis to evaluate stress and the strain gage method to evaluate postgel shrinkage and concluded that teeth restored with the flowable bulk fill followed by a microhybrid capping material led to reduced cusp deformation, postgel shrinkage, and shrinkage stress, and increased fracture resistance.[83] Therefore, in vitro evidence is still conflicting, and clinical studies are scarce. Two studies, however, seem to indicate that restorations placed with a bulk fill material did not differ from those placed with conventional placement techniques, at least after a 5-year follow-up.[84,85]

Other materials rely on optimization of the refractive index match between the inorganic filler and the organic phase, which is known to increase the depth of light transmission.[86] This is the case for at least one material (SonicFil, Kavo-Kerr, Orange, CA) that, allied with higher concentration and/or different types of initiators, has been shown to produce hardness values at 4 mm not statistically different from the top of the increment.[87] One additional feature of this material is the use of vibration to decrease the viscosity of the composite at room temperature, improving the adaptation to the cavity wall.[60] One study, however, has demonstrated inferior mechanical properties and greater susceptibility to degradation by ethanol with this material compared with a conventional microhybrid.[88] Another example of modification of the initiator technology is Tetric EvoCeram Bulk Fill (Ivoclar-Vivadent). This material uses a germanium-based photoinitiator, with maximum wavelength of absorption at 420 nm.[89] This molecule presents a much higher quantum yield than the camphorquinone–amine system, and also results in the formation of 2 active radicals, which may facilitate propagation of reactive species, even at depths where the light intensity is significantly diminished.[89] In vitro investigations have demonstrated that these materials may require at least 20 s of photoactivation to achieve levels of conversion comparable to incrementally placed conventional composites.[90] Clinical investigations have demonstrated that these bulk fill materials behaved similarly to the conventional composites they were compared with at a 5-year follow-up.[85]

Direct modifications to the chemistry of the monomer phase include the introduction of a methacrylate capable of undergoing free-radical addition fragmentation, as is the case for the Filtek Bulk Fill material (3M-ESPE, Technical profile). This is a mechanism that allows the forming crosslinked network to adapt to stress development during polymerization, significantly decreasing its final value.[91] This technology, allied with other high-molecular-weight monomers in the composition, have been shown to reduce the polymerization stress in comparison with conventional composites, even though it was not the lowest among the bulk fill materials tested.[60] The degree of conversion at 4 mm was not statistically different from that of the control, and it was comparable with the value obtained at 1 mm.[60]

One aspect that cannot be overlooked is the issue of heat generation with a larger volume of composite being polymerized at once, as is the case for bulk fill restorations. Studies have demonstrated that the temperature increases is greater for bulk fill composites compared with conventional controls, as measured in the composite itself,[92,93] but the effects of this elevated heat generation on the dental pulp have yet to be investigated. In conclusion, clinical studies with these materials are still very scarce, but the first few reports demonstrate they are at least as effective as conventional materials in the short term, as far as marginal integrity is concerned. However, in vitro studies seem to suggest that they require at least 20 s of photoactivation to produce these results.

SELF-ADHESIVE COMPOSITES AND RESIN CEMENTS

Self-adhesive cements and composites have been developed to not only streamline clinical procedures, but also to hopefully eliminate the most technique-sensitive step in the restorative procedure: the application of the adhesive system. As mentioned, the bonding to dentinal substrates is not particularly reliable, and many factors such as the degradation of the adhesive layer by the action of water percolation and of the collagen by matrix metalloproteinases contribute to decrease the long-term stability of the bonded interface.[94] In addition, potential errors in some of the clinical steps have been shown to critically affect the quality of the interface, such as the time for application of the acid (where applicable), the level of moisture of the substrate, the evaporation of solvent, the number and thickness of the bond layers, and so on.[95] Self-adhesive cements and composites rely on acidic functionalities, much as in self-etching adhesives,[96] which are theoretically capable of interacting with the tooth substrate via its mineral content to not only mildly etch the surface but also form true chemical bonds.[96] The challenge with this type of material is to promote good adaptation to the cavity preparation, and this is the reason why the commercially available products all rely on low viscosity formulations.[97] According to the manufacturers, self-adhesive flowable composites are recommended for small pit and fissure lesions, small class I and II and, in limited cases, class V restorations, where the mechanical challenge is not very pronounced. In those situations, the use of self-adhesive materials can actually be advantageous because it theoretically eliminates the adhesive step, leaving more space in the very conservative cavity preparation for the insertion of the more highly filled material to be used. At least 1 in vitro study of the interface between these materials and enamel and dentin has demonstrated an absence of etching of the surface in either substrates, demonstrating a limited interaction with smear-covered surfaces and aprismatic enamel, with a thin interaction area of only about 200 nm.[96,98] This agrees with the findings of another in vitro study that demonstrated inconsistent resin tag formation with the use of 2 commercially available

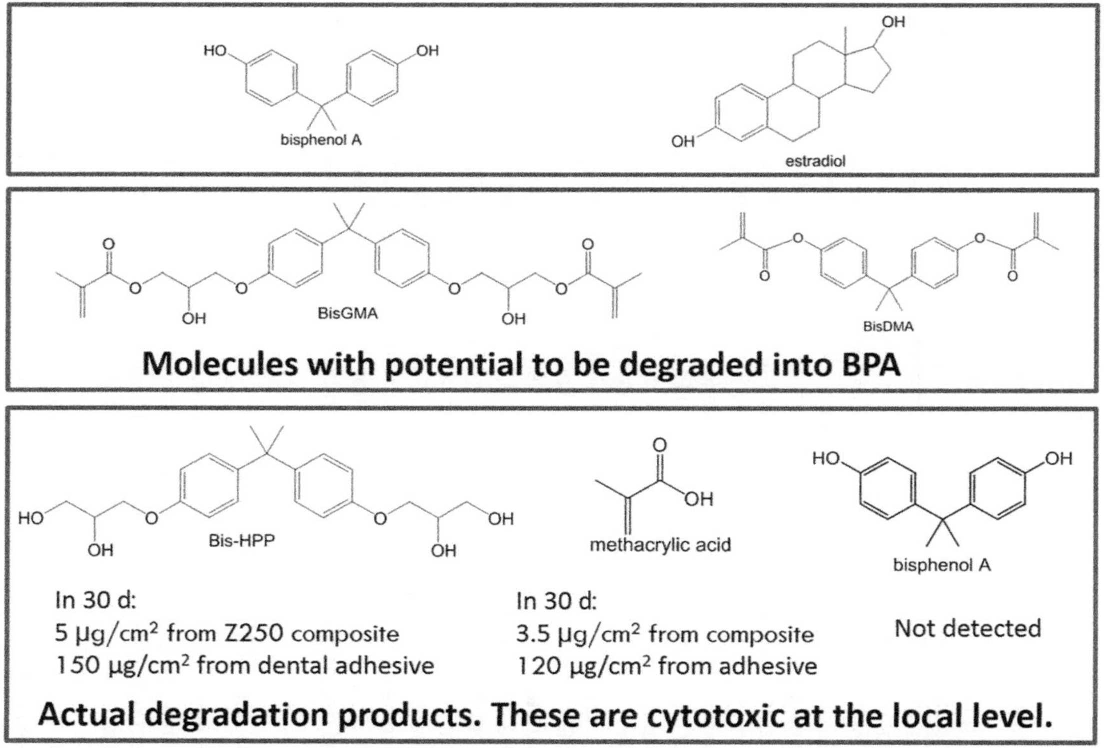
HO
OH
bisphenol A
OH
OH
estradiol
O
O
O
O
O
OH
BisGMA
OH
O
O
O
O
O
O
BisDMA
Molecules with potential to be degraded into BPA
HO
O
O
OH
OH
Bis-HPP
OH
O
OH
methacrylic acid
HO
OH
bisphenol A
In 30 d:
5 μg/cm² from Z250 composite
150 μg/cm² from dental adhesive
In 30 d:
3.5 μg/cm² from composite
120 μg/cm² from adhesive
Not detected
Actual degradation products. These are cytotoxic at the local level.

Fig. 3. Molecular structure of bisphenol A, bisphenol A diglycidyl dimethacrylate (BisGMA), bisphenol A dimethacrylate (BPADMA), and their possible degradation products.

self-adhesive composites, as reflected in a decreased shear bond strength and increased microleakage.[98,99] The prior application of acid etching seems to improve the microleakage resistance of these materials, at least in vitro.[97] Clinical studies with these materials are still scarce, but preliminary results seem to demonstrate that they are effective at reducing dental hypersensitivity, though not to any greater degree than conventional desensitizing agents.[100] When used to restore noncarious cervical lesions, 1 study found very poor results: of 40 restorations, 27 presented as clinically unacceptable after only 6 months of follow-up.[101]

TOXICITY AND THE BISPHENOL A CONTROVERSY

BPA is a high production volume chemical, in use since 1957. It is present in polycarbonate bottles and is used in can and pipe linings to prevent rusting. BPA's molecular structure is very similar to that of certain hormones (**Fig. 3**), and is therefore classified as an endocrine disruptor compound.[102] In adults, it becomes metabolized by a specific enzyme that is not present or active in fetuses or in small children. From animal studies it has been concluded that when large doses of BPA are administered to pregnant females, they produce offspring with developmental and behavioral issues.[103,104] However, a toxicology panel organized by the National Institutes of Health in 2008 failed to find such a correlation in humans, which was credited to the relatively low levels of exposure from daily plastic sources (extensive information, including the conclusions of the 2008 panel can be found at NIEHS-NIH 2008 study panel). The FDA and its counterparts in Europe and Canada have since released an update concluding that BPA levels occurring in foods are safe (FDA - BPA recommendations). There are 2 monomers used in dental composites and sealants whose molecular structure contains a BPA core: BPA diglycidyl dimethacrylate and BPA dimethacrylate (see **Fig. 3**). Although these molecules used in dental sealants and possibly composites contain the BPA core, degradation studies have failed to detect the presence of BPA byproducts from dental sealants.[105] The other degradation products can be toxic at the local level, but exposure to them is considered to be brief because they are quickly cleared by the saliva.[106] Several studies concluded that the cumulative exposure level to sealants and/or flowable composites was not associated with behavioral, psychosocial, or neuropsychological alteration,[107–109] and the American Dental Association has deemed sealants safe for use in children and adults (ADA - FDA in dental sealants).

SUMMARY AND FUTURE DIRECTIONS

Until such time in the future when regenerative therapies have completely evolved to the point that damaged dental tissues or the entire tooth can be regenerated, direct and indirect restorations will to continue to be a very important part of the clinician's armamentarium to repair the damage resulting from dental caries. Among direct restorative materials, dental composites will continue to replace amalgams, owing to esthetic demands. The past couple of decades have seen an enormous amount of progress in terms of enhancing filler and organic matrix composition, with the result being that the average life span of a composite restoration has increased significantly compared with what was expected when they were first introduced. However, as clinicians improve their techniques and researchers fine tune the composition of materials, more and more focus will likely be placed on the interaction of the material itself with its surroundings, including the mineralized tooth and soft periodontal tissues and the environment as a whole, including bacteria and components of the saliva. In other words, producing materials that can not only generate less interfacial stress and withstand the occlusal loading, but also that can resist chemical and biological degradation, will be the focus of future dental composite research. Significant efforts are currently underway to produce materials that are better able to resist enzymatic degradation, focusing on the elimination of ester-containing methacrylate monomers. In addition, materials with self-healing capabilities are also being studied. On the more biological side, remineralizing and antibacterial composites have been investigated for several years, and are getting closer to being commercially viable. Ultimately, the goal is to produce materials that are easier to use, and therefore are less technique-sensitive, and that will produce robust, long-lasting restorations. This will reduce costly replacements and will significantly advance oral health.

REFERENCES

1. Gianordoli-Neto R, Padovani GC, Mondelli J, et al. Two-year clinical evaluation of resin composite in posterior teeth: a randomized controlled study. J Conserv Dent 2016;19:306–10.

2. Karaman E, Keskin B, Inan U. Three-year clinical evaluation of class II posterior composite restorations placed with different techniques and flowable composite linings in endodontically treated teeth. Clin Oral Investig 2017;21(2):709–16.

3. Schwendicke F, Krüger H, Schlattmann P, et al. Restoration outcomes after restoring vital teeth with advanced caries lesions: a practice-based retrospective study. Clin Oral Investig 2016;20:1675–81.

4. Pfeifer CS, Ferracane JL, Sakaguchi RL, et al. Factors affecting photopolymerization stress in dental composites. J Dent Res 2008;87:1043–7.

5. Baracco B, Fuentes MV, Ceballos L. Five-year clinical performance of a silorane-vs a methacrylate-based composite combined with two different adhesive approaches. Clin Oral Investig 2016;20:991–1001.

6. Magno MB, Nascimento GCR, da Rocha YSP, et al. Silorane-based composite resin restorations are not better than conventional composites - a meta-analysis of clinical studies. J Adhes Dent 2016;18:375–86.

7. Downer MC, Azli NA, Bedi R, et al. How long do routine dental restorations last? A systematic review. Br Dental J 1999;187:432–9.

8. Casagrande L, Seminario AT, Correa MB, et al. Longevity and associated risk factors in adhesive restorations of young permanent teeth after complete and selective caries removal: a retrospective study. Clin Oral Investig 2017;21(3):847–55.

9. da Veiga AM, Cunha AC, Ferreira DM, et al. Longevity of direct and indirect resin composite restorations in permanent posterior teeth: a systematic review and meta-analysis. J Dent 2016;54:1–12.

10. Laske M, Opdam NJM, Bronkhorst EM, et al. Longevity of direct restorations in Dutch dental practices. Descriptive study out of a practice based research network. J Dent 2016;46:12–7.

11. Beck F, Lettner S, Graf A, et al. Survival of direct resin restorations in posterior teeth within a 19-year period (1996-2015): a meta-analysis of prospective studies. Dent Mater 2015;31:958–85.

12. Habib E, Wang R, Wang Y, et al. Inorganic fillers for dental resin composites: present and future. ACS Biomater Sci Eng 2016;2:1–11.

13. Kaizer MR, De Oliveira-Ogliari A, Cenci MS, et al. Do nanofill or submicron composites show improved smoothness and gloss? A systematic review of in vitro studies. Dent Mater 2014;30:e41–78.

14. Randolph LD, Palin WM, Leloup G, et al. Filler characteristics of modern dental resin composites and their influence on physico-mechanical properties. Dent Mater 2016;32:1586–99.

15. Roeder LB, Tate WH, Powers JM. Effect of finishing and polishing procedures on the surface roughness of packable composites. Oper Dent 2000;25:534–43.

16. Heintze SD, Rousson V, Hickel R. Clinical effectiveness of direct anterior restorations - A meta-analysis. Dent Mater 2015;31:481–95.

17. Vaidyanathan J, Vaidyanathan TK. Flexural creep deformation and recovery in dental composites. J Dent 2001;29:545–51.

18. Ferracane JL. Resin composite - State of the art. Dent Mater 2011;27:29–38.

19. Scholtanus JD, Zaia J, Özcan M. Compressive strength and failure types of cusp replacing direct resin composite restorations in previously amalgam-filled premolars versus sound teeth. J Adhes Sci Technol 2017;31:211–8.

20. Antonson SA, Yazici AR, Kilinc E, et al. Comparison of different finishing/polishing systems on surface roughness and gloss of resin composites. J Dent 2011; 39(Suppl 1):e9–17.

21. Da Costa J, Adams-Belusko A, Riley K, et al. The effect of various dentifrices on surface roughness and gloss of resin composites. J Dent 2010;38:e123–8.

22. Gladys S, Van Meerbeek B, Braem M, et al. Comparative physico-mechanical characterization of new hybrid restorative materials with conventional glass-ionomer and resin composite restorative materials. J Dent Res 1997;76:883–94.

23. Kakaboura A, Fragouli M, Rahiotis C, et al. Evaluation of surface characteristics of dental composites using profilometry, scanning electron, atomic force microscopy and gloss-meter. J Mater Sci Mater Med 2007;18:155–63.

24. Palaniappan S, Elsen L, Lijnen I, et al. Three-year randomised clinical trial to evaluate the clinical performance, quantitative and qualitative wear patterns of hybrid composite restorations. Clin Oral Investig 2010;14:441–58.

25. Baudin C, Osorio R, Toledano M, et al. Work of fracture of a composite resin: fracture-toughening mechanisms. J Biomed Mater Res A 2009;89:751–8.

26. Cadenaro M, Biasotto M, Scuor N, et al. Assessment of polymerization contraction stress of three composite resins. Dent Mater 2008;24:681–5.

27. Ilie N, Hickel R, Valceanu AS, et al. Fracture toughness of dental restorative materials. Clin Oral Investig 2012;16:489–98.

28. Rode KM, De Freitas PM, Lloret PR, et al. Micro-hardness evaluation of a micro-hybrid composite resin light cured with halogen light, light-emitting diode and argon ion laser. Lasers Med Sci 2009;24:87–92.

29. Ilie N, Rencz A, Hickel R. Investigations towards nano-hybrid resin-based composites. Clin Oral Investig 2013;17:185–93.

30. Öztürk-Bozkurt F, Toz-Akalin T, Gözetici B, et al. Load-bearing capacity and failure types of premolars restored with sonic activated bulk-fill-, nano-hybrid and silorane-based resin restorative materials. J Adhes Sci Technol 2016;30: 1880–90.

31. Jiang H, Lv D, Liu K, et al. Comparison of surface roughness of nanofilled and microhybrid composite resins after curing and polishing. Nan fang yi ke da xue xue bao 2014;34:727–30 [in Chinese].

32. Coelho-De-Souza FH, Gonçalves DS, Sales MP, et al. Direct anterior composite veneers in vital and non-vital teeth: a retrospective clinical evaluation. J Dent 2015;43:1330–6.

33. Loguercio AD, Lorini E, Weiss RV, et al. 12-month clinical evaluation of composite resins in class III restorations. J Adhes Dent 2007;9:57–64.

34. Lempel E, Tóth Á, Fábián T, et al. Retrospective evaluation of posterior direct composite restorations: 10-year findings. Dent Mater 2015;31:115–22.
35. Beun S, Glorieux T, Devaux J, et al. Characterization of nanofilled compared to universal and microfilled composites. Dent Mater 2007;23:51–9.
36. Ilie N, Hickel R. Investigations on mechanical behaviour of dental composites. Clinical Oral Investigations 2009;13:427–38.
37. Cetin AR, Unlu N, Cobanoglu N. A five-year clinical evaluation of direct nano-filled and indirect composite resin restorations in posterior teeth. Oper Dent 2013;38:E1–11.
38. De Andrade AKM, Duarte RM, Medeiros e Silva FDSC, et al. Resin composite class I restorations: a 54-month randomized clinical trial. Oper Dent 2014;39:588–94.
39. Yazici AR, Ustunkol I, Ozgunaltay G, et al. Three-year clinical evaluation of different restorative resins in class I restorations. Oper Dent 2014;39:248–55.
40. Pitel ML. Low-shrink composite resins: a review of their history, strategies for managing shrinkage, and clinical significance. Compend Contin Educ Dent 2013;34:578–90.
41. Feilzer AJ, de Gee AJ, Davidson CL. Setting stress in composite resin in relation to configuration of the restoration. J Dent Res 1987;66:1636–9.
42. Irie M, Suzuki K, Watts DC. Marginal gap formation of light-activated restorative materials: effects of immediate setting shrinkage and bond strength. Dent Mater 2002;18:203–10.
43. Yamamoto T, Ferracane JL, Sakaguchi RL, et al. Calculation of contraction stresses in dental composites by analysis of crack propagation in the matrix sur-rounding a cavity. Dent Mater 2009;25:543–50.
44. Ferracane JL, Hilton TJ. Polymerization stress - is it clinically meaningful? Dent Mater 2016;32:1–10.
45. Khvostenko D, Salehi S, Naleway SE, et al. Cyclic mechanical loading promotes bacterial penetration along composite restoration marginal gaps. Dent Mater 2015;31:702–10.
46. Montagner AF, Kuper NK, Opdam NJM, et al. Wall-lesion development in gaps: the role of the adhesive bonding material. J Dent 2015;43:1007–12.
47. Montagner AF, Maske TT, Opdam NJ, et al. Failed bonded interfaces submitted to microcosm biofilm caries development. J Dent 2016;52:63–9.
48. Tantbirojn D, Pfeifer CS, Braga RR, et al. Do low-shrink composites reduce poly-merization shrinkage effects? J Dent Res 2011;90:596–601.
49. Moraes RR, Garcia JW, Barros MD, et al. Control of polymerization shrinkage and stress in nanogel-modified monomer and composite materials. Dent Mater 2011;27:509–19.
50. Park JK, Lee GH, Kim JH, et al. Polymerization shrinkage, flexural and compres-sion properties of low-shrinkage dental resin composites. Dent Mater J 2014;33:104–10.
51. Yamasaki LC, De Vito Moraes AG, Barros M, et al. Polymerization development of "low-shrink" resin composites: reaction kinetics, polymerization stress and quality of network. Dent Mater 2013;29:e169–79.
52. Van Ende A, De Munck J, Mine A, et al. Does a low-shrinking composite induce less stress at the adhesive interface? Dent Mater 2010;26:215–22.
53. Boaro LCC, Gonalves F, Guimarães TC, et al. Polymerization stress, shrinkage and elastic modulus of current low-shrinkage restorative composites. Dent Mater 2010;26:1144–50.

54. Burke FJT, Crisp RJ, James A, et al. Two year clinical evaluation of a low-shrink resin composite material in UK general dental practices. Dent Mater 2011;27: 622–30.

55. Van Dijken JWV, Lindberg A. A 15-year randomized controlled study of a reduced shrinkage stress resin composite. Dent Mater 2015;31:1150–8.

56. Boulden JE, Cramer NB, Schreck KM, et al. Thiol-ene-methacrylate composites as dental restorative materials. Dent Mater 2011;27:267–72.

57. Cramer NB, Couch CL, Schreck KM, et al. Investigation of thiol-ene and thiol-ene-methacrylate based resins as dental restorative materials. Dent Mater 2010;26:21–8.

58. Park HY, Kloxin CJ, Scott TF, et al. Covalent adaptable networks as dental restorative resins: stress relaxation by addition-fragmentation chain transfer in allyl sulfide-containing resins. Dent Mater 2010;26:1010–6.

59. Lee TY, Carioscia J, Smith Z, et al. Thiol-allyl ether-methacrylate ternary systems. Evolution mechanism of polymerization-induced shrinkage stress and mechanical properties. Macromolecules 2007;40:1473–9.

60. Fronza BM, Rueggeberg FA, Braga RR, et al. Monomer conversion, microhardness, internal marginal adaptation, and shrinkage stress of bulk-fill resin composites. Dent Mater 2015;31:1542–51.

61. Kim RJY, Kim YJ, Choi NS, et al. Polymerization shrinkage, modulus, and shrinkage stress related to tooth-restoration interfacial debonding in bulk-fill composites. J Dent 2015;43:430–9.

62. Miletic V, Peric D, Milosevic M, et al. Local deformation fields and marginal integrity of sculptable bulk-fill, low-shrinkage and conventional composites. Dent Mater 2016;32:1441–51.

63. Ilie N, Hickel R. Investigations on a methacrylate-based flowable composite based on the SDR™ technology. Dent Mater 2011;27:348–55.

64. Grégoire G, Guignes P, Nasr K. Effects of dentine moisture on the permeability of total-etch and one-step self-etch adhesives. J Dent 2009;37:691–9.

65. Perdigão J, Carmo ARP, Geraldeli S. Eighteen-month clinical evaluation of two dentin adhesives applied on dry vs moist dentin. J Adhes Dent 2005;7:253–8.

66. Perdigão J, Carmo ARP, Geraldeli S, et al. Six-month clinical evaluation of two dentin adhesives applied on dry vs moist dentin. J Adhes Dent 2001;3:343–52.

67. Bicalho AA, Pereira RD, Zanatta RF, et al. Incremental filling technique and composite material-part I: cuspal deformation, bond strength, and physical properties. Oper Dent 2014;39:E71–82.

68. Price RBT, Felix CM, Whalen JM. Factors affecting the energy delivered to simulated class I and class v preparations. J Can Dent Assoc 2010;76:a94.

69. Price RB, Labrie D, Whalen JM, et al. Effect of distance on irradiance and beam homogeneity from 4 light-emitting diode curing units. J Can Dent Assoc 2011; 77:b9.

70. Boaro LCC, Meira JBC, Ballester RY, et al. Influence of specimen dimensions and their derivatives (C-factor and volume) on polymerization stress determined in a high compliance testing system. Dent Mater 2013;29:1034–9.

71. Boaro LCC, Fróes-Salgado NR, Gajewski VES, et al. Correlation between polymerization stress and interfacial integrity of composites restorations assessed by different in vitro tests. Dent Mater 2014;30:984–92.

72. Kim YJ, Kim R, Ferracane JL, et al. Influence of the compliance and layering method on the wall deflection of simulated cavities in bulk-fill composite restoration. Oper Dent 2016;41:e183–94.

73. Wang Z, Chiang MYM. System compliance dictates the effect of composite filler content on polymerization shrinkage stress. Dent Mater 2016;32:551–60.
74. Jafarpour S, El-Badrawy W, Jazi HS, et al. Effect of composite insertion technique on cuspal deflection using an in vitro simulation model. Oper Dent 2012;37:299–305.
75. Lopes GC, Baratieri LN, Monteiro S Jr, et al. Effect of posterior resin composite placement technique on the resin-dentin interface formed in vivo. Quintessence Int 2004;35:156–61.
76. Aldossary MS, Santini A. The influence of two different curing regimens on light energy transmission through bulk-fill resin composites and Vickers hardness. Am J Dent 2016;29:282–8.
77. Garoushi S, Vallittu P, Shinya A, et al. Influence of increment thickness on light transmission, degree of conversion and micro hardness of bulk fill composites. Odontology 2016;104:291–7.
78. Son SA, Park JK, Seo DG, et al. How light attenuation and filler content affect the microhardness and polymerization shrinkage and translucency of bulk-fill composites? Clin Oral Investig 2017;21(2):559–65.
79. Harlow JE, Rueggeberg FA, Labrie D, et al. Transmission of violet and blue light through conventional (layered) and bulk cured resin-based composites. J Dent 2016;53:44–50.
80. Tomaszewska IM, Kearns JO, Ilie N, et al. Bulk fill restoratives: to cap or not to cap - that is the question? J Dent 2015;43:309–16.
81. Zorzin J, Maier E, Harre S, et al. Bulk-fill resin composites: polymerization properties and extended light curing. Dent Mater 2015;31:293–301.
82. Han SH, Sadr A, Tagami J, et al. Internal adaptation of resin composites at two configurations: influence of polymerization shrinkage and stress. Dent Mater 2016;32:1085–94.
83. Rosatto CMP, Bicalho AA, Veríssimo C, et al. Mechanical properties, shrinkage stress, cuspal strain and fracture resistance of molars restored with bulk-fill composites and incremental filling technique. J Dent 2015;43:1519–28.
84. van Dijken JW, Pallesen U. Randomized 3-year clinical evaluation of class I and II posterior resin restorations placed with a bulk-fill resin composite and a one-step self-etching adhesive. J Adhes Dent 2015;17:81–8.
85. van Dijken JWV, Pallesen U. Posterior bulk-filled resin composite restorations: a 5-year randomized controlled clinical study. J Dent 2016;51:29–35.
86. Howard B, Wilson ND, Newman SM, et al. Relationships between conversion, temperature and optical properties during composite photopolymerization. Acta Biomater 2010;6:2053–9.
87. Alrahlah A, Silikas N, Watts DC. Post-cure depth of cure of bulk fill dental resin-composites. Dent Mater 2014;30:149–54.
88. Leprince JG, Palin WM, Vanacker J, et al. Physico-mechanical characteristics of commercially available bulk-fill composites. J Dent 2014;42:993–1000.
89. Moszner N, Zeuner F, Lamparth I, et al. Benzoylgermanium derivatives as novel visible-light photoinitiators for dental composites. Macromol Mater Eng 2009;294:877–86.
90. Miletic V, Pongprueksa P, de Munck J, et al. Curing characteristics of flowable and sculptable bulk-fill composites. Clin Oral Investig 2017;21(4):1201–12.
91. Park HY, Kloxin CJ, Abuelyaman AS, et al. Novel dental restorative materials having low polymerization shrinkage stress via stress relaxation by addition-fragmentation chain transfer. Dent Mater 2012;28:1113–9.

92. Guo Y, Landis FA, Wang Z, et al. Polymerization stress evolution of a bulk-fill flowable composite under different compliances. Dent Mater 2016;32(4): 578–86.

93. Kim RJY, Son SA, Hwang JY, et al. Comparison of photopolymerization temperature increases in internal and external positions of composite and tooth cavities in real time: incremental fillings of microhybrid composite vs. bulk filling of bulk fill composite. J Dent 2015;43:1093–8.

94. Pashley DH, Tay FR, Breschi L, et al. State of the art etch-and-rinse adhesives. Dent Mater 2011;27:1–16.

95. Chen C, Niu LN, Xie H, et al. Bonding of universal adhesives to dentine-old wine in new bottles? J Dent 2015;43:525–36.

96. Mine A, De Munck J, Van Ende A, et al. Limited interaction of a self-adhesive flowable composite with dentin/enamel characterized by TEM. Dent Mater 2017;33:209–17.

97. Celik EU, Kucukyilmaz E, Savas S. Effect of different surface pre-treatment methods on the microleakage of two different self-adhesive composites in class V cavities. Eur J Paediatr Dent 2015;16:33–8.

98. Makishi P, Pacheco RR, Sadr A, et al. Assessment of self-adhesive resin composites: nondestructive imaging of resin-dentin interfacial adaptation and shear bond strength. Microsc Microanal 2015;21:1523–9.

99. Brueckner C, Schneider H, Haak R. Shear bond strength and tooth-composite interaction with self-adhering flowable composites. Oper Dent 2017;42:90–100.

100. Pinna R, Bortone A, Sotgiu G, et al. Clinical evaluation of the efficacy of one self-adhesive composite in dental hypersensitivity. Clin Oral Investig 2015;19: 1663–72.

101. Çelik EU, Aka B, Yilmaz F. Six-month clinical evaluation of a self-adhesive flowable composite in noncarious cervical lesions. J Adhes Dent 2015;17:361–8.

102. Hewlett M, Chow E, Aschengrau A, et al. Prenatal exposure to endocrine disruptors: a developmental etiology for polycystic ovary syndrome. Reprod Sci 2017; 24:19–27.

103. Vandenberg LN. Non-monotonic dose responses in studies of endocrine disrupting chemicals: bisphenol A as a case study. Dose-Response 2014;12: 259–76.

104. Welshons WV, Thayer KA, Judy BM, et al. Large effects from small exposures. I. Mechanisms for endocrine-disrupting chemicals with estrogenic activity. Environ Health Perspect 2003;111:994–1006.

105. Bourbia M, Ma D, Cvitkovitch DG, et al. Cariogenic bacteria degrade dental resin composites and adhesives. J Dent Res 2013;92:989–94.

106. Lee JH, Yi SK, Kim SY, et al. Salivary bisphenol A levels and their association with composite resin restoration. Chemosphere 2017;172:46–51.

107. Azarpazhooh A, Main PA. Is there a risk of harm or toxicity in the placement of pit and fissure sealant materials? A systematic review. J Can Dent Assoc 2008;74: 179–83.

108. Fleisch AF, Sheffield PE, Chinn C, et al. Bisphenol A and related compounds in dental materials. Pediatrics 2010;126:760–8.

109. Van Landuyt KL, Nawrot T, Geebelen B, et al. How much do resin-based dental materials release? A meta-analytical approach. Dent Mater 2011;27:723–47.

Light Curing in Dentistry

Richard B.T. Price, BDS, DDS, MS, PhD

KEYWORDS

- Curing lights • Composite resin • Polymerization • Blue light hazard
- Dental curing lights

KEY POINTS

- The ability to light cure resins 'on demand' in the mouth has revolutionized dentistry.
- However, there is a widespread lack of understanding of what is required for successful light curing in the mouth.
- This article provides a brief description of light curing, resin photopolymerization, types of curing lights, interplay between light tip area and irradiance, and how to monitor light output.
- Recommendations are made to assist when selecting a curing light and guidelines are given to improve light curing technique.

The ability to light cure dental resins "on demand" in the mouth has revolutionized modern dentistry. Consequently the dental light curing unit (LCU) has become an indispensable piece of equipment in almost every dental office.[1–3] As a general recommendation, when light curing a dental resin, adhesive, sealant, or cement the clinician should aim to deliver sufficient radiant exposure at the correct wavelengths of light required by the photoinitiator(s) in the resin. It is not as just simple as using any curing light for 10 seconds, despite its routine use, the curing light and how it is should be used is not well understood by most operators.[4–6] For example, every published study that has evaluated LCUs in dental offices has shown that most curing lights are poorly maintained and deliver an inadequate light output.[7–13] In the majority of offices, the dentists did not know the irradiance from the curing light[6] and were unaware that their light was unable to adequately cure their resin restoration.[12] This deficiency is a concern because the use of resins is expected to rise with the worldwide phase-down in the use of dental amalgam as a part of the Minamata Convention.[14] It is also reported that "tooth-colored materials are inferior to amalgam as fillings, especially for posterior teeth; and that, compared to amalgam, resin composites are far more technique sensitive, have lower clinical survival rates, are more expensive, and are far more difficult to adapt to proper tooth contour.[14]" A contributing factor

Department of Dental Clinical Sciences, Dalhousie University, Halifax, Nova Scotia B3H 4R2, Canada
E-mail address: rbprice@dal.ca

Dent Clin N Am 61 (2017) 751–778
http://dx.doi.org/10.1016/j.cden.2017.06.008
0011-8532/17/© 2017 Elsevier Inc. All rights reserved.

to some of the problems associated with tooth colored resins may be because they have been undercured. This situation is highly undesirable; undercuring results in decreased bond strengths to the tooth, more bulk fractures of the resin restoration, increased wear, and an increase in the amount of leached chemicals from the resin.[15–19] This article discusses the current knowledge of dental curing lights and their use in dentistry.

RADIOMETRIC TERMINOLOGY

The International System of Units (SI) terminology should be used to describe the output from a dental LCU. Commonly used terms in dentistry to describe the output from a curing light such as "intensity," "power density," or "energy density" are not SI terms and they should not be used because they can lead to confusion. The appropriate SI radiometric terms to describe the output from a curing light are provided in **Table 1**.[3,20] In keeping with the output range from LCUs, these output values are usually reported in milli-Watts (mW) rather than Watts.

HEALTH AND SAFETY ISSUES
Electromagnetic Risk from Curing Lights

There has been some concern that electromagnetic (EM) emissions from external electrical devices such as LCUs can mimic or obscure intracardiac signals and potentially disrupt the function of implanted cardiac pacemakers.[21] However, when tested in a 2015 study, the dental curing light did not seem to interfere with pacemaker and or

Table 1
Radiometric terminology used to describe the output from a light source

Term	Units	Symbol	Notes
Radiant power, or radiant flux	Watt	W	Radiant energy per unit time (joules per second).
Radiant exitance, or radiant emittance	Watt per square centimeter	W/cm^2	Radiant power (flux) emitted from a surface, for example, the tip of a curing light. This is an averaged value over the tip area.
Irradiance (incident irradiance)	Watt per square centimeter	W/cm^2	Radiant power (flux) incident on a surface of known surface area. This is an averaged value over the surface area.
Radiant energy	Joule	J	This describes the energy from the source (Watts per second).
Radiant exposure	Joule per square centimeter	J/cm^2	This describes the energy received per unit area. Sometimes this is incorrectly described as "energy density."
Radiant energy density	Joule per cubic centimeter	J/cm^3	This is the volumetric (cm^3) energy density.
Spectral radiant power	Milli-Watt per nanometer	mW/nm	Radiant power at each wavelength (nm) of the electromagnetic spectrum.
Spectral irradiance	Milli-Watt per square centimeter per nanometer	$mW/cm^2/nm$	Irradiance received at each wavelength (nm) of the electromagnetic spectrum.

defibrillator pacing or sensing function and thus should not pose a risk to the patient.[22] In addition, companies are required to test for this potential hazard before selling electrical devices and thus there should be no risk if the dental LCU has been purchased from a reputable manufacturer.

The Blue Light Hazard

All dental curing lights can cause ocular damage from the blue light they emit. This blue light hazard is greatest at 440 nm,[23] which is within the output range from dental LCUs.[1,3] Dental professionals must be aware of and use proper protection from this blue light hazard[5,6,24] because they have a duty to protect both the patient and employees from harm. Recently, there has been concern that cumulative exposure to blue light from high-power LCUs can cause ocular damage.[24–28] Both acute and chronic exposure to this hazard can be prevented by using appropriate eye protection and although most manufacturers of dental LCUs supply some form of eye protection, these items are not used universally.[5,6,29]

Blue light is transmitted through the ocular media and absorbed by the retina. Although high levels of blue light cause immediate and irreversible retinal burning, chronic exposure to low levels of blue light can accelerate age-related macular degeneration.[30,31] Most countries follow international guidelines on exposure to optical radiation, such as those from the International Commission on Non-Ionizing Radiation Protection and the American Conference of Governmental Industrial Hygienists.[23,30] A recent study found that dental personnel using high power LCUs might exceed these American Conference of Governmental Industrial Hygienists, limits during a normal workday, unless the operator uses orange protective glasses. If they do not wear these orange 'blue blockers' and they look at the light for even just the first second of the curing cycle before averting their eyes, it may take as few as 7 curing cycles to exceed the maximum recommended daily exposure to blue light.[26] It should also be noted that the maximum recommended exposure times have been calculated for individuals with normal photosensitivity. Patients or dental personnel who have had cataract surgery or who are taking photosensitizing medications have a greater susceptibility for retinal damage. In these circumstances, ocular injury may occur after even shorter exposure times to blue light.[23,30] Using the appropriate blue light filtering glasses ('orange blue-blockers') will reduce the transmission of light of wavelengths less than 500 nm by 99%.[32] As an added benefit, when these blue light filtering glasses are used, instead of needing to look away from the bright blue light from the LCU, the operator can now safely watch what they are doing when light curing. Thus, this protection will improve the amount of light they deliver to the restoration from the LCU.[33–37]

Temperature Considerations

It is important to not arbitrarily increase the exposure time to ensure complete polymerization without understanding the potentially damaging thermal effects from the LCU. Contrary to initial claims, high-power light-emitting diode (LED) curing lights can produce significant temperature increases. When the first-generation LED lights were marketed, they were advertised as 'cool' lights that produced less of a temperature increase in the pulp compared with quartz–tungsten–halogen (QTH) lights.[38–41] This was only true because of the low power output from the initial versions of these first-generation LED curing lights. As the power output from LED units increased, the potential for generating damaging temperatures in the pulp and oral tissues also increased.[17,42–47] Thus, where the pulp is at greater risk, such as when light curing the bonding system in deep cavities where there is little overlying dentin, consideration should be given to the choice of LCU and light exposure program used.[48] It is recommended for extended curing times that the tooth be air cooled when light curing, or the operator should wait at least 2 seconds between every 10 seconds of light exposure.[49] Despite these precautions, unless the operator is careful where they aim the tip of the LCU, the heat from a powerful curing light can cause gingival or soft tissue burns.[50] **Fig. 1** provides an example of tissue burn resulting from 30 seconds of direct light exposure from a high-output LED curing light on the attached gingiva of a pig.

Budget Curing Lights and Unregulated Medical Devices

The dental profession can now purchase dental equipment, including curing lights, directly online and at a low cost, without using an approved distributor. Many of these "budget-curing lights" are unregulated and they often use small diameter (6–7 mm) light guides. As discussed elsewhere in this article, this means that although they often deliver less power, they can seem to deliver the same irradiance values as curing lights that use wider diameter tips. The light beam profiles from these budget lights can also be inferior compared with higher priced lights from major manufacturers[51,52] and the electronics in these inexpensive units may not compensate for any decrease in the output from the battery. Thus, the light output from some unregulated battery operated curing lights may decline without warning during operation.[52] Because these budget curing lights may have not been tested for safety or efficacy, the use of such unregulated devices on a patient should be discouraged and regarded as in vivo testing of a medical device on a patient who has not given informed consent.[53]

LIGHT CURING OF RESTORATIVE RESINS
Electromagnetic Energy and the Electromagnetic Spectrum

What humans perceive as "light" is EM radiation, and the colors we perceive are associated with different ranges of EM wavelengths. Our visible spectrum ranges from violet (composed of shorter wavelengths starting around 400 nm) to red, which is composed of longer wavelengths (around 700 nm) of light. Anything below 400 nm is considered to be ultraviolet A (UV) radiation. Most dental curing lights deliver light in that is between 400 and 500 nm.

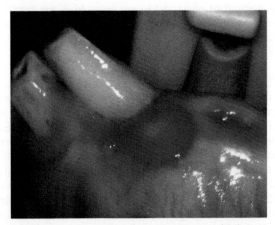

Fig. 1. Erythema resulting from exposure of pig gingiva to a high-intensity light-emitting diode curing light. (*Courtesy of* C.A.G. Arrais, DDS, MS, PhD, São Paulo, Brazil.)

The energy carried by each photon from any light source is a function of the photon's wavelength. Two photons with the same wavelength will have the same photon energy, even if 1 photon comes from a curing light and the other from the sun. What differs among the photons from the various light sources is the number of photons and the wavelength (or frequency) of these photons. The equation for the energy carried by each photon is:

$$E = \frac{hc}{\lambda}$$

Where E is the energy carried by each photon, h is Planck's constant, c is the speed of light in vacuum, and λ is the wavelength of the photon. Because both h and c are constants, changes in the wavelength λ of the photon have an inverse effect on the energy carried by each photon.

This explains why photons at the lower wavelengths of light (eg, at 400 nm) carry more energy than longer wavelengths (eg, at 500 nm). This effect is relevant when photocuring dental resins.

The Photoinitiator Molecule and Free Radical Generation

Two types of photoinitiators are used in dentistry, types I and II. These photoinitiators contain specific types of bonds that are capable of absorbing EM radiation, but only within very specific wavelength ranges. The photoinitiator then uses that energy to generate free radicals that initiate the free radical polymerization process. Type I photoinitiators have a higher quantum yield and require fewer photons to generate a free radical than do the type II initiators. This is because type II photoinitiators (eg, camphorquinone [CQ] and phenyl propanedione) also require energy for a secondary electron transfer agent, such as an amine electron accepting agent, to generate a free radical.[54] In contrast, type I initiators (eg, Lucirin TPO, and derivatives of dibenzoyl germanium such as Ivocerin) do not need additional co-initiators because they decompose directly into one or more free radicals upon receiving sufficient energy at the correct wavelength.

Fig. 2 indicates the spectral absorption profiles of 4 photoinitiators at equivalent molar concentrations and indicates the relative ability of each photoinitiator to absorb radiant energy from 320 to 510 nm. These 4 photoinitiators are all highly reactive to wavelengths of less than 330 nm, but in the range of 330 to 510 nm, it can be seen that CQ is the most sensitive to light in the blue region close to 468 to 470 nm. In the 390 to 410 nm region, type I photoinitiators such as Lucirin TPO and Ivocerin are more reactive and have a higher quantum efficiency compared with the CQ or phenyl propanedione (PPD) photoinitiators.[55–57] Initiators such as Ivocerin and phenyl propanedione are activated by EM radiation that is in both the violet and blue color ranges. For example, Ivocerin is most reactive at 408 nm, but remains very sensitive to wavelengths of light between 400 and 430 nm.[56] Thus, depending on the photoinitiators used, even small changes in the emission spectrum (wavelength) that are undetectable to the human eye, can be very relevant. Unfortunately, specific information about the photoinitiators that are used in dental resins is often a trade secret and the dentist is left guessing what initiators are present, and thus which is the best LCU to use.

High-Output Curing Lights and Stress Development During Polymerization

Recently there has been a move towards faster polymerization of dental resin–based composites. However, it is not recommended because it is thought to adversely affect the mechanical properties of the polymer network.[58,59] Although dentists wish for ever

Absorption Spectra of Initiators

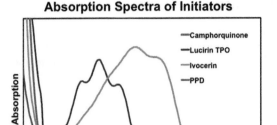

Fig. 2. Spectral absorption profiles of the most common photoinitiators used in dentistry, all at an equivalent molar concentration. PPD, phenyl propanedione.

shorter exposure times and manufacturers produce LCUs that delivered a high irradiance, there are concerns that these LCUs might generate excessive internal stresses within the resin and at the tooth–resin interface.[1] This concern surfaced because, with some dental resins and CQ photoinitiator systems, rapid photopolymerization produces shorter chain lengths because there is insufficient time for long polymer chains to form before the solid state is reached.[58] When polymerization starts, the system is still principally a viscous liquid. During further conversion from monomer to polymer, the formation of new monomer-to-monomer bonds causes shrinkage, and decreases the net volume of the system. As long as the system is a liquid, it can physically deform, and no stress is developed. However, once the resin becomes a solid, the polymerization shrinkage creates stress in the network and at the bonded interfaces. In theory, if this reaction happens at a rate that is 2 or more orders of magnitude faster, this may result in increased stress,[60] which results in increased bond failures, and more gaps between the tooth and restorative material.[61,62] Theoretically, this could all lead to premature failure of the restoration, but to date, this outcome has not been reported in a randomized controlled clinical trial.

Soft Start Exposures

In an attempt to decrease the adverse effects of polymerization shrinkage, a range of different light curing cycles have been developed. An example is the "soft start" curing mode, where a low irradiance value is initially delivered to the restoration for a short time, and then, either immediately, or over a short period of time, the light output increases to its full operating level for the remainder of the exposure time.[61,63,64] It was thought that such an exposure mode would reduce the rate at which the photocurable material reacted, delay the onset of vitrification and thus provide additional time for some stress relief to occur. Theoretically, this technique allows for the polymer chains to relax and for the partially cured resin composite to deform at its unbonded surface. This should relieve some of the polymerization contraction stresses before the gel point and vitrification stage is reached.[60,61,65–69] Another soft start method (the pulse-delay) delivers a low-level, short duration light exposure, and then the light is turned off. After waiting some 3 to 5 minutes, the final exposure is provided at the full light output. Some evidence suggests that this approach to achieve "soft start" polymerization works for certain resin composites polymerized by specific LCUs in vitro.[68,70] However, the potential correlation observed in the laboratory between improved marginal adaptation, reduced shrinkage, and a reduced polymerization contraction stress using the pulse-delay protocol has been shown to be more related to the fact that the resin received less total energy and consequently reached a lower degree of conversion than owing to the effects of any specific light exposure protocol.[1,66,71] Also, for highly crosslinked resin systems, the majority of shrinkage stress develops during and after the vitrification stage. Consequently, any stress relaxation prior to vitrification does not provide much reduction in the overall shrinkage stress.[66] Clinically, none of these attempts to control polymerization shrinkage rate and stress development have been found to provide significantly better clinical performance when compared with using a 40 seconds of continuous light exposure at 750 mW/cm^2 per increment.[72]

EVOLUTION OF DENTAL CURING LIGHTS
Ultraviolet Versus Blue Light

The initial attempts to produce light cured resins used UV radiation at about 365 nm[1] to activate the photoinitiator and thus generate free radicals.[73] Although the polymerization reaction was now under direct control of the clinician, wavelengths shorter than 400 nm are "ionizing," and could cause cataract formation or selective changes in oral bioflora.[1,74] In addition, short UV wavelengths are unable to penetrate deeply into the resin composite[1,75] and the resin increments were limited to 1-mm thick. This increased the chairside treatment time required to restore a tooth and did not result in much overall time savings when compared with self-curing resins.[76] Although when correctly used some of the UV-cured materials were very successful,[77] the use of UV light was discontinued and a different photoinitiator, CQ, and curing light were used.

Four types of blue light sources are now used to activate the photoinitiators found in dental resins: QTH, plasma arc (PAC), argon ion laser, and LED. These 4 sources produce photons of light in different ways, and deliver different emission spectra and wavelengths of light (**Fig. 3**). LED-curing lights have now come to dominate the market.[2]

Quartz–Tungsten–Halogen Lights

The early curing lights used a QTH projector bulb. The QTH bulb contains a chlorine-based halogen gas and a tungsten filament. When an electrical current passes through

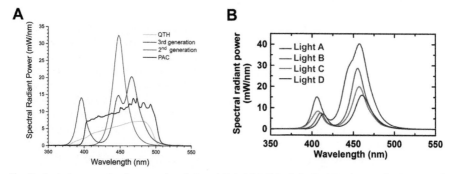

Fig. 3. Emission spectra from curing lights. (*A*) A PAC (*black line*), QTH (*green line*), second-generation (*red line*) and third-generation (*blue line*) light-emitting diode (LED) curing lights. Note the multiple emission peaks from the third-generation LED unit. (*B*) Emission spectra from 4 broad-spectrum, third-generation LED curing lights. Note that although the emission spectra are different, they all have a second emission peak below 420 nm.

the filament, the tungsten wire becomes incandescent and atoms are vaporized from its surface. This process releases a broad spectrum of radiant energy, most of which is emitted as heat in the infrared region. When the current is turned off, the filament cools, and the halogen gas redeposits the vaporized tungsten atoms onto the surface of the filament.[78] This process is called "the halogen cycle." Under ideal conditions, the QTH bulb should last about 50 hours[1,2,78] and a fan inside the unit dissipates unwanted heat away from the bulb, filters, and reflector. However, the lifespan of the bulb will be shortened if the user turns the power supply off immediately after use to stop the noise from the fan. This occurs because the halogen cycle can only occur if the bulb is allowed to cool down at a controlled rate; otherwise, the vaporized tungsten atoms are not redeposited onto the filament surface, thus shortening the lifetime of the bulb.[78]

The light from the QTH bulb is first directed toward a silverized parabolic reflector that is located behind the filament. This reflector allows some of the infrared light to pass through so that it is not reflected forward. The reflector surface becomes very hot when the light is on and vapors from solvents, cleaning agents, or moisture in the operatory air can be deposited onto the reflector surface, thus dulling or clouding its surface when it cools down. This will reduce the light output and can occur without any outward sign of failure unless the output from the light is monitored on a regular basis using a radiometer.[78]

The remaining reflected light is directed forward toward a bandpass filter that blocks out the infrared wavelengths, before it enters a fiber optic light guide. Thus, only blue light of wavelengths between approximately 400 and 500 nm reaches the proximal surface of a multistranded, bundled, glass fiber optic light guide. It has been estimated that as much as 70% of the electrical energy into the QTH bulb is converted to heat, with only 10% producing visible light and only 0.5% to 2.0% of the energy input is emitted as blue light.[79–81]

Although QTH lights deliver a broad emission spectrum (see **Fig. 3**A), the units delivered a relatively low radiant power and a low irradiance, and they required an exposure time of between 30 and 60 seconds to adequately photocure a 2-mm-thick increment of resin composite. Additionally, the majority of these lights were mains powered and the cooling fan was noisy.

Plasma Arc Lights

In an attempt to reduce light exposure times, PAC lights were introduced. These lights were promoted to deliver a high irradiance and the initial units recommended that exposure times between 3 and 5 seconds could be used to photocure a 2-mm-thick increment of resin composite. Instead of a filament, the PAC light source uses 2 tungsten electrodes that are surrounded by xenon gas. When a high voltage potential is applied, a spark is formed that ionizes the xenon gas.[1] This spark then acts as both a light emitter as well as an electrically conductive gaseous medium (a plasma) to maintain the spark. The gap between the electrodes is parallel to the long axis of a parabolic-shaped reflector that directs the emitted light forward through a sapphire window. Extreme optical filtering is used in PAC lights to prevent the emission of unwanted ionizing radiation, as well as to prevent an unacceptable temperature increase in the tooth or soft tissues.

Most PAC lights deliver a broad emission spectrum (see **Fig. 3**A), a high radiant power, and a high irradiance. However, at least 1 brand of PAC light had multiple tips to provide different light outputs and outcomes: a bleaching tip (full spectral output), a 470-nm tip for photocuring CQ-containing materials, and a 430-nm tip for photocuring materials containing the alternative initiators. The need to use specific light tips for specific situations led to confusion among clinicians, who were unsure which light tip they should use to cure the specific brand of resin they were using. Although PAC lights are excellent curing lights, they are also expensive, noisy, large, not portable, and cannot be battery operated. As a result, PAC lights have become less popular in recent years.

Argon Ion Lasers

The argon ion laser curing light was developed around the same time the initial PAC lights were introduced. The term "laser" is an acronym for **L**ight **A**mplification by **S**timulated **E**mission of **R**adiation.[78] Lasers work by delivering electrical energy to specific atoms within the unit. The electrons become "excited" and move from a low-energy orbit to a higher energy orbit around the atom's nucleus. When the electrons return to their normal or "ground" state, they emit photons that are all at the same wavelength. The specific wavelength of light from a laser is determined by the amount of energy released when the excited electron drops back to the lower orbit. The argon ion laser generates several very intense emission peaks in the blue spectral region, and it was considered to be a viable option for a high irradiance LCU.[1] However, now that high-output LED curing lights are available, laser curing lights have become less popular because they are expensive, not portable, have a narrow emission spectrum, and cannot be battery operated.

Light-Emitting Diode Technology

The next innovation in dental photocuring came in the early 1990s when it was reported that the emission spectrum from blue LEDs closely matched the absorption profile of the CQ photoinitiator used in most dental resins.[79,82] LED curing lights have many advantages because they are solid state, lightweight, battery driven, very efficient, and nonfiltered. Their emitting sources can provide a long working life when compared with filament or spark-based light sources.[1,2,82]

The semiconductor material in blue LEDs is made of a mix of gallium nitride and indium nitride that has been doped with impurities to create a p–n junction between the 2 semiconductor materials. The "p" (positive) side contains an excess of 'holes,' and the "n" (negative) side contains an excess of electrons. The color of the emitted light corresponds with the energy of the emitted photon that is in turn determined by the composition of these 2 semiconductors and their resulting "band gap" potential.[2,82] The blue light emitted from the LED has a relatively narrow bandwidth with a full width half maximum range of about 20 to 25 nm.[2,79,82]

First-Generation Light-Emitting Diode Lights

The first dental LED-based LCUs contained arrays of many individual LED emitters (cans).[1,82] Although these initial units delivered a low radiant power output, they generated great interest, because they were cordless, required little maintenance, were lightweight, and their LEDs were claimed to last for thousands of hours.

LEDs deliver a luminous efficacy that is approximately 2.5 times higher than that of the typical QTH bulb.[2] The blue wavelength output of these early LED units was in the range of maximum absorption of CQ, making these blue LEDs very efficient at producing the free radicals required for photocuring dental resins. Because these early LED units had a relatively low output, it was thought that all LED units generated 'cool blue light' and little heat in the target, something that was becoming a concern with other types of curing lights. However, the claims of low heat generation from these early LED lights were due to their low radiant power output rather than any property of the photons emitted from these LED units. These early LED units that emitted blue light from multiple, low-power LED emitters (cans), were termed first-generation LED curing lights.

Second-Generation Light-Emitting Diode Lights

Over time, LED chip design evolved to produce small light emitting pads, instead of discrete LED cans. These new LED emitters delivered a greater radiant power output so that the number of photons that were emitted within the absorption range of CQ exceeded that from high output QTH or PAC lights.[1] Thus, the recommended exposure times using the new blue LED chips became less than from QTH lights, a feature that greatly increased the marketability of LED curing lights. However, with the increase in radiant power output, the need to cool the LED emitter became critical; otherwise, the LED would overheat and destroy itself (**Fig. 4**A). For this reason, large metal heat sinks and internal cooling fans are used in some LED curing lights. Often, the metal cladding of these units is used to provide a large surface area to help dissipate the heat from the LED emitter (see **Fig. 4**B). Although these "second-generation" curing lights were more compact and more powerful than the "first-generation" of LED lights, neither the first- nor the second-generation LED lights deliver much light below 420 nm (see **Fig. 3**A).

Third-Generation Light-Emitting Diode Lights: Multiwave, Multipeak, and Polywave

As tooth whitening became popular, many dentists discovered that the shades of resin composites available at that time were too yellow and could not match the color of bleached teeth. This effect occurred primarily because the CQ photoinitiator used in the resins is bright yellow. As a result, some manufacturers incorporated co-initiators to boost the effectiveness of CQ and thus reduce the CQ concentration, whereas others started using resin compositions containing the more efficient "alternative"

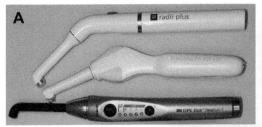
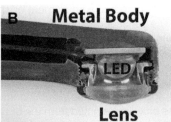
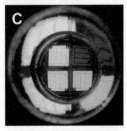

Fig. 4. Examples of curing lights and components. (*A*) Second generation light-emitting diode (LED) curing lights. (*B*) Cross-section of a curing light where the LED emitter is at the end and where the metal body acts as a heat sink. (*C*) The multiple pad style of LED emitters used in third generation LED-curing lights. Note the different color of the upper right LED emitter and the reflected light at the periphery. (*Courtesy of* [A] SDI Limited, Victoria, Australia; National Dental, Inc., Barrie, Ontario, Canada; and 3M Oral Care, St. Paul, MN, USA.)

photoinitiators that imparted less of a yellow color.[1] This change allowed manufacturers to make lighter shades of the restorative resin. These alternative photoinitiators require shorter wavelengths of light closer to violet (at or below 410 nm) light and, because second-generation LED curing lights emit very little light below 420 nm, the single peak LED lights were not very effective. They could be photocured using the broad emission spectrum from QTH and PAC curing lights.

To solve the problem caused by the narrow emission spectrum from the single peak blue-only LED units, an additional color emitter(s) was added to the blue LED pad. By incorporating several different LED color emitters into the unit, photons throughout the 380- to 500-nm spectral range could now be delivered (see **Fig. 4**C). These curing lights have been called "third-generation" LED curing lights, meaning that they emit a combination of violet and blue light. Photocuring lights of this generation have also been described as multiwave or multipeak dental curing lights, with 1 manufacturer trademarking the phrase Polywave to signify this concept within their product line.

For comparison purposes, the emission spectra from a QTH light, PAC light, a second-generation blue LED light, and a third-generation broad-spectrum LED light are shown in **Fig. 3**A. Note the narrow emission spectrum from the second generation LED unit and the large amount of spectral radiant power emitted by LED units in the 450 nm region. Note also the multiple wavelength peaks from the third generation LED units.

These broad-spectrum third-generation LED lights can activate all the photoinitiators used in dental resins. Because manufacturers rarely disclose the proprietary constituents used in their products, it is likely best to assume that if the resin manufacturer produces a polywave LED curing light, then their resins will benefit from the use of a third-generation LED curing light, for example, Ivoclar Vivadent, Heraeus Kulzer, GC, or Ultradent. Conversely, if the manufacturer only offers a single peak wavelength LCU (eg, 3M), then their resins are unlikely to benefit from the use of a third-generation LED curing light.

"Turbo" Light Guides

Conventional, glass fibered light guides come in a variety of diameters, with the proximal entrance aperture and distal exit diameters of the light guide being of the same physical size. In contrast, the entrance to a turbo light guide is made larger than the exit to increase the irradiance (the number of photons provided over the output area) (**Fig. 5**). By using hundreds of glass fibers that are larger in diameter at the proximal end (nearest to the light source) than the opposite (distal) end (nearest to the target),

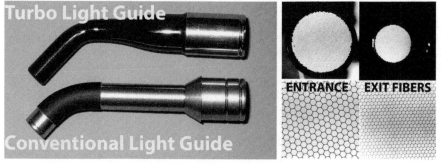

Fig. 5. Example of a conventional and a "turbo" light guide where the entrance fiber diameter is larger than the exit fiber diameter. Note how the turbo light guide tapers to the exit tip.

a large number of photons enter the light guide, but the same number (assuming no loss) of photons are emitted over a smaller area at the tip exit. This arrangement delivers the same radiant power (Watts) over a smaller area and thus increases the irradiance (mW/cm^2) delivered by these turbo light guides (**Fig. 6**). Owing to the optical design of these turbo light guides, the light beam rapidly disperses as the distance from the tip increases and the "focusing effect" of the turbo tip only increases the irradiance for a few millimeters from the tip end, beyond which the irradiance rapidly declines.[83,84]

Batteries

Most of the early LED curing lights were powered by nickel–cadmium (NiCad) batteries. These batteries can be damaged severely if they are deeply discharged, or if they are overcharged. Contemporary curing lights use a range of battery types. Smaller, high-capacity, nickel–metal hydride batteries (eg, used in the FreeLight 2, 3M and the Smartlite Focus, Dentsply) have mostly replaced these NiCad batteries. Any currently available curing units (eg, DeepCure-S, 3M and Valo, Ultradent) now use either lithium–ion, lithiun-polymer (Ivoclar Vivadent) battery technology, or 'ultracapacitors.' Generally, lithium–ion batteries are smaller than NiCad batteries, have a longer battery life, and do not suffer from any "memory effect" (this causes NiCad batteries to hold less of a charge over time). However, they may become damaged if stored without charge and are more expensive than NiCad batteries. The lithium-polymer battery can carry more charge and is thinner than a conventional Li-ion battery, but the Li-polymer batteries are more expensive. Ultracapacitors are ideally suited to power a curing light, where high bursts of power are required for only a short time. The ultracapacitors used in one brand of LED curing light (Demi Ultra, Kerr Corp, Orange, CA) can deliver a sufficient current for approximately 25, ten-second cures after which the unit must be recharged. Although these ultracapacitors cannot store the same amount of electrical energy as batteries, they can be fully recharged in as little as 40 seconds. In general, batteries used in curing lights have a limited shelf life, but they should last 2 to 3 years of normal use. To reduce the risk of the battery catching fire, always use the correct charger and follow the manufacturer's instructions. Batteries left in the light for long periods of time without recharging may become nonfunctional.

MEASURING AND REPORTING THE LIGHT OUTPUT
Radiant Exitance (Irradiance) Versus Radiant Power

Manufacturers commonly report the irradiance value (mW/cm^2) measured directly at the light tip to describe the output from their curing light. This is actually the "radiant exitance," but when measured at zero distance, such as when the curing light tip is in direct contact with a light meter or the surface of the resin, it is effectively the same as the SI term "incident irradiance." Unfortunately, this irradiance value provides very limited information about the effectiveness of the curing light, because is greatly influenced by both the diameter of the light tip and the distance between the light tip and the resin. For example, some curing lights use a tip diameter of 12 mm, compared with others that have a smaller tip diameter of 7 mm. Although a 5-mm difference in tip diameter may seem insignificant, it reduces the area of the light tip from 1.13 cm^2 (12 mm diameter), to 0.385 cm^2 (7 mm diameter). This results in an almost 3-fold increase in the radiant exitance (irradiance) at the tip, while only delivering the same amount of power. Consequently, manufacturers can produce curing lights that deliver a low radiant power output, but still deliver a high irradiance, simply by reducing the tip diameter.[85] This size may not be an issue if the dentist practices incremental filling and

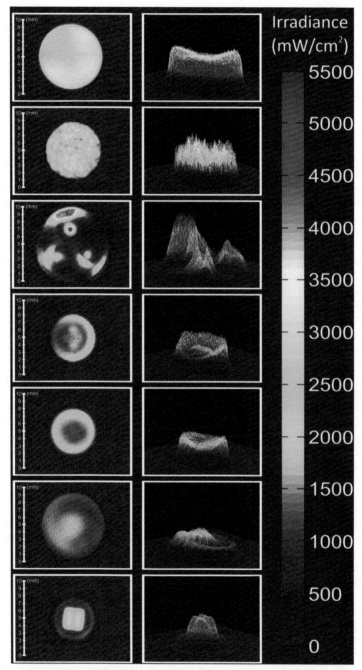

Fig. 6. Two-dimensional and 3-dimensional beam profiles of the irradiance from 7 contemporary curing lights. Note the differences in the beam diameters and the highly inhomogeneous irradiance distribution across the tips of the bottom 5 lights.

light curing, but in the era of bulk-fill composites and bulk curing, the clinician may not recognize that if they use a curing light with a small 7-mm diameter light tip, they must now use multiple exposures to fully cover a large restoration in a molar tooth. Thus, the radiant power (Watts), the active tip diameter, and the irradiance (mW/cm^2) from the curing light should all be reported.

Light Beam Uniformity

The ISO 10650:2015 standard for measuring the output from dental LCUs recommends using a laboratory-grade power meter to measure the total radiant power output. This power value is then divided by the tip area to produce a radiant exitance (irradiance) value across the light tip.[85] Because this irradiance value is obtained by dividing the total radiant power output by the total tip area, this irradiance value can only represent an averaged output value across the light tip and does not give any indication whether there are 'hot spots' of high irradiance or 'cold spots' of lower values across the light tip.

Recently, the beam profiling technique that is commonly used to examine lasers and other light sources has been adapted to measure the irradiance distribution across dental curing light tips. Several publications have now reported that the light output from many dental curing lights is not uniform and 'hot spots' of high irradiance and 'cold spots' of lower values where less light is emitted are present across the tip of many curing lights.[51,52,86–89] Examples of the light output across the emitting tips of 7 different dental LCUs are seen in the 2-dimensional and 3-dimensional images of the irradiance distribution in **Fig. 6**. Note the highly inhomogeneous irradiance distribution across the tips and the presence of 'hot spots' of high irradiance and 'cold spots' of lower values. These beam profile images clearly show that the light output at the tip may not be uniform and the extent of irradiance homogeneity depends on the design of the curing light. Thus, using a single irradiance value to describe the output from a curing light usually does not describe the irradiance across the entire light tip. Consequently, dental manufacturers should provide the beam profile for their curing light.

To highlight the clinical relevance of the beam profiles, the irradiance beam profile can be overlaid over images of tooth preparations (**Fig. 7**). These images demonstrate that for some curing lights, different locations in the restoration can receive very different amounts of light. The images also show why multiple exposures are required if the curing light has a small tip when compared with a light tip that covers the entire preparation with light. The gingival margin area is known to be a high-risk area for recurrent caries[90] and is the region that is the most difficult to reach with the curing light.[84,91] Even under ideal conditions, the resin at the bottom of these boxes will be the furthest away from the light tip, it may be in shadow, and it will receive the least amount of light. The beam profile images in **Figs. 6** and **7** illustrate that unless the operator carefully positions the light tip, the irradiance and radiant exposure received at the gingival margins of the proximal boxes from some curing lights may be inadequate to ensure adequate polymerization of the adhesive, or the resin restoration, in these regions.[3,51,52,89] Thus, although the top surface of the resin restoration may be well-polymerized, the resin at the bottom of the proximal box may well be undercured unless the exposure time is increased and the light is directed to the restoration at different angles.[18,19,84,92–94]

Curing Light Output Monitoring

Over time, the light source can degrade and the light output will decrease owing to the build up of scale on the fiber optic light probe after autoclaving,[95] breakage, or

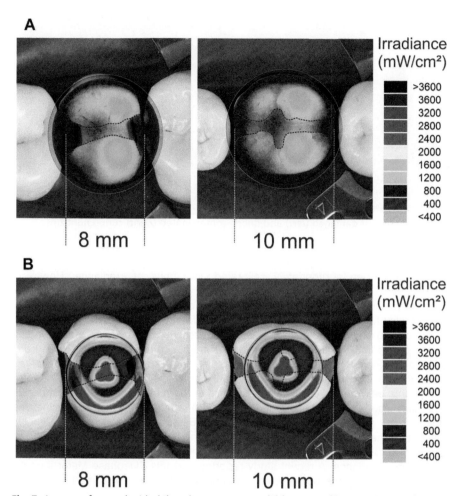

Fig. 7. Images of a good wide (*A*) and a poor narrow (*B*) beam profile, superimposed on images of a premolar and a molar tooth preparation. Both images are scaled to the same maximum irradiance value of 3600 mW/cm² and also show how an 8-mm tip diameter does not cover a molar tooth and will require multiple exposures to cover an entire molar MO restoration.

damage to the light tip,[96,97] or the presence of debris on the light tip (**Fig. 8**).[96,98] In addition, disinfectant sprays can erode the O-rings that are used to stabilize the light guide, and these liquids can bake onto the optics inside the housing, thus reducing the light output.[99] All these factors can significantly decrease the ability of the curing light to photo cure the resin. Thus, it is important that a dental radiometer be used to routinely evaluate and record the light output from the curing light.[1,100]

Handheld "Dental Radiometers"

Examples of 2 handheld dental radiometers that can be used to monitor the output from dental curing lights are displayed in **Fig. 9**. These devices often contain a small silicon photodiode detector that converts photons from the curing light into electrical

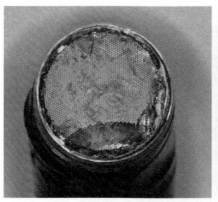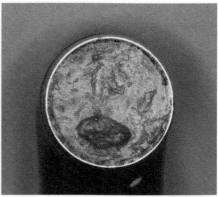

Fig. 8. Examples of damaged (*left*) and debris-contaminated (*right*) curing light tips.

current and, when appropriately calibrated, into units of irradiance. However, because the detector is usually small, and some dental radiometers only have narrow entrance apertures, most dental radiometers do not measure all of the light from the curing light.[101] Since light is rarely emitted uniformly across the entire curing light tip, depending on where the light tip is positioned over the detector area, different regions of the light tip that emit high or low irradiance values may be measured. These factors help to explain why several studies have reported that most dental radiometers are inaccurate.[101–105] In addition, because QTH, PAC, or LED dental curing lights deliver different emission spectra to the radiometer, the type of band-pass filter used within dental radiometers will affect the irradiance value reported.[101,103] A new dental radiometer, the Bluephase Meter II from Ivoclar Vivadent (Amherst, NY) contains a special filter and is able to record the radiant power up to a 13-mm diameter tip. When the tip diameter is entered, this meter also displays the irradiance. A recent study reported that this Bluephase Meter II could accurately measure the power from different output modes of 8 models of LED curing lights.[100]

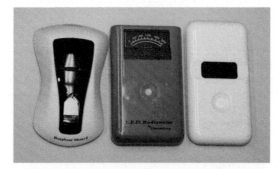

Fig. 9. Three commercial dental radiometers. The Bluephase meter II (Ivoclar Vivadent) on the left has a large entrance aperture and is able to record all the power up to light from a 13-mm diameter light tip. (*Courtesy of* Ivoclar Vivadent, Inc., Amherst, NY; Kerr Corporation, Orange, CA; and SDI Limited, Victoria, Australia.)

PRACTICAL CONSIDERATIONS FOR LIGHT CURING DENTAL RESINS IN THE MOUTH

If My Curing Light Delivers Twice the Irradiance, Can I halve the Time Spent Light Curing?

The boundary between somewhat cured and uncured resin is called the depth of cure and is often reached at a depth of 2 mm for a conventional resin composite material, and between 4 and 6 mm for a bulk fill composite if the light tip is kept close to the resin composite surface. In cases of compromised access, and darker or more opaque shades of resin, the depth of cure will be less unless longer exposure times are used. Some manufacturers recognize this fact and, for example, 1 manufacturer recommends light different exposure times of between 5 and 40 seconds to effectively light cure different shades and types of their own resin composites using the same curing light.[106] Thus, it is important not to choose just 1 exposure time, and then use the same time for all shades and situations because, depending on the location, the shade or the brand of resin, this may deliver either too much or too little energy.

In the past, it was recommended that a QTH unit should deliver a minimum irradiance of 400 mW/cm^2 for 60 seconds to adequately polymerize a 1.5 to 2-mm-thick increment of resin.[107] When the irradiance is multiplied by the exposure time, this suggests that a radiant exposure of 24 J/cm^2 should adequately polymerize the resin composite. However, true reciprocity between the duration of exposure and the irradiance does not exist.[15,108–112] Consequently, if the manufacturer recommends delivering 500 mW/cm^2 for 40 seconds or 20 J/cm^2, this does not mean that the same resin polymerization would occur if 4000 mW/cm^2 was delivered for 5 seconds, although in both cases the resin would receive the same 20 J/cm^2 of radiant exposure. However, it is possible to compensate somewhat for a lower irradiance (eg, if a less powerful light is used, or if the distance between the light tip to the top surface is increased) by prolonging the exposure time but this should be done according to the resin manufacturer's instructions for use.

Light Guide Tip Diameter

With the phase down in the use of amalgam, dentistry is now in the era of bulk-filled resins and bulk curing of large resin restorations. The diameter of the light tip can have a significant impact on the amount of light and energy delivered to the restoration.[84,113] With the dimensions of a mandibular molar being approximately 11.0 mm mesiodistally and 10.5 mm buccolingually at the crown,[114] the clinician who wishes to reduce the time spent light curing restorations should use a curing light with a light emitting tip that completely covers the entire restoration surface (**Fig. 10**). Otherwise, they will need to deliver multiple, sequential, overlapping exposures to make sure all areas of the restorative material have received adequate amounts of light.[3,51,52,89]

Distance to Target

Depending on the design and the optics of the light guide, blue light is emitted at different degrees of beam divergence. The effect of tip distance on irradiance at the target varies for different lights, because some of the light is delivered as a collimated beam and some is dispersed. The effect of increasing the distance from the tip on the decrease in the amount of light received at the target might be assumed to obey the inverse square law; however, this does not always occur. This is because the law applies to a point source of radiation emitting 360° in space (as a sphere), much like the sun. The emission from a light guide does not act as a point source.

Fig. 11 displays how the effect of increasing the tip-to-target distance can greatly differ between two different of LCUs. Much of the research on dental resins has been

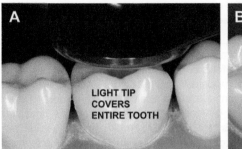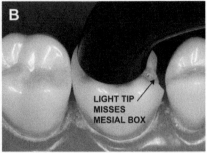

Fig. 10. (*A*) A large, wide diameter light tip can cover an entire molar tooth, whereas (*B*) a smaller, narrow diameter light tip will require multiple exposures to cover an entire molar MO restoration.

conducted in a laboratory setting, using the LCU in a fixed position very close to the resin surface. Although this may make the results look good and consistent, it is rarely possible to position the LCU tip so close to the resin in the mouth. Moreover, irradiance values stated by the manufacturers are usually only measured at the light tip. A significantly lower irradiance may be reaching the surface of the resin in the tooth that is often 2 to 8 mm away from the light tip,[115] such that some curing lights deliver only 25% or even less of the irradiance measured at the tip when the resin is at a distance of just 8 mm away from the tip.[18,84,92,93,116] Thus, the dentist should know how clinically relevant distances of 2 to 8 mm may affect the irradiance delivered by their curing light.

Xu and coworkers[18] investigated the effects of the distance from the light guide on the adhesion of composite resin to the tooth. Their investigation was prompted by the number of studies demonstrating a poor marginal seal and more microleakage at the gingival margin of these restorations when compared with the occlusal enamel margins. They reported that there was an exponential relationship between the radiant exposure and the bond strength. It was easy to halve the bond strength simply by moving the light tip 4 mm away from the tooth, thus delivering less energy to the resin. Their conclusion was that when light curing adhesives in deep proximal boxes with a curing light that delivered 600 mW/cm^2, the exposure time should be increased from 20 to 60 seconds. This would then deliver sufficient energy to ensure optimal resin

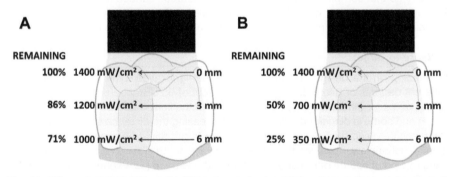

Fig. 11. Effect of distance from the light tip on the irradiance. Depending on the optical design, 2 (*A* and *B*) lights can deliver a similar irradiance at the light tip, but deliver a very different irradiance at 6 mm distance.

polymerization and bonding to the tooth. Others have also made similar recommendations to increase the exposure time for the initial increments of resin composite in the proximal boxes, even for curing lights with greater than 1000 mW/cm^2.

Size of the Curing Light and Clinical Access

Access to a restoration that is on the facial surfaces of the anterior teeth is usually not an issue. However, curing lights differ in their ability to reach all regions of the mouth. **Fig. 12** illustrates the excellent ability of a pen-style curing light such as the Valo Cordless (Ultradent Products, South Jordan, UT) to access the second molar tooth whereas another curing light could only access the second molar with the tip at a steep angle to the occlusal surface. This angle will cause shadows, affect the amount of radiant exposure delivered, and could ultimately affect the success of the resin restoration.[19,34]

Impact of Infection Control Methods

Although some fiberoptic light guides can be autoclaved, the curing light itself cannot. Thus, the use of infection control barriers that cover the entire curing light, buttons, and light guides are recommended. The barrier should fit snugly over the light tip and the seam should not impede the light output (**Fig. 13**). Some commercial barriers can reduce the radiant exitance by up to 40%[86,117–119] and latex-based barriers should be avoided because they have been reported to produce significantly lower resin conversion values. For this reason, the light output from curing lights should be recorded with the barrier over the light tip. Clear, plastic food wrap is an effective and inexpensive infection control barrier that has minimal effect on light output.[97,118,119] Disinfectant sprays can erode the O-rings used to stabilize light guides, and the residual fluid can

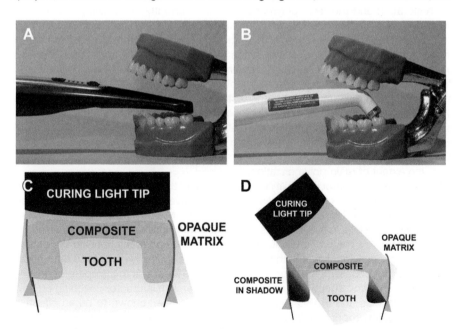

Fig. 12. Ability of different dental curing lights to access the mandibular second molar. (*A*) Light design that allows good access. (*B*) The second molar can only be accessed at an angle. (*C*) When the light tip is directly over the restoration, all regions of the composite are exposed to light. (*D*) When the light tip is held at an angle, this orientation may produce unwanted shadows and reduce the extent of resin polymerization.

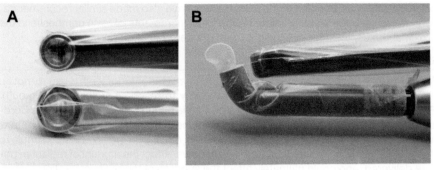

Fig. 13. The barrier should (*A*) fit snugly over the light tip and the (*B*) seam should not impede the light output.

bake onto the lens inside the light housing, thus decreasing the light output.[99] Thus, when using cold sterilizing techniques, only approved cleaning solutions should be used. If it can be detached, the light guide should be removed from time to time and the lens or filter inside the curing light housing should be checked to ensure that it, and both entrance and exit ends of the light guide, are clean and undamaged.

Effect of Training

Unless the operator is careful, the position of the light tip over the tooth can produce unwanted shadows that have an adverse effect on the amount of energy received by the restoration and the resin polymerization.[19,34] Currently, the training provided to most dentists, dental students, and dental assistants is inadequate to ensure that curing lights are being used correctly. Although there are elaborate descriptions of techniques used for material manipulation and placement, at a most critical phase of providing a successful and long-lasting restoration, usually there are only 5 words "and then you light cure."[120] It has been shown that the light curing procedure is not as simple as aiming the curing light at the restoration and turning the light on.[33,37] Both the LCU and the light delivery technique used by the operator have a significant effect on the radiant exposure delivered to the restoration. Unfortunately, it is common practice not to watch the position of the curing light tip over the tooth when light curing. This can negatively affect the amount of energy received by the restoration and, thus, the extent of resin polymerization.[17,19,33,35,121]

The amount of operator variability in how much light they deliver can be reduced and the radiant exposure delivered to restorations improved if the user has been trained how to use a curing light using a device such as the MARC Patient Simulator (Blue-Light Analytics, Halifax, Nova Scotia, Canada). Individualized hands on training on how to light cure a restoration includes learning how to correctly position the patient to improve access and ensuring that the light guide is optimally positioned throughout the light curing process.[33-37] By providing immediate feedback to the operator on how much irradiance and energy they delivered, together with instructor coaching on how to avoid mistakes, the MARC Patient Simulator has been shown to be an effective method to teach proper light curing technique. Examples of the irradiance and energy delivered when using the same curing light for 10 seconds, before and after receiving such training, are seen in **Fig. 14**. This image shows the irradiance delivered by 2 operators to a specific location over 10 seconds in the MARC Patient Simulator. The after image shows an improvement in the consistency of the irradiance delivered throughout exposure.

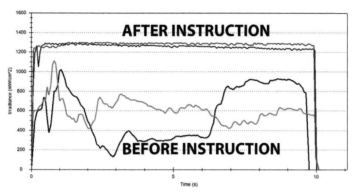

Fig. 14. Before and after images of the irradiance delivered by 2 operators to a specific location over 10 seconds in the MARC patient simulator. The results after receiving light curing instruction show great improvement in the consistency of the irradiance delivered throughout exposure.

GENERAL RECOMMENDATIONS

When making a decision about which new curing light they should purchase, the clinician should ask the following questions.

1. Has the curing light been approved for use in my country?
2. Who do I contact if I have a problem with the light, or if the patient complains about something that happened after the curing light was used?
3. What is the radiant power output (Watts) from the curing light?
4. What is the active tip size, that is, how much of the restoration will receive useful light?
5. What is the emission spectrum from the curing light? Will the wavelengths of light emitted from the light match the sensitivity of the resin that I use?
6. What is the effect of distance from the light tip on the irradiance received by the restorations?
7. Do I like the ergonomics of the curing light? Will I be able to access all restorations in the mouth with the curing light?
8. How do I disinfect the light?
9. What barriers are available and how much do they affect the light output?
10. If it is battery operated, how much does the replacement battery cost?
11. How durable is the unit. How easily will it break if dropped?

Having chosen a curing light, following these 7 clinical recommendations should help improve the use of the curing light.[94]

1. Monitor the performance of the curing light and keep a logbook of the output from the light from the date of purchase. Repair or replace the light when necessary.
2. Maximize the output from the curing light by routinely examining the light tip for damage and remove remnants of previously cured resin. Clean or replace the tip as necessary.
3. Protect the eyes of everyone in the operatory who could be exposed to the bright light, using appropriate orange (blue light blocking) safety glasses.
4. Learn how to use the curing light to maximize energy delivered to the resin.
5. Place the central axis of the tip of the curing light directly over and normal to the resin surface; the emitting end should be parallel to the resin surface being exposed.

6. Where undercuts are present that cause shadows, move the light tip around and increase the exposure time. Use supplementary buccolingual interproximal curing (but beware of overheating).
7. Beware of damaging the pulp or oral mucosa when using a powerful curing light. Use a lower power setting when curing the bonding system in deep cavities. Protect the oral mucosa from the light with gauze and either air cool or wait several seconds between each light curing cycle when using a curing light that might produce a damaging temperature increase.

ACKNOWLEDGMENTS

The author acknowledges the valuable contributions of Professor F. Rueggeberg, not only in the preparation of this article, but also for his work in highlighting the role of the curing light in dentistry.

REFERENCES

1. Rueggeberg FA. State-of-the-art: dental photocuring–a review. Dent Mater 2011;27(1):39–52.
2. Jandt KD, Mills RW. A brief history of LED photopolymerization. Dent Mater 2013;29(6):605–17.
3. Price RB, Ferracane JL, Shortall AC. Light-curing units: a review of what we need to know. J Dent Res 2015;94(9):1179–86.
4. Santini A, Turner S. General dental practitioners' knowledge of polymerisation of resin-based composite restorations and light curing unit technology. Br Dent J 2011;211(6):E13.
5. McCusker N, Bailey C, Robinson S, et al. Dental light curing and its effects on color perception. Am J Orthod Dentofacial Orthop 2012;142(3):355–63.
6. Kopperud SE, Rukke HV, Kopperud HM, et al. Light curing procedures - performance, knowledge level and safety awareness among dentists. J Dent 2017;58: 67–73.
7. Al Shaafi M, Maawadh A, Al Qahtani M. Evaluation of light intensity output of QTH and LED curing devices in various governmental health institutions. Oper Dent 2011;36(4):356–61.
8. Hao X, Luo M, Wu J, et al. A survey of power density of light-curing units used in private dental offices in Changchun City, China. Lasers Med Sci 2015;30(2): 493–7.
9. Hegde V, Jadhav S, Aher GB. A clinical survey of the output intensity of 200 light curing units in dental offices across Maharashtra. J Conserv Dent 2009;12(3): 105–8.
10. Barghi N, Fischer DE, Pham T. Revisiting the intensity output of curing lights in private dental offices. Compend Contin Educ Dent 2007;28(7):380–4 [quiz: 385–6].
11. Ernst CP, Busemann I, Kern T, et al. Feldtest zur Lichtemissionsleistung von Polymerisationsgeräten in zahnärztlichen Praxen. Dtsch Zahnarztl Zeitung 2006; 61(9):466–71.
12. El-Mowafy O, El-Badrawy W, Lewis DW, et al. Efficacy of halogen photopolymerization units in private dental offices in Toronto. J Can Dent Assoc 2005;71(8): 587.
13. Maghaireh GA, Alzraikat H, Taha NA. Assessing the irradiance delivered from light-curing units in private dental offices in Jordan. J Am Dent Assoc 2013; 144(8):922–7.

14. Meyer DM, Kaste LM, Lituri KM, et al. Policy development fosters collaborative practice: The example of the Minamata Convention on Mercury. Dent Clin North Am 2016;60(4):921–42.

15. Durner J, Obermaier J, Draenert M, et al. Correlation of the degree of conversion with the amount of elutable substances in nano-hybrid dental composites. Dent Mater 2012;28(11):1146–53.

16. Ferracane JL, Mitchem JC, Condon JR, et al. Wear and marginal breakdown of composites with various degrees of cure. J Dent Res 1997;76(8):1508–16.

17. Shortall A, El-Mahy W, Stewardson D, et al. Initial fracture resistance and curing temperature rise of ten contemporary resin-based composites with increasing radiant exposure. J Dent 2013;41(5):455–63.

18. Xu X, Sandras DA, Burgess JO. Shear bond strength with increasing light-guide distance from dentin. J Esthet Restor Dent 2006;18(1):19–27 [discussion: 28].

19. Konerding KL, Heyder M, Kranz S, et al. Study of energy transfer by different light curing units into a class III restoration as a function of tilt angle and distance, using a MARC Patient Simulator (PS). Dent Mater 2016;32(5):676–86.

20. Kirkpatrick SJ. A primer on radiometry. Dent Mater 2005;21(1):21–6.

21. Miller CS, Leonelli FM, Latham E. Selective interference with pacemaker activity by electrical dental devices. Oral Surg Oral Med Oral Pathol Oral Radiol Endod 1998;85(1):33–6.

22. Elayi CS, Lusher S, Meeks Nyquist JL, et al. Interference between dental electrical devices and pacemakers or defibrillators: results from a prospective clinical study. J Am Dent Assoc 2015;146(2):121–8.

23. American Conference of Governmental Industrial Hygienists (ACGIH). TLVs and BEIs based on the documentation for threshold limit values for chemical substances and physical agents and biological exposure indices. Cincinnati (OH), ACGIH 2015.

24. Price RB, Labrie D, Bruzell EM, et al. The dental curing light: a potential health risk. J Occup Environ Hyg 2016;13(8):639–46.

25. Bruzell Roll EM, Jacobsen N, Hensten-Pettersen A. Health hazards associated with curing light in the dental clinic. Clin Oral Investig 2004;8(3):113–7.

26. Labrie D, Moe J, Price RB, et al. Evaluation of ocular hazards from 4 types of curing lights. J Can Dent Assoc 2011;77:b116.

27. McCusker N, Lee SM, Robinson S, et al. Light curing in orthodontics; should we be concerned? Dent Mater 2013;29(6):e85–90.

28. Stamatacos C, Harrison JL. The possible ocular hazards of LED dental illumination applications. J Tenn Dent Assoc 2013;93(2):25–9 [quiz: 30–1].

29. Hill EE. Eye safety practices in U.S. dental school restorative clinics, 2006. J Dent Educ 2006;70(12):1294–7.

30. Guidelines on limits of exposure to broad-band incoherent optical radiation (0.38 to 3μm). International Commission on Non-Ionizing Radiation Protection. Health Phys 1997;73(3):539–54.

31. Ham WT Jr, Ruffolo JJ Jr, Mueller HA, et al. Histologic analysis of photochemical lesions produced in rhesus retina by short-wave-length light. Invest Ophthalmol Vis Sci 1978;17(10):1029–35.

32. Bruzell EM, Johnsen B, Aalerud TN, et al. Evaluation of eye protection filters for use with dental curing and bleaching lamps. J Occup Environ Hyg 2007;4(6):432–9.

33. Federlin M, Price R. Improving light-curing instruction in dental school. J Dent Educ 2013;77(6):764–72.

34. Price RB, McLeod ME, Felix CM. Quantifying light energy delivered to a Class I restoration. J Can Dent Assoc 2010;76:a23.
35. Seth S, Lee CJ, Ayer CD. Effect of instruction on dental students' ability to light-cure a simulated restoration. J Can Dent Assoc 2012;78:c123.
36. Mutluay MM, Rueggeberg FA, Price RB. Effect of using proper light-curing techniques on energy delivered to a class 1 restoration. Quintessence Int 2014; 45(7):549–56.
37. Price RB, Strassler HE, Price HL, et al. The effectiveness of using a patient simulator to teach light-curing skills. J Am Dent Assoc 2014;145(1):32–43.
38. Yap AU, Soh MS. Thermal emission by different light-curing units. Oper Dent 2003;28(3):260–6.
39. Hofmann N, Hugo B, Klaiber B. Effect of irradiation type (LED or QTH) on photo-activated composite shrinkage strain kinetics, temperature rise, and hardness. Eur J Oral Sci 2002;110(6):471–9.
40. Weerakoon AT, Meyers IA, Symons AL, et al. Pulpal heat changes with newly developed resin photopolymerisation systems. Aust Endod J 2002;28(3): 108–11.
41. Ozturk AN, Usumez A. Influence of different light sources on microtensile bond strength and gap formation of resin cement under porcelain inlay restorations. J Oral Rehabil 2004;31(9):905–10.
42. Matalon S, Slutzky H, Wassersprung N, et al. Temperature rises beneath resin composite restorations during curing. Am J Dent 2010;23(4):223–6.
43. Baroudi K, Silikas N, Watts DC. In vitro pulp chamber temperature rise from irradiation and exotherm of flowable composites. Int J Paediatr Dent 2009;19(1): 48–54.
44. Atai M, Motevasselian F. Temperature rise and degree of photopolymerization conversion of nanocomposites and conventional dental composites. Clin Oral Investig 2009;13(3):309–16.
45. Gomes M, DeVito-Moraes A, Francci C, et al. Temperature increase at the light guide tip of 15 contemporary LED units and thermal variation at the pulpal floor of cavities: an infrared thermographic analysis. Oper Dent 2013;38(3):324–33.
46. Leprince J, Devaux J, Mullier T, et al. Pulpal-temperature rise and polymerization efficiency of LED curing lights. Oper Dent 2010;35(2):220–30.
47. Armellin E, Bovesecchi G, Coppa P, et al. LED curing lights and temperature changes in different tooth sites. Biomed Res Int 2016;2016:1894672.
48. Mouhat M, Mercer J, Stangvaltaite L, et al. Light-curing units used in dentistry: factors associated with heat development—potential risk for patients. Clin Oral Investig 2017;21(5):1687–96.
49. Onisor I, Asmussen E, Krejci I. Temperature rise during photo-polymerization for onlay luting. Am J Dent 2011;24(4):250–6.
50. Spranley TJ, Winkler M, Dagate J, et al. Curing light burns. Gen Dent 2012; 60(4):e210–4.
51. Shimokawa CA, Turbino ML, Harlow JE, et al. Light output from six battery operated dental curing lights. Mater Sci Eng C Mater Biol Appl 2016;69:1036–42.
52. AlShaafi MM, Harlow JE, Price HL, et al. Emission characteristics and effect of battery drain in "budget" curing lights. Oper Dent 2016;41(4):397–408.
53. Shortall AC, Price RB, MacKenzie L, et al. Guidelines for the selection, use, and maintenance of LED light-curing units - part II. Br Dent J 2016;221(9):551–4.
54. Stansbury JW. Curing dental resins and composites by photopolymerization. J Esthet Dent 2000;12(6):300–8.

55. Neumann MG, Miranda WG Jr, Schmitt CC, et al. Molar extinction coefficients and the photon absorption efficiency of dental photoinitiators and light curing units. J Dent 2005;33(6):525–32.
56. Burtscher P. Ivocerin in comparison to camphorquinone. Ivoclar Vivadent Report, No. 19, July, 2013. p. 11–5.
57. Moszner N, Fischer UK, Ganster B, et al. Benzoyl germanium derivatives as novel visible light photoinitiators for dental materials. Dent Mater 2008;24(7): 901–7.
58. Burdick JA, Lovestead TM, Anseth KS. Kinetic chain lengths in highly cross-linked networks formed by the photoinitiated polymerization of divinyl mono-mers: a gel permeation chromatography investigation. Biomacromolecules 2003;4(1):149–56.
59. Feng L, Carvalho R, Suh BI. Insufficient cure under the condition of high irradi-ance and short irradiation time. Dent Mater 2009;25(3):283–9.
60. Taubock TT, Feilzer AJ, Buchalla W, et al. Effect of modulated photo-activation on polymerization shrinkage behavior of dental restorative resin composites. Eur J Oral Sci 2014;122(4):293–302.
61. Kanca J 3rd, Suh BI. Pulse activation: reducing resin-based composite contrac-tion stresses at the enamel cavosurface margins. Am J Dent 1999;12(3):107–12.
62. Randolph LD, Palin WM, Watts DC, et al. The effect of ultra-fast photopolymer-isation of experimental composites on shrinkage stress, network formation and pulpal temperature rise. Dent Mater 2014;30(11):1280–9.
63. Suh BI, Feng L, Wang Y, et al. The effect of the pulse-delay cure technique on residual strain in composites. Compend Contin Educ Dent 1999;20(2 Suppl): 4–12.
64. Feng L, Suh BI. A mechanism on why slower polymerization of a dental compos-ite produces lower contraction stress. J Biomed Mater Res B Appl Biomater 2006;78(1):63–9.
65. Bouschlicher MR, Rueggeberg FA. Effect of ramped light intensity on polymer-ization force and conversion in a photoactivated composite. J Esthet Dent 2000; 12(6):328–39.
66. Lu H, Stansbury JW, Bowman CN. Impact of curing protocol on conversion and shrinkage stress. J Dent Res 2005;84(9):822–6.
67. Chye CH, Yap AU, Laim YC, et al. Post-gel polymerization shrinkage associated with different light curing regimens. Oper Dent 2005;30(4):474–80.
68. Lopes LG, Franco EB, Pereira JC, et al. Effect of light-curing units and activation mode on polymerization shrinkage and shrinkage stress of composite resins. J Appl Oral Sci 2008;16(1):35–42.
69. Ilie N, Jelen E, Hickel R. Is the soft-start polymerisation concept still relevant for modern curing units? Clin Oral Investig 2011;15(1):21–9.
70. Dall'Magro E, Correr AB, Costa AR, et al. Effect of different photoactivation tech-niques on the bond strength of a dental composite. Braz Dent J 2010;21(3): 220–4.
71. Inoue K, Howashi G, Kanetou T, et al. Effect of light intensity on linear shrinkage of photo-activated composite resins during setting. J Oral Rehabil 2005;32(1): 22–7.
72. van Dijken JW, Pallesen U. A 7-year randomized prospective study of a one-step self-etching adhesive in non-carious cervical lesions. The effect of curing modes and restorative material. J Dent 2012;40(12):1060–7.

73. Buonocore MG, Davila J. Restoration of fractured anterior teeth with ultraviolet-light-polymerized bonding materials: a new technique. J Am Dent Assoc 1973; 86(6):1349–54.
74. Birdsell DC, Bannon PJ, Webb RB. Harmful effects of near-ultraviolet radiation used for polymerization of a sealant and a composite resin. J Am Dent Assoc 1977;94(2):311–4.
75. Cook WD. Factors affecting the depth of cure of UV-polymerized composites. J Dent Res 1980;59(5):800–8.
76. Tirtha R, Fan PL, Dennison JB, et al. In vitro depth of cure of photo-activated composites. J Dent Res 1982;61(10):1184–7.
77. Wilder AD Jr, May KN Jr, Bayne SC, et al. Seventeen-year clinical study of ultraviolet-cured posterior composite class I and II restorations. J Esthet Dent 1999;11(3):135–42.
78. Rueggeberg F. Contemporary issues in photocuring. Compend Contin Educ Dent Suppl 1999;(25):S4–15.
79. Fujibayashi K, Shimaru K, Takahashi N, et al. Newly developed curing unit using blue light-emitting diodes. Dent Jpn (Tokyo) 1998;34:49–53.
80. Yaman BC, Efes BG, Dorter C, et al. The effects of halogen and light-emitting diode light curing on the depth of cure and surface microhardness of composite resins. J Conserv Dent 2011;14(2):136–9.
81. Shortall AC, Price RB, MacKenzie L, et al. Guidelines for the selection, use, and maintenance of LED light-curing units - Part 1. Br Dent J 2016;221(8):453–60.
82. Mills RW, Jandt KD, Ashworth SH. Dental composite depth of cure with halogen and blue light emitting diode technology. Br Dent J 1999;186(8):388–91.
83. Curtis JW Jr, Rueggeberg FA, Lee AJ. Curing efficiency of the turbo tip. Gen Dent 1995;43(5):428–33.
84. Price RB, Derand T, Sedarous M, et al. Effect of distance on the power density from two light guides. J Esthet Dent 2000;12(6):320–7.
85. ISO 10650 Dentistry-Powered polymerization activators (ISO 10650:2015). Geneva (Switzerland): International Standards Organization; 2015. p. 14.
86. Vandewalle KS, Roberts HW, Rueggeberg FA. Power distribution across the face of different light guides and its effect on composite surface microhardness. J Esthet Restor Dent 2008;20(2):108–17 [discussion: 18].
87. Price RB, Labrie D, Rueggeberg FA, et al. Irradiance differences in the violet (405 nm) and blue (460 nm) spectral ranges among dental light-curing units. J Esthet Restor Dent 2010;22(6):363–77.
88. Michaud PL, Price RB, Labrie D, et al. Localised irradiance distribution found in dental light curing units. J Dent 2014;42(2):129–39.
89. Price RB, Labrie D, Rueggeberg FA, et al. Correlation between the beam profile from a curing light and the microhardness of four resins. Dent Mater 2014; 30(12):1345–57.
90. Mjör IA. Clinical diagnosis of recurrent caries. J Am Dent Assoc 2005;136(10): 1426–33.
91. Yearn JA. Factors affecting cure of visible light activated composites. Int Dent J 1985;35(3):218–25.
92. Price RB, Labrie D, Whalen JM, et al. Effect of distance on irradiance and beam homogeneity from 4 light-emitting diode curing units. J Can Dent Assoc 2011; 77:b9.
93. Corciolani G, Vichi A, Davidson CL, et al. The influence of tip geometry and distance on light-curing efficacy. Oper Dent 2008;33(3):325–31.

94. Price RB, Shortall AC, Palin WM. Contemporary issues in light curing. Oper Dent 2014;39(1):4–14.

95. Rueggeberg FA, Caughman WF, Comer RW. The effect of autoclaving on energy transmission through light-curing tips. J Am Dent Assoc 1996;127(8):1183–7.

96. Poulos JG, Styner DL. Curing lights: changes in intensity output with use over time. Gen Dent 1997;45(1):70–3.

97. McAndrew R, Lynch CD, Pavli M, et al. The effect of disposable infection control barriers and physical damage on the power output of light curing units and light curing tips. Br Dent J 2011;210(8):E12.

98. Strydom C. Dental curing lights–maintenance of visible light curing units. SADJ 2002;57(6):227–33.

99. Strassler HE, Price RB. Understanding light curing, part II. Delivering predictable and successful restorations. Dent Today 2014;1–8 [quiz: 9]. Available at: https://www.dentalcetoday.com/courses/165%2FPDF%2FDT_June_14_174_fnl.pdf. Accessed January 3, 2017.

100. Shimokawa CA, Harlow JE, Turbino ML, et al. Ability of four dental radiometers to measure the light output from nine curing lights. J Dent 2016;54:48–55.

101. Price RB, Labrie D, Kazmi S, et al. Intra- and inter-brand accuracy of four dental radiometers. Clin Oral Investig 2012;16(3):707–17.

102. Leonard DL, Charlton DG, Hilton TJ. Effect of curing-tip diameter on the accuracy of dental radiometers. Oper Dent 1999;24(1):31–7.

103. Roberts HW, Vandewalle KS, Berzins DW, et al. Accuracy of LED and halogen radiometers using different light sources. J Esthet Restor Dent 2006;18(4):214–22 [discussion: 23–4].

104. Kameyama A, Haruyama A, Asami M, et al. Effect of emitted wavelength and light guide type on irradiance discrepancies in hand-held dental curing radiometers. Scientific World Journal 2013;2013:647941.

105. Marovic D, Matic S, Kelic K, et al. Time dependent accuracy of dental radiometers. Acta Clin Croat 2013;52(2):173–80.

106. SmartLite maX Curing Card. Form #544161. Milford (DE): DENTSPLY International Inc; 2010.

107. Rueggeberg FA, Caughman WF, Curtis JW Jr. Effect of light intensity and exposure duration on cure of resin composite. Oper Dent 1994;19(1):26–32.

108. Musanje L, Darvell BW. Polymerization of resin composite restorative materials: exposure reciprocity. Dent Mater 2003;19(6):531–41.

109. Selig D, Haenel T, Hausnerova B, et al. Examining exposure reciprocity in a resin based composite using high irradiance levels and real-time degree of conversion values. Dent Mater 2015;31(5):583–93.

110. Leprince JG, Hadis M, Shortall AC, et al. Photoinitiator type and applicability of exposure reciprocity law in filled and unfilled photoactive resins. Dent Mater 2011;27(2):157–64.

111. Hadis M, Leprince JG, Shortall AC, et al. High irradiance curing and anomalies of exposure reciprocity law in resin-based materials. J Dent 2011;39(8):549–57.

112. Wydra JW, Cramer NB, Stansbury JW, et al. The reciprocity law concerning light dose relationships applied to BisGMA/TEGDMA photopolymers: theoretical analysis and experimental characterization. Dent Mater 2014;30(6):605–12.

113. Nitta K. Effect of light guide tip diameter of LED-light curing unit on polymerization of light-cured composites. Dent Mater 2005;21(3):217–23.

114. Ash MM, Nelson SJ, Ash MM. Dental anatomy, physiology, and occlusion. 8th edition. Philadelphia: W.B. Saunders; 2003.

115. Catelan A, de Araujo LS, da Silveira BC, et al. Impact of the distance of light curing on the degree of conversion and microhardness of a composite resin. Acta Odontol Scand 2015;73(4):298–301.
116. Vandewalle KS, Roberts HW, Andrus JL, et al. Effect of light dispersion of LED curing lights on resin composite polymerization. J Esthet Restor Dent 2005; 17(4):244–54 [discussion: 54–5].
117. Coutinho M, Trevizam NC, Takayassu RN, et al. Distance and protective barrier effects on the composite resin degree of conversion. Contemp Clin Dent 2013; 4(2):152–5.
118. Scott BA, Felix CA, Price RB. Effect of disposable infection control barriers on light output from dental curing lights. J Can Dent Assoc 2004;70(2):105–10.
119. Sword RJ, Do UN, Chang JH, et al. Effect of curing light barriers and light types on radiant exposure and composite conversion. J Esthet Restor Dent 2016; 28(1):29–42.
120. Strassler HE. Successful light curing- not as easy as it looks. Oral Health 2013; 103(7):18–26.
121. Price RB, Felix CM, Whalen JM. Factors affecting the energy delivered to simulated class I and class v preparations. J Can Dent Assoc 2010;76:a94.

Dental Impression Materials and Techniques

Amit Punj, BDS, DMD[a],*, Despoina Bompolaki, DDS, MS[b], Jorge Garaicoa, DDS, MS[b]

KEYWORDS

- Dental impressions • Digital impressions • Conventional impressions
- Dental materials

KEY POINTS

- Dental impressions are an integral part of patient management from diagnosis to treatment and understanding their properties and manipulation is vital to practicing clinicians.
- Digital dentistry is well established and rapidly evolving, and therefore it is incumbent on dentists to familiarize themselves with this technology and adopt it in contemporary practice.
- Conventional impression techniques are still being widely used in many practices and reviewing current materials and procedures enhances clinicians' confidence and improves patient outcomes.

INTRODUCTION

Imagine fabricating a fixed or removable dental prosthesis directly in the patient's mouth and subjecting it to extreme temperatures and harsh chemicals, and working in a confined cavity. Although the oral structures have evolved to be highly resilient, they are severely challenged when facing the abnormal forces required to construct an indirect dental restoration. Impression making is the first part of this process by creating a negative form of the teeth and tissues into which gypsum or other die materials can be processed to create the working analogues. This process is as much an art as it is a science. Painters and sculptors who create beautiful works of art cannot achieve this without understanding the properties and handling characteristics of the paint or clay that they use. Similarly, dental practitioners should understand the properties of the materials and methods to manipulate these materials safely and effectively to capture the exact form of the oral tissues.

Disclosure: The authors have nothing to disclose.
[a] Department of Restorative Dentistry, OHSU School of Dentistry, 2730 Southwest Moody Avenue, Room 10N078, Portland, OR 97201, USA; [b] Department of Restorative Dentistry, OHSU School of Dentistry, 2730 Southwest Moody Avenue, Room 10N076, Portland, OR 97201, USA
* Corresponding author.
E-mail address: punj@ohsu.edu

Dent Clin N Am 61 (2017) 779–796
http://dx.doi.org/10.1016/j.cden.2017.06.004
0011-8532/17/© 2017 Elsevier Inc. All rights reserved.

dental.theclinics.com

HISTORICAL PERSPECTIVE

In the mid–seventeenth century, early references to making impressions in wax to reproduce parts of jaws and teeth were recorded by a German military surgeon, Gottfried Purman. Then, in the eighteenth century, there were reports of an impression technique that involved pressing a piece of bone or ivory on the oral tissues that were painted with a coloring material and then carving out the fitting surface at the chairside.[1] Philip Pfaff in 1756 was the first to make an impression of an edentulous jaw with 2 pieces of wax and then join them and making a cast using plaster of Paris.[1] Other impression materials used were zinc oxide eugenol impression paste and compound, although their applications were limited by their inability to surpass undercuts without distorting or fracturing.[2] Reversible hydrocolloids were introduced in 1925, followed by the irreversible hydrocolloids becoming available in 1941.[3] The disadvantage of the hydrocolloids is shrinkage caused by the loss of water, leading to inaccuracy. In 1953, polysulfide was used as an impression material along with condensation reaction silicones, but they both show significant shrinkage over a period of several hours, mainly because of the evaporation of low-molecular-weight by-products.[3,4] In the late 1960s, polyether was proposed as an alternative polymer because of its improved mechanical properties and low shrinkage.[4] In the 1970s, polyvinyl siloxane (PVS) appeared on the market and became very popular, in part because of its high dimensional stability.

CLASSIFICATION OF IMPRESSION MATERIALS

Impression materials can be classified according to their composition, setting reaction, and setting properties, but a commonly used system is based on the properties after the material has set (**Fig. 1**).

At present, the most popular types of impression materials for removable, fixed, and implant prosthodontics are irreversible hydrocolloids, polyethers, and PVSs. A summary of the properties of elastomeric impression materials is shown in (**Table 1**).

IRREVERSIBLE HYDROCOLLOIDS (ALGINATE)

Alginate impression materials are used for full-arch impressions because of their low cost and good wetting properties,[2] making them a popular choice to fabricate diagnostic casts. They can also be used for impression of partial removable dental prosthesis frameworks and for the fabrication of immediate/interim complete or partial

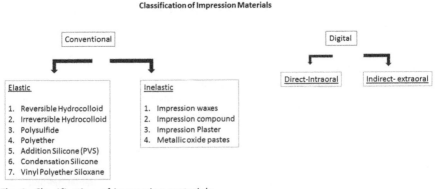

Fig. 1. Classification of impression materials.

Table 1				
Physical and mechanical properties of elastomeric impression materials				
Properties	**PVS**	**Polyether**	**Condensation Silicone**	**Polysulfide**
Working time	Short to moderate	Short	Short	Moderate to long
Setting time	Short to moderate	Short	Short to moderate	Moderate to long
Setting shrinkage	Very Low	Low	Moderate to high	High
Elastic recovery	Very high	High	High	Moderate
Flexibility during removal	Low to moderate	Low to moderate	Moderate	High
Tear strength	Low to moderate	Moderate	Low to moderate	Moderate to high
Wettability by gypsum	Good to very good	Very good	Poor	Moderate
Detail reproduction	Excellent	Excellent	Excellent	Excellent

Adapted from Powers J, Wataha J. Impression materials. In: Powers J, Wataha J, editors. Dental materials foundations and applications. 11th edition. St Louis (MO): Elsevier; 2016; with permission.

denture prostheses. The hydrophilic nature of the material allows it to be used in the presence of saliva and blood with a moderate ability to reproduce details. Its poor dimensional stability caused by loss of water creates distortion and shrinkage if it is not poured within 10 minutes,[5,6] and it can be poured only once because of distortion and low tear strength. This material is flexible and easy to remove from the mouth compared with other materials if they flow into undercuts. They are easy to use and easy to mix with sufficient setting time to be handled and placed in the oral cavity.[6]

POLYETHERS

Polyethers were introduced in the late 1960s. The setting reaction for these materials is via cationic polymerization by opening of the reactive ethylene imine terminal rings to unite molecules with no by-product formation. These material are hydrophilic, allowing them to be used in a moist environment. Their good wetting properties also allow gypsum casts to be made more easily.[7] Newer polyether impression materials are slightly more flexible than the older products, making them easier to remove from the mouth.[8] Because of the nature of the material absorbing water, the impression should not be submerged in water for a period of time because it could lead to distortion.[8] These materials are available in low, medium, and high viscosities and can be used as a single-phase material or with a syringe-and-tray technique. The most popular method of dispensing this material is via a motorized mixing unit.

POLYVINYL SILOXANES

The chemical reaction for PVS (or addition silicone) involves a base paste containing hydrosilane-terminated molecules reacting with an accelerator paste containing siloxane oligomers with vinyl end groups and a platinum catalyst. Although there is no by-product formed, there is often a secondary reaction that can release hydrogen in the presence of hydroxyl groups, commonly found in impurities from the oligomerization reaction of the siloxane molecule. It is therefore recommended to wait at least 60 minutes before pouring a PVS impression, although some manufacturers claim that they can be poured immediately.[7,8] PVS impression material is one of the most favored impression materials in dentistry because of excellent properties and availability in different viscosities ranging from extralight body to putty. Impressions made from this material produce great detail reproduction and can be poured multiple times because of their high tear strength and high elastic recovery. Caution should be taken to avoid contact of the material with latex rubber dams or latex gloves, which may leave a sulfur or sulfur compound that inhibits polymerization of the material.[9,10] Moreover, gingival retraction soaked cords containing sulfur may also contribute to the inhibition.[11]

VINYL SILOXANETHER (VINYL POLYETHER SILOXANE)

A new impression material that combines the properties of polyether and PVS, vinyl siloxanether or vinyl polyether siloxane, was introduced in the dental market in 2009 (Identium, Kettenbach Co, Eschenburg, Germany).[12] This material has been reported to combine the ease of removal of PVS with the hydrophilicity (wetting properties) of polyether,[13] making it a promising material for difficult situations in which moisture control are present, such as narrow, deep gingival crevices.[3] However, literature on the accuracy of this new material is still scarce.[14]

HYDROPHILIC POLYVINYL SILOXANE

Traditionally, PVS is a hydrophobic material and proper moisture control is of paramount importance in order to obtain a clinically acceptable impression. Many newer PVS impression materials have been advertised as hydrophilic, suggesting that they can perform adequately under moist or wet conditions. These products contain intrinsic surfactants that improve their wettability and facilitate the pouring process with gypsum materials. However, so-called hydrophilic PVS seems to remain hydrophobic when it is still in the liquid, unpolymerized state and its wetting abilities are compromised in the presence of moisture. As a result, their surface detail reproduction is inconsistent when moisture control is not maintained.[6,7,15]

FAST-SET ELASTOMERIC MATERIALS

Fast-set impression materials have been advocated in order to reduce chair time and facilitate the impression process, qualities that can be especially important when treating patients with severe gag reflexes. The literature on the accuracy of these materials is limited; one study showed that fast-set polyether was more accurate than fast-set PVS, but both materials produced casts with negligible difference in dimensions compared with the master cast, therefore both were regarded as being clinically acceptable.[16] The same study indicated that fast-set PVS materials may require pouring with a high-expansion dental stone and use of additional die relief, in order to minimize adjustments of the intaglio surface and achieve better marginal fit. This method does not seem necessary for fast-set polyether materials.

ALGINATE SUBSTITUTE MATERIALS

Alginate substitute materials, which were introduced in the dental market in the 1980s, are low-cost medium-body PVS materials that possess better mechanical properties than traditional alginate.[17,18] These materials are cheaper than traditional PVS but more expensive than alginate; most of them require a custom tray and an automix delivery system, which provides a uniform consistency and precise setting times, facilitating the impression procedure.

Alginate substitute materials have been reported to offer improved detail reproduction, tear strength, and dimensional stability.[17,18] Their manufacturers claim that the biggest drawbacks of traditional alginate are the need for immediate pouring and no chance for second pours, drawbacks that are not associated with these products. Another advantage of using this type of material is that impressions can be sent to the laboratory and digitized to create virtual casts.

Table 2, **Table 3**, and **Table 4**, accompanied by **Fig. 2**, **Fig. 3** and **Fig. 4**, summarize the current best clinical practices in impression making for fixed implant and removable restorative procedures.

DISINFECTION OF CONVENTIONAL IMPRESSIONS

Dental impressions are exposed to blood, saliva, or both[25]; therefore, dental offices and commercial laboratories need to follow coordinated protocols to eliminate the risks of cross-contamination.[26,27] To maximize effectiveness, disinfection should take place immediately on removal from the mouth.[27] Over the past 25 years, numerous reports have studied the effect of disinfection procedures on the surface properties and dimensional stability of dental impression materials.[28–31] These studies indicate that disinfection procedures do not have a clinically significant effect on impression quality and/or accuracy.

Disinfection protocols consist of 2 steps. The first step includes rinsing the impression with tap water immediately after removal from the patient's mouth. This process significantly reduces the number of blood-borne pathogens that can be transferred to the stone casts. The second step includes spraying the impression with an appropriate disinfecting agent or immersing it in a chemical solution for a specified amount of time. Care should be taken when disinfecting water-based materials or polyethers, because extended immersion times (>30 minutes) can have a negative impact on impression quality.[6,32]

Recent studies have investigated the effect of disinfecting agents on the hydrophilicity of PVS, which is attributed to the removal of added surfactants from the material.[33,34] These nonionic surfactants are added to improve the quality of the

Table 2	
Impressions for fixed prosthodontics (see Fig. 2)	
Clinical Scenarios	**Indicated Materials/Techniques**
Need for increased accuracy and surface detail reproduction	PVS or polyether, light body consistency using a 1-step technique with putty, heavy or medium body as tray material[6,19]
Presence of undercuts	Block out using a resin modified glass ionomer material before final impression using an elastomeric impression material, to maximize elastic recovery of the impression material and minimize distortion on removal from the mouth[6]
Moisture control issues	Good isolation, consider medicaments[19] or use hydrophilic materials such as reversible hydrocolloid[6]
Need for increased working time (multiple units)	Use automixed materials; avoid hand mixing. Refrigerate PVS impression material to increase working time[4]
Long, thin preparations	Avoid polyether because of high rigidity. Consider pouring dies using epoxy resin die material[7] or scanning the final impression to create digital cast analogue and eliminate the need for pouring

Table 3
Impressions for implant prosthodontics (see Fig. 3)

Clinical Scenarios	Indicated Materials/Techniques
Completely edentulous, implant/abutment level impression	Splinted impression copings, open tray technique with PVS or polyether[20]
Partially edentulous, implant/abutment level impression	Splinted open tray impression coping or closed tray with PVS or polyether[21]
Three or fewer implants	Open or closed tray PVS or polyether[22]

impression and stone cast; however, disinfection procedures may result in their loss and can subsequently compromise the impression surface and cast quality.[34] A recent study[35] showed that chlorine-based disinfecting agents are less effective in removing nonionic surfactants from PVS impression materials compared with quaternary ammonium–based agents. The investigators recommended using a wetting agent to counteract the loss of surfactants and reduce the hydrophobicity of PVS before pouring the impression. In general, prolonged disinfection times should be avoided because of their adverse effects on contact angle and material wettability.

GINGIVAL DISPLACEMENT

Excellent marginal fit and proper restoration contours are both prerequisites for optimal periodontal tissue health. The former is ensured by capturing the uninterrupted finish line during the final impression process; the latter is significantly facilitated when the unprepared tooth structure below the restoration margin is captured in the impression. In order for both these prerequisites to be present, adequate gingival displacement is necessary. The ideal amount of gingival displacement has been reported to be 0.2 mm, which provides sufficient thickness of impression material and prevents distortion or tearing on removal.[36,37]

For more than 40 years, various techniques for gingival displacement have been described in the literature.[38] Mechanical methods (use of retraction cords or injectable agents[39,40]), chemical methods (use of hemostatic medicaments[39,40]), surgical methods (copper band retraction,[41] rotary curettage,[42] electrosurgery,[43,44] soft tissue laser[45]), or combinations of these[39] have been extensively described. According to recent surveys, the most commonly used technique is a combination of mechanical and chemical displacement, with the use of gingival displacement cords of various sizes and hemostatic agents such as aluminum chloride and ferric sulfate.[46] This technique has been thoroughly described in the literature.[39,40]

In a survey, a significant number of general dentists (28%) reported using cordless techniques for gingival displacement. Those techniques include syringing a

Table 4
Impressions for removable prosthodontics (see Fig. 4)

Clinical Scenarios	Indicated Materials/Techniques
Complete dentures	Selective pressure technique, using a combination of elastic and rigid impression materials in a custom tray[23]
Partial dentures	Irreversible hydrocolloid material in a rigid stock tray or elastomeric impression material in a custom tray[24]

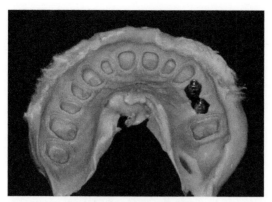

Fig. 2. PVS impression in a custom tray for fixed prosthodontics.

synthetic polymer material into the unretracted gingival sulcus; on contact with the crevicular fluid, this material expands and provides the desired gingival displacement with minimal time and trauma. Conventional and cordless gingival displacement techniques have been reported to have similar efficacy and both have minimal effect on periodontal tissue health.[47,48] However, a recent study showed that cordless techniques were less stressful for the patients, and also produced lower posttreatment levels of proinflammatory cytokines in the crevicular fluid compared with conventional techniques.[47] Cordless techniques have also been reported to be less time consuming and easier to use compared with displacement cords.[48]

One study reported that cordless techniques generate more than 10 times less pressure on the gingival tissues compared with conventional techniques, which include the use of displacement cords.[49] This significantly lower pressure indicates that cordless techniques potentially cause less trauma to the periodontal tissues; however, it could also signify a reduced efficacy at achieving adequate gingival displacement, which clinically translates to a less successful impression. The highest pressures were generated with the use of Expasyl (Acteon, Mt Laurel, NJ), a pastelike material used for gingival retraction.

In a study comparing the effects of conventional and cordless gingival displacement techniques on the periodontal health of healthy subjects, use of Expasyl resulted in slower healing and significant increase of the gingival index compared with a different PVS expanding material (Magic FoamCord, Coltène/Whaledent, Cuyahoga Falls, OH) or with conventional displacement cords.[50]

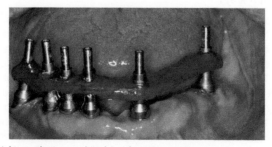

Fig. 3. Splinted pick-up abutment level implant impression.

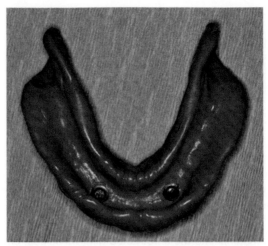

Fig. 4. PVS final impression for an implant retained overdenture using a custom tray that was border molded with modeling compound.

TRAY SELECTION
Custom Versus Stock Trays

Custom trays allow uniform impression material thickness, minimizing distortion and material waste, and are also more comfortable for patients.[6] Custom trays have been shown to produce impressions of higher accuracy; however, newer PVS materials can still provide a quality single-unit impression when used with nonrigid stock trays.[51] Custom trays are still indicated for clinical situations in which multiple teeth are being restored or when the arch form and size do not allow the use of a stock tray.

Use of nonrigid plastic trays may result in flexure of the side walls of the tray during the impression procedure; subsequent tray rebound on removal from the mouth produces an inaccurate cast and, ultimately, poor restoration fit. In contrast, use of rigid (metal) stock trays requires additional care to block out any existing undercuts on adjacent teeth or areas where the material could flow and cause problems on removal, such as pontic sites. If clinicians fail to take such precautions, the rigidity of contemporary impression materials may create an unpleasant clinical situation in which the metal tray is locked into the mouth; its removal requires a significant amount of time and effort, causing severe discomfort to the patient as well.

Dual-arch Impression Trays

The dual-arch impression method became popular in the late 1980s.[52] It is a closed-mouth technique that allows dentists to capture the preparation, opposing teeth, and occluding surfaces in a single-step procedure. This technique is more comfortable for the patients and requires less time and material, making it a popular technique among dentists. In 2008, 1403 impressions that were submitted to a dental laboratory to fabricate fixed indirect restorations over a 3-month period were examined to provide data with regard to tray selection, captured teeth, and overall impression quality. The study revealed that 73.1% of the submitted impressions were made using the dual-arch impression technique. However, the investigators noted that the recommendations for the use of this method were not followed in a large portion of the cases.[53]

Dual-arch impression trays should be used for single-unit prostheses or short span (up to 3-unit) fixed dental prostheses. Both adjacent teeth, as well as the antagonist of the prepared abutment, should be intact. Occlusal requirements for optimal results when using this technique include a stable maximum intercuspation with absence of interferences, canine guidance or other type of posterior disclusion, angle class I occlusion, and intact dentition (Braley class I).[54] When using the dual-arch technique, care should be taken so that the canine is registered on the impression in order to eliminate the potential of occlusal interferences in the final restoration.

There are many types of dual-arch trays available (full or partial arch, metal or plastic, possessing side walls or sideless), and selection is based on clinical parameters, such as arch form and size or position of the teeth.[41] A small number of studies are available on accuracy of metal versus plastic partial dual-arch trays; plastic trays have been found to provide better accuracy compared with metal trays[55,56] and have also been reported as being more comfortable for the patients.[56] However, other studies found metal dual-arch trays to be more accurate compared with plastic ones, because they have less flexure during the impression process.[57,58]

With regard to choice of material when using the dual-arch technique, a recent study showed that PVS provides better impressions compared with polyether (fewer surface defects and voids/bubbles).[59] When using the dual-arch technique, clinicians should choose a stiff material that can maintain its shape easily, because the support provided by the dual-arch impression trays is limited compared with traditional full-arch trays. This difference becomes even more critical when using partial dual-arch trays without side support. International Organization for Standardization (ISO) type 0 (putty) or type 1 (heavy body) materials should be used for the tray and type 3 (light or extralight body) materials should only be used for capturing the prepared tooth.

Literature is scarce in terms of accuracy of dual-arch impressions compared with the conventional complete-arch technique.[55,56,60–62] The limited published studies on this matter indicate that this technique has comparable accuracy with traditional complete-arch impressions. These were all well-controlled studies, which underlines the importance of following closely the exact recommendations and guidelines when using this technique, in order to achieve similar results in a dental office setting.

DELIVERY SYSTEMS OF IMPRESSION MATERIALS

Elastomeric impression materials typically consist of separate base and catalyst pastes, which are mixed immediately before impression making. Automix systems, in the form of disposable intraoral syringes, dispensers with attached cartridges, or automatic mixing machines, have become popular and have replaced hand mixing. Automatic mixing is easier than hand mixing and yields an impression material with fewer voids and improved homogeneity.[63,64] It has been shown that automixed alginate has improved tensile strength and surface detail reproduction that is even comparable with elastomeric materials.[65] Automixing of impression materials also affects their rheological properties, producing materials that are less viscous and flow better, a property that is clinically relevant and desirable in many clinical situations.[66]

DIGITAL IMPRESSIONS

The Mid-twentieth century saw a rapid movement in digital technology sweeping across different industries worldwide from the military to aviation and ultimately to the health care field. Most of modern dentistry is already immersed in digital dentistry, and it is likely that most practitioners use some aspect of digital dentistry in their dental offices. Everything from electronic health records and digital imaging to manufacturing of ceramic crowns in the office or in laboratories involves a digital interface. Dr Francois Duret from France pioneered optical impressions in 1971. In the early 1980s, Professor Mörmann from Switzerland was the first to patent and design a handheld intraoral scanner, which was the first-generation Chairside Economical Restoration of Esthetic Ceramics (CEREC). The initial reputation of the systems was less than optimal because the margins were difficult to capture, digitize, and reproduce with a high level of accuracy.[67]

The advantages and disadvantages of digital impression are summarized in **Box 1** and **Box 2**. Computer-aided design (CAD)/computer-aided manufacturing (CAM) technologies are advancing rapidly; so much so that every few years there is new software and hardware being introduced in the market (visit dentsplysirona.com to view a contemporary CAD/CAM unit). Note that the technology is changing so rapidly that the evidence in the literature may be based on an older iteration and it is difficult to find long-term data on a particular system or technology.

The basic process of creating a digital work flow is shown in **Fig. 5**. Each brand of optical impression system has its own niche and most commercially available systems yield clinically acceptable results. The conundrum for most dentists wanting to get involved with CAD/CAM dentistry is the decision about which system to invest in. The following are some suggestions that can help in making choices:

1. Type of practice: does the practice do a lot of single-unit and a small number of multiple-unit indirect restorations? Does the practice do orthodontic procedures or implants?
2. Budget: does the practice want to invest in just the scanning unit or does it want to include the software and chairside milling device also?
3. Customer support: does the desired system offer support and technical expertise in a timely manner?

Box 1
Advantages of intraoral scanning

1. Real-time visualization and evaluation
2. Easy to correct, manipulate, or recapture images
3. Segmental image capture
4. Archival digitally, therefore no need to store physical casts
5. No wastage of impression material and therefore environmentally friendly
6. Economical, considering no use of impression trays, adhesives, or gypsum
7. Do not need to disinfect before sending information to the laboratory
8. No damage or wear and tear of the stone casts
9. Swift communication with the laboratory via the Internet
10. Self-assessment for tooth preparations
11. File transfer capabilities to merge with other files like DICOM (Digital Imaging and Communications in Medicine) images using sophisticated software
12. Increased patient satisfaction
13. Some systems have color scanning, shade selection, and still photograph image-taking capabilities

Data from Zimmermann M, Mehl A, Mörmann WH, et al. Intraoral scanning systems – a current overview. Int J Comput Dent 2015;18(2):101–29.

Box 2
Disadvantages of intraoral scanning

1. Initial cost of equipment and software maintenance fees
2. Learning curve can be difficult for some individuals
3. Scan bodies needed for implant systems that are compatible with the design software
4. Difficult to capture occlusion information for complex prosthodontics treatments
5. Closed systems restrict options for transferring STL (standard tessellation language) files
6. Cannot capture subgingival margins if obscured with blood, saliva, or tissue
7. Unable to accurately capture images of the edentulous arches
8. Scanning patterns need to be followed as per manufacturer's recommendations

Data from Zimmermann M, Mehl A, Mörmann WH, et al. Intraoral scanning systems – a current overview. Int J Comput Dent 2015;18(2):101–29.

---

4. Is the practice comfortable with a system that requires the use of the light dusting spray to capture images?
5. What are the yearly maintenance and software fees and warranties?
6. What size impression wand and field-of-view sensor would be most suitable for the practice?
7. How big is the foot print of the unit? Does the office have the space for storage of the scanner and mill?

Units that only scan and capture optical images and send data via the Internet to laboratories are suitable for practices that do not want to offer same-day crowns and prefer to have a laboratory design and complete the restorations. Offices that want to complete the work flow in-house need to buy the appropriate software to handle orthodontics, implants, and indirect restorations. Customer support is very important because initially there is a steep learning curve and, when faced with hardware or software issues, there should be swift and efficient support from the manufacturer. Although studies have shown that a light dusting of titanium dioxide powder improves the image capture capabilities,[68] some practitioners and patients find it objectionable.

It is important to be familiar with the terms used in CAD/CAM dentistry for better understanding and communication (**Box 3**).

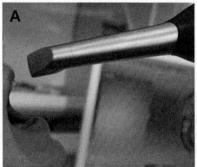 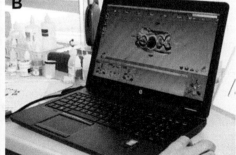

Fig. 5. Digital workflow: (*A*) scan, (*B*) design, and mill (visit http://www.planmeca.com/ CADCAM/CADCAM-for-dental-clinics/planmeca-planmill-40/ to view the PlanMill 40).

Box 3
Terms used in computer-aided design/computer-aided manufacturing dentistry

1. Three-dimensional (3D) file formats: file formats are used for creating and storing 3D data files. The STL file format is commonly used for many open-platform dental scanning and design systems.

2. 3D scanner: a device that analyzes a real-world object to collect data on its shape and/or other attributes, such as color or texture.

3. Active triangulation: a method to determine the 3D geometry of real-world objects. In this method, the light or laser source is positioned at a fixed distance from a sensor or camera. As light/laser is reflected from the scanned object, it falls on the camera. The position of points on the object can be calculated using the angle of the reflected light.

4. CAD/CAM dentistry: using computer technologies to design and produce different types of dental restorations, including crowns, veneers, inlays and onlays, fixed prostheses, dental implant restorations, and orthodontics.

5. Closed architecture: software or hardware restricted to a specific company's digital equipment or digital workflow.

6. DICOM: standard for handling, storing, printing, and transmitting information in medical imaging; for example, cone-beam computed tomography file.

7. Image capture: the process of 3D scanning to record digital information about the shape of an object with equipment that uses a laser or light to measure the distance between the scanner and the object.

8. Image stitching: the process of combining multiple photographic images with overlapping fields of view to produce a segmented panorama or high-resolution image.

9. Impression wand: handheld device used for intraoral digital scanning.

10. Intraoral scanning: the process of scanning and capturing the intraoral cavity for translation into a digital file format, such as STL.

11. Open architecture: a digital process or work flow that can be performed on various digital platforms, as opposed to closed architecture processes. These workflows can only be performed on a specific platform. STL is an example of open architecture.

12. Optical scanners: devices that use light projection or laser beams to obtain a 3D digital replica of an object.

13. Scan body: scannable object used to accurately translate the position of an implant into a digital file for use in the digital design of an implant abutment.

14. STL: file format native to the stereolithography CAD software created by 3D Systems.

Data from Grant GT, Campbell SD, Masri RM, et al. Glossary of digital dental terms: American College of Prosthodontists. J Prosthodont 2016;25(S2):S2–9.

The following are some of the features of the most commonly used systems in the United States:

CEREC (Sirona, Dentsply)

This system has been around for the longest time. The Omnicam unit is the latest version, and is available as a cart system that includes the camera and computer, all of which can be connected or simply transmit files to a milling system. The device works on the principle of triangulation (defined in **Box 3**) but yields three-dimensional (3D) full-color video scans without the need for using imaging powder. This device is a closed system in that the software is only compatible with the company's milling unit and the image files cannot be exported and used with other milling systems. The work flow can be achieved directly at the chairside or sent to a laboratory using CEREC Connect software. This system can be used for restorative dentistry, implants, as well as orthodontics.

Planscan (Planmeca, USA)

Similar to Sirona's CEREC, this system has an acquisition unit, design software, and milling device. This device is a powder-free system that obtains individual sequential images in color using blue laser technology. The scanner is available as a USB version that connects to a laptop. This device is an open system wherein .stl files can be exported to other systems for milling. This device is predominantly used for restorative dentistry.

True Definition Scanner (3M ESPE, United States)

This is an open system that uses a light dusting of titanium dioxide powder on the teeth to acquire intraoral images. The imaging wand is one of the smallest on the market and image capture is based on wave-front sampling technology. The margins of a preparation can be visualized in a 3D format but this scanner does not feature a snipping tool, which is a feature that allows clinicians to perform a preoperative overview scan and, once the preparation is begun, only the affected teeth need to be scanned.[69] Another feature is that there is no color rendition. A new portable version has been introduced with a screen the size of a popular tablet. This imaging acquisition unit can capture images that can be used in orthodontics, restorative dentistry, and implant dentistry. There is no proprietary design software or mill assigned to this system and therefore images are sent via a cloud-based platform to an auxiliary CAD software and milling unit.

Trios 3 (3 Shape, Denmark)

This system is available as a cart version as well as a handheld, USB version. The imaging wand comes with 2 different grip designs and allows powder-free scanning that works on the principle of confocal microscopy and displays 3D color images. Recently, a more economical black and white version has been introduced, Trios 3 Mono. This device is an open system and .stl files can be exported to other systems for designing and milling. A unique feature is shade determination. This system can be used in orthodontics, restorative dentistry, and implantology.

iTero Element (Align Technology, United States)

This scanner is based on the principle of confocal laser scanning microscopy and uses no powder to capture images. A color display is now available and the unit comes as a cart or a USB version with touch screens. This device is an open system and can be used for orthodontics, restorative dentistry, and implantology.

CS 3600 (Carestream, United States)

The newest version of this scanner is faster than its predecessor and acquires images using the triangulation principle in high-definition 3D color. This powder-free system has a feature that allows clinicians to fill in missing information from the scan. This scanner is an open system and available in a USB version. It is suitable for implantology, restorative dentistry, and orthodontics.

The reason why some systems are better indicated for certain applications has to do with the specific software that was developed for use with a given hardware. For example, the CS3600 system operates with software that contains features useful for implantology, restorative dentistry, or orthodontics, whereas other systems are more suitable for specific applications.

Current evidence for Intraoral Scanners

The state of the science at this time proclaims that, for single units and quadrant dentistry, the intraoral scanners are highly accurate and even better than conventional impressions for manufacturing indirect restorations.[70,71] There is still insufficient data in the literature about complete-arch scans. Ender and colleagues[72] reported that conventional impression materials were more precise than digital systems for complete-arch impressions. In another study, Cho and colleagues[73] reported that the accuracy of the entire cast area of a conventional cast was significantly better than a printed stereolithographic model, although there was no difference for a single-crown or partial fixed dental prosthesis. Arguably, the learning curve for digital impression techniques can be steeper for some dentists; however, there is a study that reports that it was the preferred technique for dental students.[74] An in vitro study reported that digital impression making was less time consuming and more efficient than the conventional method and that patients preferred it.[75,76]

Future of impression technology

Digital devices are here to stay and will only increase in use in the near future. Technology is rapidly growing and equipment is becoming more affordable. Impression wands and units are becoming smaller, more user friendly, and capable of capturing color images at increasing speeds. Most systems do not require powder to capture intraoral images and the open-platform interface can be exported to integrate with other imaging modalities, like cone-beam computed tomography (CBCT), facial laser scans, or 3D photographic images. These files can then be combined and used for diagnosis or 3D printed to create life-sized analogues or become part of the patient's health record. The applications for this technology are voluminous and it can be used in orthodontics, oral and maxillofacial surgery, and maxillofacial prosthodontics.[77] The line between digital impressions and imaging technology is already getting blurred and in the future, with low-dose and ultralow-dose CBCT scans, there may be a possibility of designing and milling restorations from imaging procedures only.[77] One of the disadvantages of current optical impression systems is the inability to penetrate soft tissue and acquire data through blood and saliva. Sonography, particularly ultrasonography and optical coherence tomography, which are radiation-free methods and used widely in medicine, has shown promise in the dental field.[78,79] Scanning devices of the future should be able to differentiate between hard and soft tissues, and blood and saliva, and be able to take rapid, accurate, and stress-free images for diagnosis and treatment without the need for merging files, as is currently done.

REFERENCES

1. Ward G. Impression materials and impression taking: an historical survey. Br Dent J 1961;110(4):118–9.
2. Rubel BS. Impression materials: a comparative review of impression materials most commonly used in restorative dentistry. Dent Clin North Am 2007;51(3):629–42, vi.
3. Schulein TM. Significant events in the history of operative dentistry. J Hist Dent 2005;53(2):63–72.
4. Hamalian TA, Nasr E, Chidiac JJ. Impression materials in fixed prosthodontics: influence of choice on clinical procedure. J Prosthodont 2011;20(2):153–60.

5. Combe EC, Burke FJ, Douglas WH. Dental biomaterials, 1st edition. Boston: Kluwer; 1999.
6. Donovan TE, Chee WW. A review of contemporary impression materials and techniques. Dent Clin North Am 2004;48(2):vi–vii, 445-470.
7. Sakaguchi RL, Powers JM. Craig's restorative dental materials. Philadelphia (PA): Elsevier Health Sciences; 2012.
8. Powers J, Wataha J. Dental materials foundations and applications. 11th edition. St. Louis (MO): Elsevier; 2017.
9. Reitz CD, Clark NP. The setting of vinyl polysiloxane and condensation silicone putties when mixed with gloved hands. J Am Dent Assoc 1988; 116(3):371–5.
10. Noonan JE, Goldfogel MH, Lambert RL. Inhibited set of the surface of addition silicones in contact with rubber dam. Oper Dent 1985;10(2):46–8.
11. Boening KW, Walter MH, Schuette U. Clinical significance of surface activation of silicone impression materials. J Dent 1998;26(5–6):447–52.
12. Enkling N, Bayer S, Jöhren P, et al. Vinylsiloxanether: a new impression material. clinical study of implant impressions with vinylsiloxanether versus polyether materials. Clin Implant Dent Relat Res 2012;14(1):144–51.
13. Walker MP, Alderman N, Petrie CS, et al. Correlation of impression removal force with elastomeric impression material rigidity and hardness. J Prosthodont 2013; 22(5):362–6.
14. Stober T, Johnson GH, Schmitter M. Accuracy of the newly formulated vinyl siloxanether elastomeric impression material. J Prosthet Dent 2010;103(4):228–39.
15. Petrie CS, Walker MP, O'Mahony AM, et al. Dimensional accuracy and surface detail reproduction of two hydrophilic vinyl polysiloxane impression materials tested under dry, moist, and wet conditions. J Prosthet Dent 2003;90(4): 365–72.
16. Wadhwani CP, Johnson GH, Lepe X, et al. Accuracy of newly formulated fast-setting elastomeric impression materials. J Prosthet Dent 2005;93(6):530–9.
17. Baxter R, Lawson N, Cakir D, et al. Evaluation of outgassing, tear strength, and detail reproduction in alginate substitute materials. Oper Dent 2012;37(5):540–7.
18. Nassar U, Hussein B, Oko A, et al. Dimensional accuracy of 2 irreversible hydrocolloid alternative impression materials with immediate and delayed pouring. J Can Dent Assoc 2012;78(78):c2.
19. Rosenstiel SF, Land MF, Fujimoto J. Contemporary fixed prosthodontics. St. Louis (MO): Elsevier Health Sciences; 2015.
20. Papaspyridakos P, Hirayama H, Chen CJ, et al. Full-arch implant fixed prostheses: a comparative study on the effect of connection type and impression technique on accuracy of fit. Clin Oral Implants Res 2016;27(9):1099–105.
21. Papaspyridakos P, Chen C-J, Gallucci GO, et al. Accuracy of implant impressions for partially and completely edentulous patients: a systematic review. Int J Oral Maxillofac Implants 2014;29(4):836–45.
22. Lee H, So JS, Hochstedler J, et al. The accuracy of implant impressions: a systematic review. J Prosthet Dent 2008;100(4):285–91.
23. Salinas TJ. Treatment of edentulism: optimizing outcomes with tissue management and impression techniques. J Prosthodont 2009;18(2):97–105.
24. Carr AB, Brown DT. McCracken's removable partial prosthodontics. St. Louis (MO): Elsevier Health Sciences; 2015.
25. Choi Y-R, Kim K-N, Kim K-M. The disinfection of impression materials by using microwave irradiation and hydrogen peroxide. J Prosthet Dent 2014;112(4): 981–7.

26. Owen CP, Goolam R. Disinfection of impression materials to prevent viral cross contamination: a review and a protocol. Int J Prosthodont 1993;6(5):480–94.

27. Estafanous EW, Palenik CJ, Platt JA. Disinfection of bacterially contaminated hydrophilic PVS impression materials. J Prosthodont 2012;21(1):16–21.

28. Bock JJ, Werner Fuhrmann RA, Setz J. The influence of different disinfectants on primary impression materials. Quintessence Int 2008;39(3):e93–8.

29. Demajo JK, Cassar V, Farrugia C, et al. Effectiveness of disinfectants on antimicrobial and physical properties of dental impression materials. Int J Prosthodont 2015;29(1):63–7.

30. Walker MP, Rondeau M, Petrie C, et al. Surface quality and long-term dimensional stability of current elastomeric impression materials after disinfection. J Prosthodont 2007;16(5):343–51.

31. Yilmaz H, Aydin C, Gul B, et al. Effect of disinfection on the dimensional stability of polyether impression materials. J Prosthodont 2007;16(6):473–9.

32. Kotsiomiti E, Tzialla A, Hatjivasiliou K. Accuracy and stability of impression materials subjected to chemical disinfection–a literature review. J Oral Rehabil 2008; 35(4):291–9.

33. Milward PJ, Waters MG. The effect of disinfection and a wetting agent on the wettability of addition-polymerized silicone impression materials. J Prosthet Dent 2001;86(2):165–7.

34. Blalock JS, Cooper JR, Rueggeberg FA. The effect of chlorine-based disinfectant on wettability of a vinyl polysiloxane impression material. J Prosthet Dent 2010; 104(5):333–41.

35. Kang YS, Rueggeberg F, Ramos V. Effects of chlorine-based and quaternary ammonium-based disinfectants on the wettability of a polyvinyl siloxane impression material. J Prosthet Dent 2017;117(2):266–70.

36. Laufer BZ, Baharav H, Langer Y, et al. The closure of the gingival crevice following gingival retraction for impression making. J Oral Rehabil 1997;24(9): 629–35.

37. Laufer B-Z, Baharav H, Cardash HS. The linear accuracy of impressions and stone dies as affected by the thickness of the impression margin. Int J Prosthodont 1994;7(3):247–52.

38. Benson B, Bomberg T, Hatch R, et al. Tissue displacement methods in fixed prosthodontics. J Prosthet Dent 1986;55(2):175–81.

39. Donovan TE, Chee WW. Current concepts in gingival displacement. Dent Clin North Am 2004;48(2):433–44.

40. Baba NZ, Goodacre CJ, Jekki R, et al. Gingival displacement for impression making in fixed prosthodontics: contemporary principles, materials, and techniques. Dent Clin North Am 2014;58(1):45–68.

41. Darby H, Darby LH. Copper-band gingival retraction to produce void-free crown and bridge impressions. J Prosthet Dent 1973;29(5):513–6.

42. Tupac RG, Neacy K. A comparison of cord gingival displacement with the gingitage technique. J Prosthet Dent 1981;46(5):509–15.

43. Flocken JE. Electrosurgical management of soft tissues and restorative dentistry. Dent Clin North Am 1980;24(2):247–69.

44. Wilhelmsen NR, Ramfjord SP, Blankenship JR. Effects of electrosurgery on the gingival attachment in rhesus monkeys. J Periodontol 1976;47(3):160–70.

45. Scott A. Use of an erbium laser in lieu of retraction cord: a modern technique. Gen Dent 2005;53(2):116–9.

46. Ahmed SN, Donovan TE. Gingival displacement: survey results of dentists' practice procedures. J Prosthet Dent 2015;114(1):81–5.e1-2.

47. Sarmento H, Leite F, Dantas R, et al. A double-blind randomised clinical trial of two techniques for gingival displacement. J Oral Rehabil 2014;41(4):306–13.

48. Acar Ö, Erkut S, Özçelik TB, et al. A clinical comparison of cordless and conventional displacement systems regarding clinical performance and impression quality. J Prosthet Dent 2014;111(5):388–94.

49. Bennani V, Inger M, Aarts JM. Comparison of pressure generated by cordless gingival displacement materials. J Prosthet Dent 2014;112(2):163–7.

50. Al Hamad KQ, Azar WZ, Alwaeli HA, et al. A clinical study on the effects of cordless and conventional retraction techniques on the gingival and periodontal health. J Clin Periodontol 2008;35(12):1053–8.

51. Thongthammachat S, Moore BK, Barco MT, et al. Dimensional accuracy of dental casts: influence of tray material, impression material, and time. J Prosthodont 2002;11(2):98–108.

52. Schwartz R, Davis R. Accuracy of second pour casts using dual-arch impressions. Am J Dent 1992;5(4):192–4.

53. Mitchell ST, Ramp MH, Ramp LC, et al. A preliminary survey of impression trays used in the fabrication of fixed indirect restorations. J Prosthodont 2009;18(7): 582–8.

54. Kaplowitz GJ. Trouble-shooting dual arch impressions. J Am Dent Assoc 1996; 127(2):234–40.

55. Wöstmann B, Rehmann P, Balkenhol M. Accuracy of impressions obtained with dual-arch trays. Int J Prosthodont 2009;22(2):158–60.

56. Ceyhan JA, Johnson GH, Lepe X, et al. A clinical study comparing the three-dimensional accuracy of a working die generated from two dual-arch trays and a complete-arch custom tray. J Prosthet Dent 2003;90(3):228–34.

57. Breeding LC, Dixon DL. Accuracy of casts generated from dual-arch impressions. J Prosthet Dent 2000;84(4):403–7.

58. Larson TD, Nielsen MA, Brackett WW. The accuracy of dual-arch impressions: a pilot study. J Prosthet Dent 2002;87(6):625–7.

59. Johnson GH, Mancl LA, Schwedhelm ER, et al. Clinical trial investigating success rates for polyether and vinyl polysiloxane impressions made with full-arch and dual-arch plastic trays. J Prosthet Dent 2010;103(1):13–22.

60. Cox J. A clinical study comparing marginal and occlusal accuracy of crowns fabricated from double-arch and complete-arch impressions. Aust Dent J 2005; 50(2):90–4.

61. Cox JR, Brandt RL, Hughes HJ. A clinical pilot study of the dimensional accuracy of double-arch and complete-arch impressions. J Prosthet Dent 2002;87(5): 510–5.

62. Cayouette MJ, Burgess JO, Jones RE Jr, et al. Three-dimensional analysis of dual-arch impression trays. Quintessence Int 2003;34(3):189–98.

63. Soh G, Chong Y. Relationship of viscosity to porosities in automixed elastomeric impressions. Clin Mater 1991;7(1):23–6.

64. Lim KC, Chong YH, Soh G. Effect of operator variability on void formation in impressions made with an automixed addition silicone. Aust Dent J 1992;37(1): 35–8.

65. Dreesen K, Kellens A, Wevers M, et al. The influence of mixing methods and disinfectant on the physical properties of alginate impression materials. Eur J Orthod 2013;35(3):381–7.

66. Inoue K, Song Y, Kamiunten O, et al. Effect of mixing method on rheological properties of alginate impression materials. J Oral Rehabil 2002;29(7):615–9.

67. Miyazaki T, Hotta Y, Kunii J, et al. A review of dental CAD/CAM: current status and future perspectives from 20 years of experience. Dent Mater J 2009;28(1):44–56.
68. Fasbinder DJ. Digital dentistry: innovation for restorative treatment. Compend Contin Educ Dent 2010;31(4):2–11.
69. Zimmermann M, Mehl A, Mörmann W, et al. Intraoral scanning systems-a current overview. Int J Comput Dent 2014;18(2):101–29.
70. Ender A, Zimmermann M, Attin T, et al. In vivo precision of conventional and digital methods for obtaining quadrant dental impressions. Clin Oral Investig 2016; 20(7):1495–504.
71. Chochlidakis KM, Papaspyridakos P, Geminiani A, et al. Digital versus conventional impressions for fixed prosthodontics: a systematic review and meta-analysis. J Prosthet Dent 2016;116(2):184–90.e12.
72. Ender A, Attin T, Mehl A. In vivo precision of conventional and digital methods of obtaining complete-arch dental impressions. J Prosthet Dent 2016;115(3): 313–20.
73. Cho S-H, Schaefer O, Thompson GA, et al. Comparison of accuracy and reproducibility of casts made by digital and conventional methods. J Prosthet Dent 2015;113(4):310–5.
74. Lee SJ, MacArthur RX, Gallucci GO. An evaluation of student and clinician perception of digital and conventional implant impressions. J Prosthet Dent 2013;110(5):420–3.
75. Patzelt SB, Lamprinos C, Stampf S, et al. The time efficiency of intraoral scanners: an in vitro comparative study. J Am Dent Assoc 2014;145(6):542–51.
76. Schepke U, Meijer HJ, Kerdijk W, et al. Digital versus analog complete-arch impressions for single-unit premolar implant crowns: operating time and patient preference. J Prosthet Dent 2015;114(3):403–6.e1.
77. Masri R, Driscoll C. Clinical applications of digital dental technology. Hoboken (NJ): John Wiley; 2015.
78. Vollborn T, Habor D, Pekam FC, et al. Soft tissue-preserving computer-aided impression: a novel concept using ultrasonic 3D-scanning. Int J Comput Dent 2013;17(4):277–96.
79. Hsieh Y-S, Ho Y-C, Lee S-Y, et al. Dental optical coherence tomography. Sensors (Basel) 2013;13(7):8928–49.

Dental Ceramics for Restoration and Metal Veneering

Yu Zhang, PhD[a],*, J. Robert Kelly, DDS, PhD[b]

KEYWORDS

- Dental ceramics • All-ceramic restorations • Metal-ceramic restorations • Porcelain
- Glass-ceramics • Zirconia • Ceramic-polymer interpenetrating network

KEY POINTS

- A facile understanding of the development, composition, microstructure, properties, and indications of various classes of ceramic dental materials.
- Knowledge of the rationale behind the choice and usage of dental ceramics to maximize esthetics and durability.
- Successful ceramic restorations depend on the balancing of multiple factors.

INTRODUCTION

According to the American College of Prosthodontists, 178 million people in the United States, which represents 55% of the US population, are missing at least 1 tooth and this number is expected to grow over the next 2 decades because of an aging population. Teeth play a critically important role in human life because loss of function reduces people's ability to eat a balanced diet, with negative consequences for systemic health. Loss of esthetics can also negatively affect social function. Both function and esthetics can be restored with dental crowns and fixed dental prostheses (FDPs). Ceramics have become increasingly popular as restorative materials because of their esthetics, inertness, and biocompatibility. Of the crowns and fixed prostheses currently produced in the United States, 80.2% are all-ceramic restorations, 16.9% are porcelain fused to metal (PFM), 2.2% are full-cast, and 0.7% are resin-based composite (RBC).[1] Demands for more esthetic and metal-free restorations, as well as soaring metal prices, are likely to increase further the number of all-ceramic prostheses.[2]

Disclosure: The authors have nothing to disclose.
[a] Department of Biomaterials and Biomimetics, NYU College of Dentistry, 433 First Avenue, Room 810, New York, NY 10010, USA; [b] Department of Biomedical Engineering, University of Connecticut Health Center, Mailstop 1615, 263 Farmington Avenue, Farmington, CT 06030-1615, USA
* Corresponding author.
E-mail address: yz21@nyu.edu

However, a major clinical concern is that ceramics are brittle and subject to fracture.[3,4] The financial drivers for developing fracture-resistant and esthetic ceramics are high: the European crown and FDP market approached $2 billion in 2007[5]; the global crown and FDP market was estimated to be $25 billion in 2010 and more than $30 billion in 2015.[6] This article provides an overview of the background and the current knowledge base associated with dental ceramics for restoration and metal veneering, including a historical review of the development of ceramic restorations and their limitations. It also includes a summary of the current state of the art of porcelain, glass-ceramics, and polycrystalline ceramics. In addition, materials design considerations for dental prostheses are discussed.

THE HISTORY OF DENTAL CERAMICS

Shortly after the introduction of porcelain into Europe in the early eighteenth century, Alexis Duchateau, a Parisian apothecary, introduced ceramics to dentistry when he successfully replaced his ivory dentures with porcelain. With the help of a Parisian dentist, Nicholas Dubois de Chemant, Duchateau, working in concert with a new, high-technology porcelain manufacturer in 1774, created a complete set of porcelain dentures. They must have been very well made because they lasted Duchateau the rest of his life. The development of porcelain dentures was revolutionary in terms of esthetics and oral hygiene, and was recognized as such by Edward Jenner (developer of the smallpox vaccine) and the Faculty of Medicine Paris: they "…united the qualities of beauty, solidity and comfort with the exigencies of hygiene.[7]" Because the then-popular ivory-based or wood-based dentures, often using cadaver teeth, were all porous, they absorbed oral fluids and eventually became badly stained and highly un-hygienic. Also, these early porcelain dentures were dysfunctional because patients had to remove them in order to eat. In addition, those complete porcelain dentures were only intended for edentulous patients, requiring the removal of the remaining teeth from patients' mouths, which was a painful procedure before the discovery of anesthesia by Horace Wells in the middle of the nineteenth century.

Porcelain inlays, onlays, and crowns were introduced by Charles Land[8] in 1886, which ultimately led to the creation of esthetic and functional ceramic restorations. However, the original dental porcelain contained a high feldspathic glass content and was extremely brittle and weak ($\sigma \sim$ 60 MPa; σ stands for strength).[9,10] Therefore, despite the esthetic advantage, the early porcelain restorations were not widely applied in dentistry.[11] Dental ceramics have become increasingly popular as restorative materials because of improvements in strength and the increased goodness of fit with development of pressing and computer-assisted design (CAD)/computer-assisted manufacturing (CAM) processes. The timeline of the development of dental ceramics from the inception of initial porcelain materials to modern ceramic compositions, along with processing technologies, is shown in **Fig. 1**. The main compositions and pertinent mechanical properties of various dental ceramic materials, representative of major material classes and developments, are shown in **Table 1**.

Since Weinstein and colleagues[12,13] solved the problem of the coefficient of thermal expansion (CTE) mismatch between the porcelain veneer and metal framework in 1962, great improvements have been made in PFM systems. Until very recently, it was estimated that 70% to 80% of fixed prostheses produced in the United States were PFM (Ivoclar Vivadent, 3M ESPE, Jensen Dental, Marotta Dental Studio, and Glidewell Laboratories, personal communication, 2011). In contrast, the dental community has long recognized that to realize the full potential of dental prostheses, all-ceramic restorations are necessary. Several strategies have been developed to

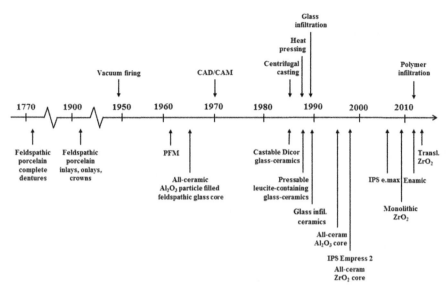

Fig. 1. The timeline of the development of dental ceramics and their processing technologies.

improve the strength and fit of dental ceramics over the past 50 years. Other improvements in longevity have involved the use of high elastic moduli cores and buildup materials and cements to protect single crowns against bulk fracture.

One well-grounded approach to strengthening porcelain is to add uniformly dispersed filler particles to the glass matrix, a technique referred to as dispersion strengthening. One of the most successful particle fillers used in dental ceramics is leucite, a crystalline mineral possessing an index of refraction similar to that of feldspathic glasses.[14] Commercial dental ceramics containing leucite as a strengthener include IPS Empress ($\sigma \sim 138$ MPa) (Ivoclar Vivadent, Schaan, Liechtenstein) and Finesse All-Ceramic ($\sigma \sim 125$ MPa) (Dentsply International). Particle strengthening can also be achieved by heat-treating the glass to facilitate the precipitation and subsequent growth of crystallites within the glass, a process termed ceraming. Dental ceramics produced using the ceraming process are called glass-ceramics. Several commercial products, such as Dicor ($\sigma \sim 229$ MPa) (Dentsply International), IPS Empress II ($\sigma \sim 350$ MPa) (Ivoclar Vivadent), and more recently IPS e.max Press ($\sigma \sim 400$ MPa) and IPS e.max CAD ($\sigma \sim 480$ MPa) (Ivoclar Vivadent) are in this category. The leucite-strengthened porcelains and the glass-ceramics are translucent, so single-layer (monolithic) restorations can be made from these materials. The drawback is that only moderate strength increases can be achieved via the particle strengthening techniques. Therefore, monolithic ceramic restorations experience high failure rates, ranging from 4% to 6% for Dicor molar crowns[15,16] and 3% to 4% per year for IPS Empress crowns.[17,18]

The traditional approach to the fracture problem of monolithic glass-ceramic restorations is to use a layer structure with esthetic but weak porcelain veneers fused onto strong but opaque ceramic cores. The history of the development of higher-strength ceramic cores involves an increase in crystalline content (from ~40 vol % to 99.9 vol%) accompanied by a reduction in glass content. The first successful strengthened core ceramic was made of feldspathic glass filled with ~40 vol% (vol

Table 1
Properties of various dental ceramic materials

Material	Crystalline Phase (vol%)	Modulus E (GPa)	Hardness H (GPa)	Toughness T (MPa·m$^{1/2}$)	Strength σ (MPa)
Porcelain					
Feldspathic ceramic (Vita Mark II)	Albite (<20)	72	6.2	1.2	122
Veneer for ceramic (Lava Ceram)	Leucite (6)	80	5.2	1.1	85
Veneer for metal (d.SIGN)	Leucite/apatite (25)	68	5.9	1.1	104
Glass-Ceramic					
Mica glass-ceramic (Dicor MGC)	Fluormica (70)	69	6.0	1.2	229
Leucite glass-ceramic (IPS Empress CAD)	Leucite (35–45)	65	6.2	1.3	140
Lithium Disilicate–Ceramic					
(IPS Empress 2)	Lithium disilicate (65)	96	5.5–6.3	2.9–3.2	306–420
(IPS e.max CAD)	Lithium disilicate (70)	95	5.8	2.3	480
(IPS e.max Press)	Lithium disilicate (70)	95	5.8	2.8	400
Ceramic-Glass Interpenetrating Network					
Glass-infiltrated spinel	Spinel (68)	185	—	2.5	350
Glass-infiltrated alumina	Alumina (68)	274	11.8	3.6	548
Glass-infiltrated zirconia	Zirconia-toughened alumina (67)	245	13.1	3.5	700
Polycrystalline Ceramic					
Alumina (dense, fine grain)	Alumina (>99)	372	19.6	3.1	572
Zirconia (Lava Plus)	3 mol% Y-TZP (>99)	210	14.0	4.0	1200
Zirconia (Zpex smile)	Cubic/tetragonal zirconia (>99)	210	13.4	2.4	485
Ceramic-Resin Interpenetrating Network					
Resin-infiltrated porcelain (Enamic)	Feldspathic ceramic (75)	30	1.7	1.3	159
Tooth					
Dentin	Hydroxyapatite (50)	18	0.6	3.1	34–98
Enamel	Hydroxyapatite (95)	94	3.2	0.8	12–42

%, percentage by volume) of alumina particles.[19] The alumina fillers increased the flexural strength of the ceramic to ~120 MPa with a trade-off in translucency; hence veneering was required. In 1983, Coors Biomedical (Golden, CO) developed Cerestore all-ceramic restorations with a ceramic core containing ~60 wt% of Al_2O_3, 9 wt% of MgO, a barium aluminosilicate glass at 13 wt% (wt%, percentage by weight), and enough silicone (12 wt%) and kaolin clay (4 wt%) to impart sufficient plasticity for transfer molding at 160°C.[20] It was reported that the alumina reacted with magnesia to form magnesium aluminate spinel, expanding to become net shaped. It is highly unlikely that this reaction occurred given the low firing temperature of 1300°C and short firing time. Subsequent analysis showed that the net-shape ability occurred because of oxidation of the silicone base releasing gaseous products and leading to the crown blowing up like a loaf of bread contained within its mold.[21] However, following universal problems with fractured restorations, the manufacturer withdrew the system. A similar product from the same era, the Hi-Ceram restorative system (Vita Zahnfabrik, Bad Säckingen, Germany) with its core material containing around the same amount of alumina as the Cerestore core, also failed to meet the requirements for posterior restorations.[22] The Hi-Ceram system was replaced by In-Ceram (Vita Zahnfabrik) in 1990. The In-Ceram restoration had a core that was fabricated by lightly sintering an alumina powder compact and then infiltrating the still-porous alumina matrix with a low-viscosity glass containing lanthanum, which reduced viscosity and increased the index of refraction of the infiltration glass. In contrast with Hi-Ceram, in which ~60 vol% alumina particles were added to a glass matrix, In-Ceram alumina was derived from high-temperature glass infiltration of an alumina scaffold, resulting in an alumina-glass interpenetrating network structure. The final product contained ~70 vol% of alumina and had a flexural strength of ~550 MPa.[23] Products along the same line are In-Ceram spinel and In-Ceram zirconia (toughened alumina). The former has a higher translucency but lower strength, whereas the latter has a higher strength but lower translucency, relative to In-Ceram alumina. In 1993, Procera (Nobel Biocare, Göteborg, Sweden) presented a new all-ceramic restoration concept[24] in which the fully dense core material contained 99.9 vol% alumina and displayed a flexural strength of 572 MPa. Several years later, even stronger yttria-stabilized tetragonal zirconia polycrystal (Y-TZP) ceramic was introduced to dentistry as a core material with a flexural strength more than 1200 MPa.

Despite significant improvements in the performance of dental ceramics, the structural stability of all-ceramic systems remains less reliable than that of PFM systems, in which only nonbiological complications are considered.[25] Clinical studies have revealed that the primary cause of failure for lithium disilicate and alumina restorations are fracture in both veneer and framework, whereas that for zirconia-based restorations is cohesive fracture of the veneering porcelain.[26] In an effort to circumvent the problem of veneer chipping and fracture, translucent glass-ceramic materials and, more recently, so-called cubic zirconias have been developed for monolithic restoration applications. However, these translucent ceramic materials are considerably weaker than the traditional dental tetragonal zirconia (Y-TZP), and thus cannot be used to replace the strong but more opaque Y-TZP.

THE STATE-OF-THE-ART DENTAL CERAMICS
Porcelain

Dental ceramics that best mimic the optical properties of natural teeth are predominantly glassy materials, which derive principally from feldspar-quartz-kaolin triaxial porcelain compositions.[21,27] Many technological advances have contributed to the use of porcelain in fixed prosthodontics, such as the development of the vacuum firing technology in 1949, the invention of the high-speed handpiece, the discovery of elastomeric impression materials, and the advent of pressing and CAD/CAM technologies in the 1980s.[28] From a materialistic viewpoint, porcelain compositions have evolved from the original hard-paste Meissen porcelain, which contained a high clay content and thus required a high firing temperature, to the modern soft-paste porcelains that are composed of mostly feldspar with no kaolin or quartz and possess excellent translucency. However, dental porcelains with the most desirable esthetics also tend to have the lowest strength and resistance to crack propagation, which severely limits their clinical indications.[29–32] One major breakthrough came in 1962, when the Weinsteins, with the help of Koenig[27], developed a leucite-containing porcelain composition that could be fired directly onto common dental alloys.[21] Leucite is a rock-forming mineral that is composed of potassium aluminosilicate. At room temperature, leucite possesses a tetragonal structure. However, the crystal structure undergoes a tetragonal to cubic phase transformation at 625°C. This phase transformation is accompanied by a volume expansion of 1.2%, resulting in a high CTE ($20–25 \times 10^{-6}/°C$).[33] In contrast, feldspar glass has a low CTE ($\sim 8 \times 10^{-6}/°C$). Therefore, by varying the proportions of leucite and feldspar glass, porcelain frits with average CTEs matching those ($12–14 \times 10^{-6}/°C$) of dental alloys can be produced. A matching CTE between porcelain veneer and metal alloy coping prevents the development of deleterious thermal stresses on cooling from firing temperatures. Dental manufactures have also discovered that having the porcelain with a slightly lower CTE than the metal (typically differing from $<1 \times 10^{-6}/°C$) can place the porcelain in slight compression, thus increasing the fracture resistance of the restoration. The leucite content for tailoring the CTE of porcelain can vary from several weight percent when coupled with ceramic frameworks to 17 to 25 wt% when matched with common metal alloys. Leucite is also an effective material for the dispersion strengthening of feldspar glass, because a large amount of leucite (up to 35–50 wt%) can be incorporated without significantly compromising its translucency because the refractive index of leucite (n = 1.51) is very close to that of the feldspar glass (n = 1.52–1.53). In addition, owing to preferential etching of leucite crystals relative to the glass matrix, the leucite-containing feldspar glasses can be acid etched to create micromechanical features for resin bonding, thus making the restorations more fracture resistant. The microstructures of several commercial leucite-containing feldspathic ceramics used as veneers for ceramics and metals, as well as dispersion-strengthened monolithic glass-ceramics, are shown in **Fig. 2**.

Leucite feldspathic porcelain materials remain as some of the most esthetic and widely used dental ceramics. Their clinical indications include inlays, onlays, partial crowns, and crowns, as well as veneers for ceramics and metals. Clinical studies have shown that feldspathic porcelain restorations have excellent long-term success rates when bonded to and supported by primarily enamel structures. For example, the survival rate of inlays and onlays is 92% at 8 years,[34] veneers 94% at 12 years,[35] and crowns 95% at 11 years.[36] These findings suggest that this class of materials is ideal for cases in which a significant amount of healthy tooth structure and enamel remain.[29]

The PFM technology has made it possible to fabricate more structurally demanding dental restorations, such as crowns and FDPs. PFM restorations are ideal for cases in which minimal to no tooth structures remain[29] and splinted restorations are required.[37] The esthetic qualities of PFM are at their best when a high-gold-content framework material (eg, Captek) is used.[29] However, the trade-off is that the low modulus of the high-gold framework provides little support to the porcelain veneer, resulting in a greater tendency for veneer fracture and chipping.[38]

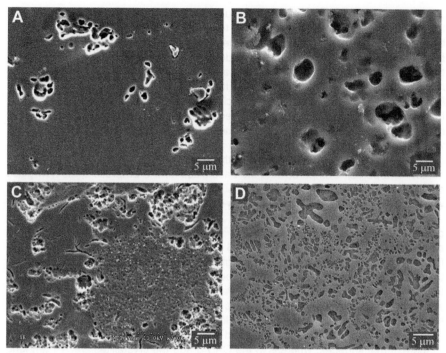

Fig. 2. Microstructures of leucite-containing feldspathic ceramics. Images were taken using secondary electrons in a scanning electron microscope (SEM). Feldspathic overlay porcelains for zirconia: (*A*) Lava Ceram and (*B*) Vita VM9. Porcelain overlay for metal: (*C*) d.SIGN. A dispersion strengthened glass-ceramic: (*D*) Empress CAD. Acid-etched surface revealing craters once occupied by leucite crystals and microcracks in the glassy matrix. Note: the leucite content increases from porcelain veneers for ceramic to metal to dispersion-strengthened glass-ceramic.

Glass-Ceramics

Glass-ceramics are much stronger and tougher but also have lower translucency relative to porcelain. The strengthening and toughening of glass-ceramics are achieved by a ceraming process, in which crystals are precipitated under controlled heat treatments from homogeneous glass through the nucleation and growth processes. The material Dicor was the first glass-ceramic material used for the fabrication of dental restorations. It consisted of fluormica crystals in the form of individual sheets or plates embedded in a glass matrix. Its microstructure, analogous to a house of cards, provides an interlocking mechanism for strengthening. However, because of its poor mechanical performance in clinical applications, Dicor was withdrawn from the market. Some current leucite-reinforced glasses are also produced via the ceraming process. However, currently the most widely used and, arguably, the strongest and toughest dental glass-ceramics are made with lithium disilicate reinforcement.

The first dental lithium disilicate ceramic was fabricated from a base glass composition (SiO_2-Li_2O-Al_2O_3-K_2O-P_2O_5-ZnO-La_2O_3) plus some additives for color and fluorescence. A homogeneous base glass ingot, containing a limited amount of lithium metasilicate, was heated until it reached a viscous state, and then pressed into a mold. Through a judiciously controlled heat treatment, a glass-ceramic containing ~70 vol% of elongated lithium disilicate crystals could be precipitated from the base glass to produce an interlocked microstructure. The resulting material possessed a flexural strength of 350 MPa and fracture toughness 2.9 MPa m$^{1/2}$, which were more than twice those of leucite-based glass-ceramics. The material was commercialized for dental framework use and marketed under the trade name IPS Empress 2. However, this material had high clinical failure rates at 9% to 50% after 24 to 60 months, with a higher tendency of framework fracture in the connector area of short-span posterior FDPs.[39–41] These findings indicate insufficient flexural strength of the IPS Empress 2 framework for multiunit prostheses. Subsequently, a new and improved lithium disilicate glass-ceramic (IPS e.max) with a much higher flexural strength (400–480 MPa) was developed. The improvements were made through the refinement of the base glass composition as well as by improving the quality of the initial glass ingot (with fewer defects and pores). Compared with the base glass for IPS Empress 2, the new glass composition (SiO_2-Li_2O-Al_2O_3-K_2O-P_2O_5-ZrO_2) contained up to 4 wt% ZrO_2 additives, whereas it had diminished ZnO and La_2O_3 contents (<0.1 wt%).

The IPS e.max glass-ceramics come in 2 forms, Press and CAD (**Fig. 3**), reflecting differences in processing conditions.[42,43] The IPS e.max Press ingots are heat-pressed at 920°C for 20 minutes. The IPS e.max CAD ingots are first heat treated to form the intermediate lithium metasilicate glass-ceramics, which are easier to machine to shape. These glass-ceramics are then heated to 840°C for 7 minutes, during which the lithium metasilicate glass-ceramic is transformed to a chemically more stable and esthetically pleasing lithium disilicate glass-ceramic. Lithium disilicate Press and CAD have a glass matrix containing ~70% elongated, needlelike crystals. In the Press grade the crystallites are ~4 μm long and ~0.6 μm wide and aligned perpendicular to the external surfaces, whereas in the CAD grade the crystallites are ~1 μm long and ~0.4 μm wide and more randomly oriented. The Press grade has slightly higher toughness because of the greater impedance to crack propagation by the larger grains (ie, crystals). However, it also has slightly lower strength because these same grains introduce larger starting flaws into the structure (see **Table 1**). Lithium disilicate glass-ceramics are indicated for veneers, anterior crowns, and posterior inlays and onlays. However, when fabricated to monolithic restorations and luted with resin cements, they are also suitable for single-unit, full-coverage crowns for molar teeth. In addition, the large elongated grains in lithium disilicate Press are thought to improve the fracture toughness by crack bridging and deflection, especially in the connector areas of an FDP, in which elongated crystals are preferentially oriented parallel to

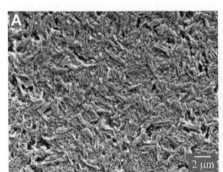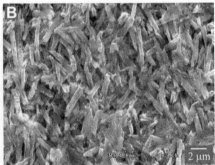

Fig. 3. Microstructures of lithium disilicate glass-ceramics. (A) CAD and (B) Press. Images were taken on an acid-etched surface using secondary electrons in an SEM, revealing elongated lithium disilicate crystallites. Note in the Press material (B), the preferential orientation of the coarse elongated lithium disilicate crystallites.

the tensile surface. Such a logs-on-the-river structure can effectively improve the fracture resistance of the restoration. Long-term clinical data support the use of lithium disilicates as single restorations anywhere in the mouth[44] and as short-span FDPs in the anterior region.[45]

Polycrystalline Ceramics

Recent advances have created stronger and tougher ceramics, predominantly Y-TZP (**Fig. 4**). However, Y-TZP has severe clinical deficiencies owing to its low translucency. The opacity of zirconia becomes a problem, especially when placing an anterior crown or short-span FDPs in the presence of natural teeth. In that case, the reflectance and light scattering do not appear natural. In order to create space for a porcelain veneer thick enough to cover an opaque zirconia core and to match the optical properties of the adjacent natural dentition, a substantial reduction of existing tooth structure is required. In addition, clinical research and practice have revealed that although zirconia frameworks are very fracture resistant, chipping[46–53] and delamination[54,55] of the porcelain veneer are frequent problems. In 25 clinical trials on a variety of brands and makes of zirconia-based crowns and FDPs, chips and delaminations were consistently reported at 6% to 10% in 3 to 5 years in single crowns and 20% to 32% in 5 to 10 years in FDPs.[51–53,56–75] In contrast, crowns and FDPs with metal frameworks revealed substantially lower fracture rates, ranging from 2.7% to 6% up to 15 years.[76–79] One of the primary reasons for the poor clinical performance of porcelain-veneered zirconia bilayer prostheses is the low thermal conductivity of the zirconia core relative to the metal coping, which could result in a large temperature gradient in the porcelain veneer on cooling, and thus residual thermal stresses become locked into the material system.[80] Although it is evident that the high chipping/fracture rate is caused predominantly by these residual stresses, a comprehensive knowledge of the governing material (elastic modulus and CTE), design (veneer/core thickness ratio), and processing (cooling rate) parameters remains largely absent.[80–84] Thus, this continues to be an active research area.

In an effort to avoid veneer chipping and delamination, monolithic zirconia is often used in full-arch restorations, posterior crowns, and FDPs.[85–88] In all these cases, the opacity of Y-TZP zirconia remains a serious issue, although the white, opaque, monolithic Y-TZP restorations may be suitable for bleached teeth.

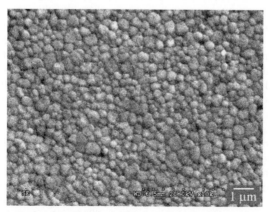

Fig. 4. Scanning electron micrograph, showing a typical fine-grained microstructure of high-strength dental zirconias (Y-TZP). Specimen surface was polished and thermally etched.

After a decade of research and development, progress has been made in improving the translucency of Y-TZP by reducing porosity, decreasing grain size, and eliminating any alumina added as a sintering aid.[89] However, close examinations have revealed that, unless they are thin (ie, <0.5 mm), so-called commercial translucent Y-TZP restorative materials remain largely opaque.[90] Eliminating porosity and impurities alone is not sufficient to significantly improve the translucency of Y-TZP. Tetragonal zirconia is birefringent, meaning that the index of refraction is anisotropic in different crystallographic directions.[89,91] This property causes reflection and refraction at grain boundaries, thus reducing light transmittance. Theory predicts that to make a Y-TZP ceramic sufficiently translucent while preserving strength, a sub–100-nm grain size is necessary, so that light may penetrate without substantial scattering.[89,91–93] However, it is technologically challenging to achieve densification without substantial grain growth beyond the critical 100-nm size.

The current approach to this problem is to introduce an optically isotropic cubic zirconia phase into an ordinarily tetragonal material (eg, DDcubeX^2 by Dental Direkt Materials and Zpex Smile by Tosoh Corporation). However, biphasic tetragonal/cubic zirconia is weaker and more brittle compared with its tetragonal counterpart. For instance, the flexural strength and fracture toughness of Zpex Smile (609 MPa and 2.4 MPa m$^{1/2}$) are only slightly more than one-half of that of Y-TZP. They are more like a dental alumina material (Procera alumina, Nobel Biocare),[33,94] and are also subject to low-temperature degradation. In general, increasing yttria content leads to a larger amount of cubic phase and thus greater translucency. The trade-off is that strength and toughness diminish as the cubic content increases, which has led to the development of several translucent dental zirconia materials containing various amounts of cubic phase. For example, the Katana ultratranslucent zirconia material has a flexural strength of 557 MPa, whereas their supertranslucent and high-translucent zirconias have flexural strengths of 748 and 1125 MPa, respectively. These translucent zirconia pucks also feature multilayered color with a lighter shade in the occlusal one-third thickness and a darker shade at the gingival one-third, sandwiching 2 thinner transition layers. However, the mechanical integrity of these multilayered structures has yet to be evaluated.

New Classes of Materials

The current esthetic and highly fracture-resistant restorative materials are either high-crystalline ceramics or heavily particle-filled resin composites. The elastic properties of these materials are not compatible with enamel or dentin substrates. Therefore, there is a greater tendency for restoration fracture to occur when a much stiffer ceramic material is used, and for underlying tooth fracture to occur when a low-modulus resin composite material is used.[95] In addition, the current advent of great interest in minimally invasive dentistry and chairside 1-visit restorations has resulted in the widespread usage of CAD/CAM technology. Ceramic restorative materials are susceptible to machining damage, especially when the restoration or part of the restoration is thin (eg, marginal chipping).[96,97]

Recently, a new class of material, ceramic-polymer interpenetrating network (CPIN) material (Vita Enamic), has been developed. The impetus for developing the CPIN material is to tailor the material properties, such as elastic modulus, strength, toughness, and hardness, through judicious control of its composition and microstructure. The Enamic material consists of 86 wt% (75 vol%) of a feldspathic ceramic matrix into which an organic phase of dimethacrylate resin containing urethane dimethacrylate and triethylene glycol dimethacrylate is infiltrated.[98] The fabrication process of this material involves 2 steps: first, a porous presintered ceramic network is produced and conditioned by a coupling agent; then, the network structure is infiltrated with the monomers by capillary action.[99,100] The resulting microstructure has a hybrid structure with interpenetrating networks of ceramic and polymer (**Fig. 5**), mimicking the interlocking of prism bands in natural teeth. The flexural strength, elastic modulus, hardness, and fracture toughness of the Enamic material have been evaluated by several investigators,[99,100] and has similar properties to natural tooth structures (see **Table 1**). Compared with ceramic restorative materials, Enamic has reliable millability and edge stability in terms of its ability to be fast milled into thin (<0.5 mm) restorations with excellent precision.[101] A full-contour posterior crown takes a little more than 5 minutes to mill, and eliminates the need for postmilling firing. The material is also easy to adjust and polish. Thus, it is an ideal material for chairside 1-visit restorations.

The three-dimensional (3D) interconnected dual-network structure of CPIN differs from the RBC materials, in which only the resin matrix is continuous. The most recent generation of laboratory-fabricated millable RBC blocks (eg, Lava Ultimate from 3M and Cerasmart from GC) are heavily particle-filled resins cured at a high temperature and pressure. The filler particles in Lava Ultimate are composed of dispersed silica (~20 nm) and zirconia (4–11 nm) nanoparticles, as well as silica/zirconia nanoparticle clusters (0.6–10 μm) (**Fig. 6**). The rationale behind the usage of nanoclusters is that, compared with the traditional hard micrometer-sized filler particles, the nanoparticle clusters (analogous to a bunch of grapes) may not be as effective in terms of crack deflection and strengthening, but they are very effective for polish retention. The large nanoclusters break down to nanoparticles on mastication, leading to a smooth wear surface. However, the nanoclusters inevitably consist of defects and voids, which can soak up oral fluids, resulting in the discoloration and degradation of the RBC. Although the filler loading (80–90 wt% or 65–77 vol%) in the millable RBCs is similar to that of CPIN, their elastic properties and fracture behavior are different. In the case of CPIN materials, the interconnectivity of the ceramic phase provides stiffness and hardness that are necessary for the resistance to plastic deformation and wear. In contrast, the ductile polymer network is able to effectively distribute stresses in all directions.[102] As a result, the 3D interpenetrating dual-network materials possess enhanced resistances to a variety of breakdown phenomena, including contact and flexural damage as well as fatigue crack growth and wear.[98,101–104]

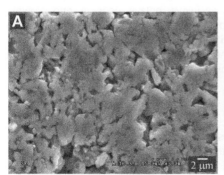
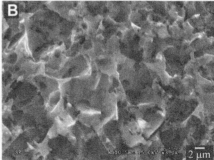

Fig. 5. Microstructure of Vita Enamic observed using secondary electrons in an SEM. (*A*) A polished and then thermally etched surface, revealing a ceramic network structure consisting of ~25 vol% porosity following selective removal of the polymer phase. (*B*) A polished and then acid-etched surface, showing the polymer network after selective removal of the surface ceramic material.

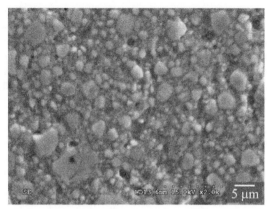

Fig. 6. Scanning electron micrograph of an RBC, Lava Ultimate. The material surface was polished down to 1 μm before imaging.

The CPIN material also differs from another interpenetrating network material (ie, In-Ceram alumina) in which alumina powders consisting of both coarse and fine particles are slip cast to ~70% density. The cast objects are sintered at 1000°C to 1200°C to facilitate the formation of necks between the individual particles, and to prevent significant shrinkage of the components. This effect is achieved by the presence of the coarse grains, which prevent contraction and result in an interconnected porous structure throughout the object. The porous structure is then infiltrated with a low-viscosity lanthanum-containing glass at 950°C to 1000°C, during which infiltrating glass completely wets the alumina scaffold under the influence of capillary forces. The resultant material consisted of a 3D alumina (~70 vol%) and glass interpenetrating network structure. However, because both alumina and glass are brittle materials, only limited toughening mechanics (ie, crack deflection) may be achieved and no significant stress distribution can occur.

It seems desirable to develop a new restorative material that combines the elastic modulus of RBC, which is much lower than that of dentin and even more so than enamel, with the long-lasting esthetics of ceramics. This new CPIN material may offer a unique biomimetic alternative to traditional composites and ceramics. Clinically, Vita Enamic is suitable for single-tooth restorations such as inlays, onlays, veneers, and crowns, including implant-supported crowns and posterior restorations. There are no credible clinical data available concerning the longevity of Enamic restorations at this time. However, laboratory studies have shown that Enamic has excellent resistance to wear and fatigue damage relative to traditional ceramic restorative materials.[98,101]

MATERIALS DESIGN CONSIDERATIONS

Because the clinical performance, in particular the fracture resistance, of dental restorations is influenced by a host of variables, the restoration design and materials selection involve balancing several factors that are considered later. In addition, for reader convenience, some of the commonly observed clinical fracture modes are sketched in **Fig. 7**.

Material Properties

Fracture in ceramics is governed by toughness and strength, and to a lesser extent by elastic modulus and hardness.[105] For crownlike structures, increasing strength simply

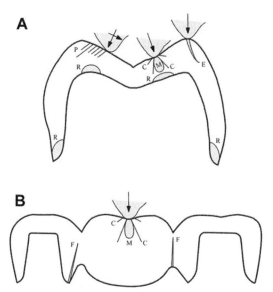

Fig. 7. Various fracture modes in all-ceramic (*A*) crown and (*B*) FDP structures: axisymmetric cone (C) and median (M) cracks; partial cone (P) cracks; edge chipping (E) cracks; radial (R) cracks at cementation surfaces; flexure (F) cracks at connectors. Linear-trace cracks (C, P, E, F) extend out of the plane of diagram, shaded (R, M) cracks extend within the plane of diagram. *The arrows* indicates the directions of load. (*Modified from* Zhang Y, Sailer I, Lawn BR. Fatigue of dental ceramics. J Dent 2013;41(12):1136; with permission.)

increases the resistance to crack initiation in these structures, whereas increasing toughness increases the resistance to crack propagation.[106–109] In many clinical trials covering numerous ceramic systems, fracture toughness of the core ceramic tracks well with clinical success. This fact was taken into consideration when designing a new ceramic classification system based on known clinical indications now in the international standard ISO (International Organization for Standardization) 6872. In addition, strength may be more relevant to FDP structures, in which failure can occur by slow crack growth from a surface flaw, usually on the gingival side of connectors (see **Fig. 7**B). A higher modulus reduces layer flexure on a dentin base, decreasing the failure trends for flexural radial fracture (see **Fig. 7**A).[3,110] Increased hardness diminishes the susceptibility to quasiplastic deformation (contact-induced plastic deformation in brittle materials, which is a precursor of median cracks) and wear at the top surface, and therefore suppresses contact damage (see **Fig. 7**A). Note that zirconia has higher toughness and strength than alumina but lower modulus and hardness. Zirconia is also subject to other forms of long-term degradation; for example, "aging" from hydrothermal degradation associated with phase transformations.[111–114] Porcelains are most vulnerable to damage, whereas glass-ceramics such as lithium disilicate occupy a middle ground. Accordingly, choice of material is a compromise, and requires a fundamental materials science understanding.

Microstructure

Ultimately, material properties are determined by the underlying microstructure.[115] Current dental ceramic technology borrows heavily from the science of materials fabrication, involving a complexity of starting powder preparation, processing additives, and sintering treatments. Veneering ceramics are generally leucite-containing feldspathic porcelains, with the leucite in the form of crystallites to toughen the structure as well as to create a material thermally compatible with the ceramic framework.[28,116,117] Glass-ceramics are likewise formed by heat-treatment crystallization of glass compositions. The key to superior properties is the choice of constituent starting powders and heat treatments. Lithium disilicates comprise the most recent and most durable of the glass-ceramics.[42,118] Up to 70 vol% needle-like crystallites result in moderately high strengths and toughness by virtue of their crack-containment properties.[119] Alumina ceramics have been prepared in a variety of microstructures, but are now supplanted by zirconias. Zirconia properties are governed by many factors, including transformation phases (which confer toughness) and grain size.[120] Translucent zirconias are fabricated via refinement of processing routes, beginning with ultrafine equiaxed powders with yttrium stabilizer, reduction or elimination of light-scattering sintering aids and porosities, and higher sintering temperatures.[121] Judicious microstructural control holds the key to future dental materials development.

Residual Stresses

Residual stresses can develop in a porcelain veneer from CTE mismatch between the veneer and ceramic framework, and from rapid cooling during processing, especially in frameworks with low thermal diffusivities.[80,83,84,122–128] In some layer structures, thermal stresses may be beneficial; for example, by placing a weak outer porcelain veneer into compression. However, thermal stresses must average out to zero across any layer section, so that compression in one part of a prosthesis must inevitably be counterbalanced by tension elsewhere.[110] Moreover, these stresses are never uniform across the section, so any given layer may experience compression at one surface but tension at the other. Monolithic prostheses are not subject to the same concerns, although even there some stresses can arise from rapid cooling during processing, owing to the presence of substantial thermal gradients. Such stresses can have a profound influence on service lifetime.[110]

Monolithic Versus Veneered Structures

Porcelain-veneered ceramics have superior esthetics but are more vulnerable to fracture, especially chipping. Veneered crowns and FDPs still constitute mainstream dental practice, but are gradually being supplanted by monolithic prostheses fabricated from more resilient ceramics. Full-contour monoliths are much less susceptible to either occlusal surface or cementation fracture damage. The key to the advance of monoliths is improved esthetics. In modern-day zirconias, this is being achieved by fabricating more translucent microstructures or by infiltrating glass into outer surfaces to produce graded structures.[129–135]

Layer Thickness

In accord with intuition, thicker layers provide greater protection against fracture, partly because they diminish flexure and membrane stresses at any given occlusal load (a thickness squared relationship) and partly because they increase the distance cracks have to propagate before encountering a weak internal interface (veneered structures) or opposite surface (monoliths). The influence is strongest for radial cracks at the intaglio surface, with greater fatigue life with increased net layer thickness (see **Fig. 7**A).[106,107,136] In veneered structures, the critical bite forces to produce flexural radial cracks at the intaglio surface are only mildly sensitive to relative veneer-to-core thickness.[137,138] This allows the veneer/core thickness ratio to be tailored to optimize the residual stress profile while retaining the flexural strength of the veneered restoration.

Tooth Contact Conditions

Changes in contact geometry primarily affect the ease and extent of occlusal surface damage.[139] Sharper, harder contacts in axial loading distribute the load over smaller areas, increasing local stresses and thereby making it easier to initiate cone cracks (see **Fig. 7**).[139] Such contacts are also likely to promote wear and abrasion damage and to initiate median cracks.[140] However, once these cracks grow away from the contact into the far field, they become less influenced by the nature of the con-tact.[106,107,109] Radial cracks (especially at the margins) are fairly insensitive to con-tact conditions. Off-axis contacts can enhance the failure process by initiating partial cones (sliding contacts) or edge chipping (near-edge contacts) (see **Fig. 7**A). From a design aspect, it is advisable to avoid sharp cusps near the edges of crowns, to prevent incurring damage in the first place. Sharp cusps are also more prone to quasiplastic deformation and wear. Contacts with soft materials relative to tooth modulus or hardness (eg, normal food items) or with blunt objects may sup-press initiation of occlusal surface damage altogether by spreading the load over a greater area.[141]

Tooth Size and Shape

The geometry of prosthesis, most notably the dispositions of different cuspal shapes and connector configurations, plays a governing role in fracture resistance. Essen-tially, the greater the curvature (ie, the smaller the radius) of a contacting surface, the lower the bite force to initiate cracks associated with layer flexure.[142] Also, the smaller the crown height, the lower the force to drive longitudinal cracks around a side wall.[143] Clearly, these geometric factors are governed by the spatial restrictions imposed by opposing and adjacent dentition.

Substrate Modulus

The modulus of tooth dentin is about one-fifth that of enamel and an even smaller frac-tion than that of most ceramics used in crowns and FDPs.[144] A compliant substrate is an additional source of enhanced flexure,[145–148] and hence of radial fracture.[149–152] The modulus of cements or adhesives used to bond the dental prostheses to the un-derlying tooth structure is a factor of 2 to 5 times lower still, further degrading the load-bearing capacity,[145,148,153,154] and even thin cement layers (eg, <0.1 mm) can sub-stantially enhance crown flexure. The use of high-modulus buildup materials and dental cements seems to be a useful strategy for minimizing flexural fractures.[145]

Surface State

It is evident that some precautions need to be taken in the preparation of prosthesis surfaces to stop cracks forming in the first place. Surface treatments can lead to the introduction of flaws that diminish strength. Aggressive sandblasting procedures with hard, coarse, abrasive particles under high air pressure used to provide greater adhesion at the cementation surfaces of crowns are in this category.[155–157] Likewise, the use of coarse diamond burs to grind down crown cusps in order to adjust the occlusal surfaces enhances the prospect of crack initiation. In contrast, although they compromise the load-bearing capacity of a restoration, prematurely initiated cracks from such damage may arrest within the structure, with little consequent effect on the final fracture condition.[142]

SUMMARY

Ceramic restorations are developed for esthetics, biocompatibility, and chemical durability. The composition, microstructure, and properties of ceramic materials determine the clinical indications of various classes of dental ceramics. Other factors that influence material selection include restoration designs (monolithic or layered structure), layer thickness, residual stresses, tooth contact conditions, tooth size and shape, elastic modulus of the adhesives and substrate (enamel or dentin), and surface state. Successful application of ceramic restorations ultimately depends on material selection, manufacturing technique, and restoration design.

REFERENCES

1. Christensen GJ. Is the rush to all-ceramic crowns justified? J Am Dent Assoc 2014;145(2):192–4.
2. Chan C. US markets for crowns and bridges 2011. Toronto (Canada): Millennium Research Group; 2010. p. 142025.
3. Lawn BR, Deng Y, Thompson VP. Use of contact testing in the characterization and design of all-ceramic crownlike layer structures: a review. J Prosthet Dent 2001;86(5):495–510.
4. Griggs JA. Recent advances in materials for all-ceramic restorations. Dent Clin North Am 2007;51(3):713–27, viii.
5. European markets for crowns & bridges 2008. Toronto: Millennium Research Group; 2007.
6. Palmer R. Dentistry without borders. dlpmagazinecom 2010.
7. Wynbrandt J. The Excruciating History of Dentistry: Toothsome Tales & Oral Oddities from Babylon to Braces. New York: St. Martin's Press, Macmillan Publishing; 2000.
8. Land CH. Porcelain dental art: no. II. Dent Cosmos 1903;45(8):615–20.
9. McLean JW. The science and art of dental ceramics. Chicago: Quintessence Publishing; 1979.
10. Binns D. The chemical and physical properties of dental porcelain. Chicago: Quintessence Publishing; 1983.
11. van Noort R. Introduction to dental materials. 2nd edition. London: Mosby; 2002. p. 231–46.
12. Weinstein M, Katz S, Weinstein AB, inventors; US patent 3,052,982. 1962.
13. Weinstein M, Weinstein AB, inventors; US patent 3,052,983. 1962.
14. Denry IL. Recent advances in ceramics for dentistry. Crit Rev Oral Biol Med 1996;7(2):134–43.
15. Malament KA, Socransky SS. Survival of Dicor glass-ceramic dental restorations over 14 years: part I. Survival of Dicor complete coverage restorations and effect of internal surface acid etching, tooth position, gender and age. J Prosthet Dent 1999;81:23–32.
16. Sjogren G, Lantto R, Tillberg A. Clinical evaluation of all-ceramic crowns (Dicor) in general practice. J Prosthet Dent 1999;81:277–84.
17. Fradeani M, Aquilano A. Clinical experience with Empress crowns. Int J Prosthodont 1997;10(3):241–7.
18. Sjogren G, Lantto R, Granberg A, et al. Clinical examination of leucite-reinforced glass-ceramic crowns (Empress) in general practice: a retrospective study. Int J Prosthodont 1999;12:122–8.
19. McLean JW, Hughs TH. The reinforcement of dental porcelain with ceramic oxides. Br Dent J 1965;119:251–67.

20. Sozio RB, Riley EJ. The shrink-free ceramic crown. J Prosthet Dent 1983;69: 1982–5.
21. Kelly JR. Ceramics in restorative and prosthetic dentistry. Annu Rev Mater Sci 1997;27:443–68.
22. Bieniek KW, Marx R. Die mechanische belastbarkeit neuer vollkeramischer kronen- und bruckenmaterialen. Schweitz Monatsschr Zahnmed 1994;104: 284–9.
23. Probster L, Diehl J. Slip-casting alumina ceramics for crown and bridge restorations. Quintessence Int 1992;23(1):25–31.
24. Anderson M, Oden A. A new all-ceramic crown. A dense-sintered, high-purity alumina coping with porcelain. Acta Odontol Scand 1993;51:59–64.
25. Goodacre CJ, Bernal G, Rungcharassaeng K, et al. Clinical complications in fixed prosthodontics. J Prosthet Dent 2003;90(1):31–41.
26. Conrad HJ, Seong WJ, Pesun IJ. Current ceramic materials and systems with clinical recommendations: a systematic review. J Prosthet Dent 2007;98(5): 389–404.
27. Kelly JR. Dental ceramics: current thinking and trends. Dent Clin North Am 2004;48(2):513–30.
28. Kelly JR, Benetti P. Ceramic materials in dentistry: historical evolution and current practice. Aust Dent J 2011;56(Suppl 1):84–96.
29. McLaren EA, Figueira J. Updating classifications of ceramic dental materials: a guide to material selection. Compend Contin Educ Dent 2015;36(6):400–5 [quiz: 406, 416].
30. Peterson IM, Pajares A, Lawn BR, et al. Mechanical characterization of dental ceramics by hertzian contacts. J Dent Res 1998;77(4):589–602.
31. Peterson IM, Wuttiphan S, Lawn BR, et al. Role of microstructure on contact damage and strength degradation of micaceous glass-ceramics. Dent Mater 1998;14(1):80–9.
32. Scherrer SS, Kelly JR, Quinn GD, et al. Fracture toughness (K_{Ic}) of a dental porcelain determined by fractographic analysis. Dent Mater 1999;15(5):342–8.
33. Denry IL, Holloway JA. Ceramics for dental applications: a review. Materials 2010;3(1):351–68.
34. Kramer N, Frankenberger R. Clinical performance of bonded leucite-reinforced glass ceramic inlays and onlays after eight years. Dent Mater 2005;21(3): 262–71.
35. Fradeani M, Redemagni M, Corrado M. Porcelain laminate veneers: 6- to 12-year clinical evaluation–a retrospective study. Int J Periodontics Restorative Dent 2005;25(1):9–17.
36. Fradeani M, Redemagni M. An 11-year clinical evaluation of leucite-reinforced glass-ceramic crowns: a retrospective study. Quintessence Int 2002;33(7): 503–10.
37. Malament KA. Reflections on modem dental ceramics. Dent Today 2015;34(11): 10, 12.
38. Kim B, Zhang Y, Pines M, et al. Fracture of porcelain-veneered structures in fatigue. J Dent Res 2007;86(2):142–6.
39. Esquivel-Upshaw JF, Anusavice KJ, Young H, et al. Clinical performance of a lithia disilicate-based core ceramic for three-unit posterior FPDs. Int J Prosthodont 2004;17(4):469–75.
40. Marquardt P, Strub JR. Survival rates of IPS empress 2 all-ceramic crowns and fixed partial dentures: results of a 5-year prospective clinical study. Quintessence Int 2006;37(4):253–9.

41. Taskonak B, Sertgoz A. Two-year clinical evaluation of lithia-disilicate-based all-ceramic crowns and fixed partial dentures. Dent Mater 2006;22(11):1008–13.

42. Holand W, Schweiger M, Watzke R, et al. Ceramics as biomaterials for dental restoration. Expert Rev Med Devices 2008;5(6):729–45.

43. Zhang Y, Lee JJ, Srikanth R, et al. Edge chipping and flexural resistance of monolithic ceramics. Dent Mater 2013;29(12):1201–8.

44. Gehrt M, Wolfart S, Rafai N, et al. Clinical results of lithium-disilicate crowns after up to 9 years of service. Clin Oral Investig 2013;17(1):275–84.

45. Kern M, Sasse M, Wolfart S. Ten-year outcome of three-unit fixed dental prostheses made from monolithic lithium disilicate ceramic. J Am Dent Assoc 2012; 143(3):234–40.

46. Al-Amleh B, Lyons K, Swain M. Clinical trials in zirconia: a systematic review. J Oral Rehabil 2010;37(8):641–52.

47. Christensen GJ. Porcelain-fused-to-metal versus zirconia-based ceramic restorations, 2009. J Am Dent Assoc 2009;140(8):1036–9.

48. Denry I, Kelly JR. State of the art of zirconia for dental applications. Dent Mater 2008;24(3):299–307.

49. Sailer I, Feher A, Filser F, et al. Five-year clinical results of zirconia frameworks for posterior fixed partial dentures. Int J Prosthodont 2007;20(4):383–8.

50. Sailer I, Pjetursson BE, Zwahlen M, et al. A systematic review of the survival and complication rates of all-ceramic and metal-ceramic reconstructions after an observation period of at least 3 years. Part II: Fixed dental prostheses. Clin Oral Implants Res 2007;18(Suppl 3):86–96.

51. Larsson C, Vult Von Steyern P. Implant-supported full-arch zirconia-based mandibular fixed dental prostheses. Eight-year results from a clinical pilot study. Acta Odontol Scand 2013;71(5):1118–22.

52. Ortorp A, Kihl ML, Carlsson GE. A 5-year retrospective study of survival of zirconia single crowns fitted in a private clinical setting. J Dent 2012;40(6):527–30.

53. Schmitter M, Mussotter K, Rammelsberg P, et al. Clinical performance of long-span zirconia frameworks for fixed dental prostheses: 5-year results. J Oral Rehabil 2012;39(7):552–7.

54. Liu Y, Liu G, Wang Y, et al. Failure modes and fracture origins of porcelain veneers on bilayer dental crowns. Int J Prosthodont 2014;27(2):147–50.

55. Pang Z, Chughtai A, Sailer I, et al. A fractographic study of clinically retrieved zirconia-ceramic and metal-ceramic fixed dental prostheses. Dent Mater 2015;31(10):1198–206.

56. Sax C, Hammerle CH, Sailer I. 10-year clinical outcomes of fixed dental prostheses with zirconia frameworks. Int J Comput Dent 2011;14(3):183–202.

57. Larsson C, Vult von Steyern P, Nilner K. A prospective study of implant-supported full-arch yttria-stabilized tetragonal zirconia polycrystal mandibular fixed dental prostheses: three-year results. Int J Prosthodont 2010;23(4):364–9.

58. Tsumita M, Kokubo Y, Ohkubo C, et al. Clinical evaluation of posterior all-ceramic FPDs (Cercon): a prospective clinical pilot study. J Prosthodont Res 2010;54(2):102–5.

59. Schmitter M, Mussotter K, Rammelsberg P, et al. Clinical performance of extended zirconia frameworks for fixed dental prostheses: two-year results. J Oral Rehabil 2009;36(8):610–5.

60. Bornemann G, Rinke S, Huels A. Prospective clinical trial with conventionally luted zirconia-based fixed partial dentures – 18-month results. J Dent Res 2003;82:B117.

61. Raigrodski AJ, Yu A, Chiche GJ, et al. Clinical efficacy of veneered zirconium dioxide-based posterior partial fixed dental prostheses: five-year results. J Prosthet Dent 2012;108(4):214–22.

62. Salido MP, Martinez-Rus F, del Rio F, et al. Prospective clinical study of zirconia-based posterior four-unit fixed dental prostheses: four-year follow-up. Int J Prosthodont 2012;25(4):403–9.

63. Pelaez J, Cogolludo PG, Serrano B, et al. A four-year prospective clinical evaluation of zirconia and metal-ceramic posterior fixed dental prostheses. Int J Prosthodont 2012;25(5):451–8.

64. Schmitt J, Holst S, Wichmann M, et al. Zirconia posterior fixed partial dentures: a prospective clinical 3-year follow-up. Int J Prosthodont 2009;22(6):597–603.

65. Raigrodski AJ, Chiche GJ, Potiket N, et al. The efficacy of posterior three-unit zirconium-oxide-based ceramic fixed partial dental prostheses: a prospective clinical pilot study. J Prosthet Dent 2006;96(4):237–44.

66. Pospiech P, Rountree P, Nothdurft F. Clinical evaluation of zirconia-based all-ceramic posterior bridges: two-year results. J Dent Res 2003;82:114.

67. Crisp RJ, Cowan AJ, Lamb J, et al. A clinical evaluation of all-ceramic bridges placed in UK general dental practices: first-year results. Br Dent J 2008;205(9): 477–82.

68. Ohlmann B, Rammelsberg P, Schmitter M, et al. All-ceramic inlay-retained fixed partial dentures: preliminary results from a clinical study. J Dent 2008;36(9): 692–6.

69. Sorrentino R, De Simone G, Tete S, et al. Five-year prospective clinical study of posterior three-unit zirconia-based fixed dental prostheses. Clin Oral Investig 2012;16(3):977–85.

70. Ortorp A, Kihl ML, Carlsson GE. A 3-year retrospective and clinical follow-up study of zirconia single crowns performed in a private practice. J Dent 2009; 37(9):731–6.

71. Tinschert J, Schulze KA, Natt G, et al. Clinical behavior of zirconia-based fixed partial dentures made of DC-Zirkon: 3-year results. Int J Prosthodont 2008; 21(3):217–22.

72. Vult von Steyern P, Carlson P, Nilner K. All-ceramic fixed partial dentures designed according to the DC-Zirkon technique. A 2-year clinical study. J Oral Rehabil 2005;32(3):180–7.

73. Molin MK, Karlsson SL. Five-year clinical prospective evaluation of zirconia-based Denzir 3-unit FPDs. Int J Prosthodont 2008;21(3):223–7.

74. Larsson C, Vult von Steyern P, Sunzel B, et al. All-ceramic two- to five-unit implant-supported reconstructions. A randomized, prospective clinical trial. Swed Dent J 2006;30(2):45–53.

75. Edelhoff D, Florian B, Florian W, et al. HIP zirconia fixed partial dentures–clinical results after 3 years of clinical service. Quintessence Int 2008;39(6):459–71.

76. Valderhaug J. A 15-year clinical evaluation of fixed prosthodontics. Acta Odontol Scand 1991;49(1):35–40.

77. Walton TR. A 10-year longitudinal study of fixed prosthodontics: clinical characteristics and outcome of single-unit metal-ceramic crowns. Int J Prosthodont 1999;12(6):519–26.

78. Walton TR. An up to 15-year longitudinal study of 515 metal-ceramic FPDs: Part 1. Outcome. Int J Prosthodont 2002;15(5):439–45.

79. Walton TR. An up to 15-year longitudinal study of 515 metal-ceramic FPDs: Part 2. Modes of failure and influence of various clinical characteristics. Int J Prosthodont 2003;16(2):177–82.

80. Swain MV. Unstable cracking (chipping) of veneering porcelain on all-ceramic dental crowns and fixed partial dentures. Acta Biomater 2009;5(5):1668–77.

81. Al-Amleh B, Neil Waddell J, Lyons K, et al. Influence of veneering porcelain thickness and cooling rate on residual stresses in zirconia molar crowns. Dent Mater 2014;30(3):271–80.

82. Baldassarri M, Stappert CF, Wolff MS, et al. Residual stresses in porcelain-veneered zirconia prostheses. Dent Mater 2012;28(8):873–9.

83. Belli R, Monteiro S Jr, Baratieri LN, et al. A photoelastic assessment of residual stresses in zirconia-veneer crowns. J Dent Res 2012;91(3):316–20.

84. Mainjot AK, Schajer GS, Vanheusden AJ, et al. Residual stress measurement in veneering ceramic by hole-drilling. Dent Mater 2011;27(5):439–44.

85. Beuer F, Stimmelmayr M, Gueth JF, et al. In vitro performance of full-contour zirconia single crowns. Dent Mater 2012;28(4):449–56.

86. Christensen R. Focus on: monolithic crowns. Dent Today 2013;32(3):22.

87. Rinke S, Fischer C. Range of indications for translucent zirconia modifications: clinical and technical aspects. Quintessence Int 2013;44(8):557–66.

88. Stober T, Bermejo JL, Rammelsberg P, et al. Enamel wear caused by monolithic zirconia crowns after 6 months of clinical use. J Oral Rehabil 2014;41(4):314–22.

89. Zhang HB, Li ZP, Kim BN, et al. Effect of alumina dopant on transparency of tetragonal zirconia. J Nanomater 2012;269064.

90. Tong H, Tanaka CB, Kaizer MR, et al. Characterization of three commercial Y-TZP ceramics produced for their high-translucency, high-strength and high-surface area. Ceram Int 2016;42(1 Pt B):1077–85.

91. Klimke J, Trunec M, Krell A. Transparent tetragonal yttria-stabilized zirconia ceramics: influence of scattering caused by birefringence. J Am Ceram Soc 2011;94(6):1850–8.

92. Zhang Y. Making yttria-stabilized tetragonal zirconia translucent. Dent Mater 2014;30(10):1195–203.

93. Anselmi-Tamburini U, Woolman JN, Munir ZA. Transparent nanometric cubic and tetragonal zirconia obtained by high-pressure pulsed electric current sintering. Adv Funct Mater 2007;17(16):3267–73.

94. Zeng K, Oden A, Rowcliffe D. Evaluation of mechanical properties of dental ceramic core materials in combination with porcelains. Int J Prosthodont 1998;11(2):183–9.

95. Zhang Y, Mai Z, Barani A, et al. Fracture-resistant monolithic dental crowns. Dent Mater 2016;32(3):442–9.

96. Giannetopoulos S, van Noort R, Tsitrou E. Evaluation of the marginal integrity of ceramic copings with different marginal angles using two different CAD/CAM systems. J Dent 2010;38(12):980–6.

97. Tsitrou EA, Northeast SE, van Noort R. Brittleness index of machinable dental materials and its relation to the marginal chipping factor. J Dent 2007;35(12):897–902.

98. El Zhawi H, Kaizer MR, Chughtai A, et al. Polymer infiltrated ceramic network structures for resistance to fatigue fracture and wear. Dent Mater 2016;32(11):1352–61.

99. Coldea A, Swain MV, Thiel N. Mechanical properties of polymer-infiltrated-ceramic-network materials. Dent Mater 2013;29(4):419–26.

100. Della Bona A, Corazza PH, Zhang Y. Characterization of a polymer-infiltrated ceramic-network material. Dent Mater 2014;30(5):564–9.

101. Swain MV, Coldea A, Bilkhair A, et al. Interpenetrating network ceramic-resin composite dental restorative materials. Dent Mater 2016;32(1):34–42.

102. Feng XQ, Mai YW, Qin QH. A micromechanical model for interpenetrating multiphase composites. Comput Mater Sci 2003;28(3–4):486–93.

103. Coldea A, Fischer J, Swain MV, et al. Damage tolerance of indirect restorative materials (including PICN) after simulated bur adjustments. Dent Mater 2015; 31(6):684–94.

104. Coldea A, Swain MV, Thiel N. Hertzian contact response and damage tolerance of dental ceramics. J Mech Behav Biomed Mater 2014;34:124–33.

105. Lawn BR. Fracture of brittle solids. 2nd edition. Cambridge: Cambridge University Press; 1993.

106. Bhowmick S, Zhang Y, Lawn BR. Competing fracture modes in brittle materials subject to concentrated cyclic loading in liquid environments: bilayer structures. J Mater Res 2005;20(10):2792–800.

107. Hermann I, Bhowmick S, Zhang Y, et al. Competing fracture modes in brittle materials subject to concentrated cyclic loading in liquid environments: trilayer structures. J Mater Res 2006;21(2):512–21.

108. Lawn BR, Bhowmick S, Bush MB, et al. Failure modes in ceramic-based layer structures: a basis for materials design of dental crowns. J Am Ceram Soc 2007;90(6):1671–83.

109. Zhang Y, Bhowmick S, Lawn BR. Competing fracture modes in brittle materials subject to concentrated cyclic loading in liquid environments: monoliths. J Mater Res 2005;20(8):2021–9.

110. Hermann I, Bhowmick S, Lawn BR. Role of core support material in veneer failure of brittle layer structures. J Biomed Mater Res B Appl Biomater 2007;82(1): 115–21.

111. Chevalier J. What future for zirconia as a biomaterial? Biomaterials 2006;27: 534–43.

112. Chevalier J, Cales B, Drouin JM. Low-temperature aging of Y-TZP ceramics. J Am Ceram Soc 1999;82(8):2150–4.

113. Chevalier J, Olagnon C, Fantozzi G. Crack propagation and fatigue in zirconia-based composites. Compos Part A Appl Sci and Manuf 1999;30(4):525–30.

114. Kim JW, Covel NS, Guess PC, et al. Concerns of hydrothermal degradation in CAD/CAM zirconia. Journal of Dental Research 2010;89(1):91–5.

115. Giordano R, McLaren EA. Ceramics overview: classification by microstructure and processing methods. Compend Contin Educ Dent 2010;31(9):682–4, 686, 688 passim; [quiz 698, 700].

116. Denry IL, Mackert JR Jr, Holloway JA, et al. Effect of cubic leucite stabilization on the flexural strength of feldspathic dental porcelain. J Dent Res 1996;75(12): 1928–35.

117. Mackert JR Jr, Evans AL. Effect of cooling rate on leucite volume fraction in dental porcelains. J Dent Res 1991;70(2):137–9.

118. Culp L, McLaren EA. Lithium disilicate: the restorative material of multiple options. Compend Contin Educ Dent 2010;31(9):716–20, 722, 724-715.

119. Chai H, Lee JJ, Lawn BR. On the chipping and splitting of teeth. J Mech Behav Biomed Mater 2011;4(3):315–21.

120. Hannink RHJ, Kelly PM, Muddle BC. Transformation toughening in zirconia-containing ceramics. J Am Ceram Soc 2000;83(3):461–87.

121. Stawarczyk B, Ozcan M, Hallmann L, et al. The effect of zirconia sintering temperature on flexural strength, grain size, and contrast ratio. Clin Oral Investig 2013;17(1):269–74.

122. Baldassarri M, Zhang Y, Thompson VP, et al. Reliability and failure modes of implant-supported zirconium-oxide fixed dental prostheses related to veneering techniques. J Dent 2011;39(7):489–98.

123. Benetti P, Kelly JR, Della Bona A. Analysis of thermal distributions in veneered zirconia and metal restorations during firing. Dent Mater 2013;29(11):1166–72.

124. Mainjot AK, Schajer GS, Vanheusden AJ, et al. Influence of cooling rate on residual stress profile in veneering ceramic: measurement by hole-drilling. Dent Mater 2011;27(9):906–14.

125. Mainjot AK, Schajer GS, Vanheusden AJ, et al. Influence of zirconia framework thickness on residual stress profile in veneering ceramic: measurement by hole-drilling. Dent Mater 2012;28(4):378–84.

126. Mainjot AK, Schajer GS, Vanheusden AJ, et al. Influence of veneer thickness on residual stress profile in veneering ceramic: measurement by hole-drilling. Dent Mater 2012;28(2):160–7.

127. Meira JB, Reis BR, Tanaka CB, et al. Residual stresses in Y-TZP crowns due to changes in the thermal contraction coefficient of veneers. Dent Mater 2013; 29(5):594–601.

128. Tholey MJ, Swain MV, Thiel N. Thermal gradients and residual stresses in veneered Y-TZP frameworks. Dent Mater 2011;27(11):1102–10.

129. Ren L, Janal MN, Zhang Y. Sliding contact fatigue of graded zirconia with external esthetic glass. J Dent Res 2011;90(9):1116–21.

130. Zhang Y. Overview: damage resistance of graded ceramic restorative materials. J Eur Ceram Soc 2012;32(11):2623–32.

131. Zhang Y, Chai H, Lawn BR. Graded structures for all-ceramic restorations. J Dent Res 2010;89(4):417–21.

132. Zhang Y, Kim JW. Graded structures for damage resistant and aesthetic all-ceramic restorations. Dent Mater 2009;25(6):781–90.

133. Zhang Y, Kim JW. Graded zirconia glass for resistance to veneer fracture. J Dent Res 2010;89(10):1057–62.

134. Zhang Y, Ma L. Optimization of ceramic strength using elastic gradients. Acta Mater 2009;57:2721–9.

135. Zhang Y, Sun MJ, Zhang DZ. Designing functionally graded materials with superior load-bearing properties. Acta Biomater 2012;8(3):1101–8.

136. Bhowmick S, Melendez-Martinez JJ, Zhang Y, et al. Design maps for failure of all-ceramic layer structures in concentrated cyclic loading. Acta Mater 2007; 55(7):2479–88.

137. Deng Y, Miranda P, Pajares A, et al. Fracture of ceramic/ceramic/polymer trilayers for biomechanical applications. J Biomed Mater Res A 2003;67(3): 828–33.

138. Dibner AC, Kelly JR. Fatigue strength of bilayered ceramics under cyclic loading as a function of core veneer thickness ratios. J Prosthet Dent 2016; 115(3):335–40.

139. Bhowmick S, Melendez-Martinez JJ, Hermann I, et al. Role of indenter material and size in veneer failure of brittle layer structures. J Biomed Mater Res B Appl Biomater 2007;82(1):253–9.

140. Ren L, Zhang Y. Sliding contact fracture of dental ceramics: principles and validation. Acta Biomater 2014;10(7):3243–53.

141. Qasim T, Ford C, Bush MB, et al. Margin failures in brittle dome structures: relevance to failure of dental crowns. J Biomed Mater Res B Appl Biomater 2007; 80(1):78–85.

142. Qasim T, Bush MB, Hu X, et al. Contact damage in brittle coating layers: influence of surface curvature. J Biomed Mater Res B Appl Biomater 2005;73(1): 179–85.

143. Barani A, Keown AJ, Bush MB, et al. Role of tooth elongation in promoting fracture resistance. J Mech Behav Biomed Mater 2012;8:37–46.

144. Xu HH, Smith DT, Jahanmir S, et al. Indentation damage and mechanical properties of human enamel and dentin. J Dent Res 1998;77(3):472–80.

145. Zhang Y, Kim JW, Bhowmick S, et al. Competition of fracture mechanisms in monolithic dental ceramics: flat model systems. J Biomed Mater Res B Appl Biomater 2009;88(2):402–11.

146. Scherrer SS, de Rijk WG, Belser UC, et al. Effect of cement film thickness on the fracture resistance of a machinable glass-ceramic. Dent Mater 1994;10(3): 172–7.

147. Scherrer SS, de Rijk WG. The fracture resistance of all-ceramic crowns on supporting structures with different elastic moduli. Int J Prosthodont 1993;6(5): 462–7.

148. Ma L, Guess PC, Zhang Y. Load-bearing properties of minimal-invasive monolithic lithium disilicate and zirconia occlusal onlays: finite element and theoretical analyses. Dent Mater 2013;29(7):742–51.

149. Zhang Y, Lawn B. Long-term strength of ceramics for biomedical applications. J Biomed Mater Res B Appl Biomater 2004;69(2):166–72.

150. Lee KS, Jung Y-G, Peterson IM, et al. Model for cyclic fatigue of quasiplastic ceramics in contact with spheres. J Am Ceram Soc 2000;83(9):2255–62.

151. Lawn BR, Pajares A, Zhang Y, et al. Materials design in the performance of all-ceramic crowns. Biomaterials 2004;25(14):2885–92.

152. Kim JW, Bhowmick S, Chai H, et al. Role of substrate material in failure of crown-like layer structures. J Biomed Mater Res B Appl Biomater 2007;81(2):305–11.

153. Chai H, Lawn BR. Role of adhesive interlayer in transverse fracture of brittle layer structures. J Mater Res 2000;15(4):1017–24.

154. Kim JH, Miranda P, Kim DK, et al. Effect of an adhesive interlayer on the fracture of a brittle coating on a supporting substrate. J Mater Res 2003;18(1):222–7.

155. Zhang Y, Lawn BR, Malament KA, et al. Damage accumulation and fatigue life of particle-abraded ceramics. Int J Prosthodont 2006;19(5):442–8.

156. Zhang Y, Lawn BR, Rekow ED, et al. Effect of sandblasting on the long-term performance of dental ceramics. J Biomed Mater Res B Appl Biomater 2004;71(2): 381–6.

157. Guess PC, Zhang Y, Kim JW, et al. Damage and reliability of Y-TZP after cementation surface treatment. J Dent Res 2010;89(6):592–6.

Dental Cements for Luting and Bonding Restorations
Self-Adhesive Resin Cements

 CrossMark

Adriana P. Manso, DDS, MSc, PhD, Ricardo M. Carvalho, DDS, PhD*

KEYWORDS

- Self-adhesive resin cements • Dental cements • Luting cement • Cementation

KEY POINTS

- Self-adhesive resin cements are current popular luting materials with advantages over traditional luting cements: ease of use and improved properties.
- The chemistry of the materials dictates their behavior. Acidic monomers need to be neutralized during setting to prevent compromising curing, increased sorption and expansion and lowering overall properties.
- There is not enough clinical evidence to draw robust conclusions about its performance. Early, short-term studies suggest performance similar to conventional cements and traditional luting cements.

INTRODUCTION

In the last two decades, the increased demand for esthetics in dentistry has resulted in significant improvements in metal-free restorations, from indirect resin composites to various categories of ceramic materials. Nevertheless, the clinical performance of those esthetic restorative materials relies largely on the luting/bonding procedure. Among the desired features of a luting material for a metal-free restoration are optical characteristics similar to natural dentition, improved mechanical properties to strengthen the final restoration, and ability to bond to multiple substrates. The customarily used conventional luting cements, such as zinc phosphate and glass-ionomer, do not meet these expectations. With the introduction of metal-free indirect restorations, there was an imminent need to develop alternative luting materials. The first resin-based or conventional resin cements introduced to the market required the use of dental adhesives to promote bonding to enamel and dentin. Several studies

Supported by UBC Start-Up grants to A.P. Manso and R.M. Carvalho.
Department of Oral Biological and Medical Sciences, Division of Biomaterials, Faculty of Dentistry, The University of British Columbia, 368-2199 Wesbrook Mall, Vancouver, British Columbia V6T 1Z3, Canada
* Corresponding author. Faculty of Dentistry, The University of British Columbia, 368-2199 Wesbrook Mall, Vancouver, British Columbia V6T 1Z3, Canada.
E-mail address: rickmc@dentistry.ubc.ca

Dent Clin N Am 61 (2017) 821–834
http://dx.doi.org/10.1016/j.cden.2017.06.006
0011-8532/17/© 2017 Elsevier Inc. All rights reserved.

demonstrated that the use of conventional resin cements can improve mechanical properties of metal-free indirect restorations when compared with other luting cements,[1] and this has been directly related to long-term clinical success.[2] However, incompatibility issues between simplified adhesive systems having acidic and hydrophilic characteristics and self- and dual-cured resin cements were reported at the early stage of development of the new resin cements.[3–5] This incompatibility was responsible for directly compromising bond strengths, potentially reducing retention and support for the restorations.

Most clinical procedures involving resin-based luting materials occur under unfavorable circumstances, such as altered and/or deep dentin, subgingival preparations, and sometimes with challenging field isolation. Combined, all these limiting factors can have a significant impact on the adhesive application and subsequent performance when resin cements requiring prebonding are used. However, their use is justified if one considers all the benefits offered by a resin luting material, such as improved mechanical properties, lower solubility, and reinforcement of all-ceramic restorations in comparison with the traditional luting cements.[6,7] Commercially available self-adhesive resin cements (**Table 1**) combine the easy application of conventional luting materials with the improved mechanical properties and bonding capability of the conventional resin cements. The presence of functional acidic monomers, dual cure setting mechanism, and fillers capable of neutralizing the initial low pH of the cement are essential clinically relevant elements of the material that should be understood when selecting the ideal luting material for each particular clinical situation. This review addresses the most relevant aspects of self-adhesive resin cements and their potential impact on clinical performance. The article focuses only on self-adhesive resin cements as the "modern" luting material, because extensive information on traditional

Table 1
Self-adhesive resin cements listed by alphabetical order

Cement	Manufacturer
BeautiCem SA	Shofu Inc
Bifix SE	Voco
BisCem	Bisco Inc
Breeze	Pentron
Calibra Universal	Dentsply
Clearfil SA	Kuraray Noritake Dental
Embrace WetBond	Pulpdent Corporation
G-Cem	GC Corporation
G-Cem LinkAce	GC Corporation
iCem	Heraeus-Kulzer
Maxcem Elite	Kerr
Monocem	Shofu
Panavia SA	Kuraray Noritake Dental
RelyX Unicem	3M/ESPE
RelyX Unicem 2	3M/ESPE
SeT	SDI
Smart Cem 2	Dentsply
SpeedCEM Plus	Ivoclar Vivadent

The list is not intended to cover all products available. Any omission is unintentional.

luting cements and conventional resin cements are covered in several previous publications.[6–8] The clinical performance of self-adhesive resin cements has also been included in this review. Although a limited number of clinical studies are available to establish solid clinical evidence, the information presented aims to provide clinical guidance in the dynamic environment of material development.

CHEMISTRY AND CURING MECHANISM

In general terms, a self-adhesive resin cement is, by nature, a self-etching material during the initial stages of its chemical reaction. Its low pH and high hydrophilicity at early stages after mixing yields good wetting of tooth structure and promotes surface demineralization, similar to what occurs with self-etching adhesives.[9] As the reaction progresses, the acidity of the cement is gradually neutralized because of the reaction with the apatite from dental substrates[10,11] and with the metal oxides present in the basic, acid-soluble inorganic fillers.[9,12,13] In parallel, as the hydrophilic and acidic monomers are consumed by the chemical reactions in situ, the cement becomes more hydrophobic, which is highly desirable in a fully set resin cement to minimize water sorption, hygroscopic expansion, and hydrolytic degradation.[14] Self-adhesive resin cements demonstrate different levels of pH neutralization during their setting reaction. In general, the least pH-neutralization has been observed with the most hydrophilic cements. Additionally, unconsumed, residual acidic monomers can have an impact on the polymerization reaction of the cement, especially by inhibiting the action of the amine accelerator required for the camphor quinone–amine photo initiator system present in essentially all current cement systems[15] (**Fig. 1**).

Self-adhesive resin cements must be presented as two-part materials, usually in separate, individual syringes or in the more popular dual-barrel syringe dispensers. In either case, the components must be separated because of the possibility of premature acid-base interaction between acidic monomers and the ion-leachable glass fillers, the need to separate the self-curing chemical components, and the need to isolate the tertiary amine used in the photo curing mechanism from the acidic monomers.[9] The main constituents of any self-adhesive resin cement are the predominant functional acidic monomers (**Table 2**), conventional di-methacrylate monomers (eg, bis-GMA, UDMA, and TEGDMA), filler particles, and activator-initiator systems. The manufacturer's challenge is to create an adequate balance between the acidic/hydrophilic monomers and the conventional/hydrophobic monomers to promote the required initial self-adhesion from the former and ultimately the desired long-term stability for optimal clinical performance from the polymer produced by the latter.

Current self-adhesive resin cements are dual-cure resin materials that rely on light-cure and chemical-cure activation to convert monomers into polymers. However, the two curing mechanisms are not necessarily integrated and do not always follow the assumption that light-curing supplements self-curing or vice versa.[16] It has been suggested that the early vitrification (polymer network formation) induced by light activation could interfere with the self-polymerization, thus compromising the overall degree of conversion of dual-cure resin cements.[17] More recently, it has been confirmed that insufficient light exposure to self-adhesive resin cement could result in incomplete polymerization, to a level even lower than that of self-curing alone. The authors speculated that because the self-cure mechanism proceeds more slowly, the early vitrification brought on by the initial light activation minimizes the extent of the subsequent self-polymerization of the dual-cure resin cements because of restricted molecular mobility.[18] This has profound clinical implication because it suggests that some

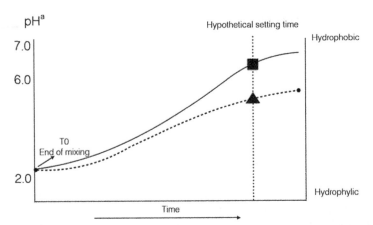

Fig. 1. Schematic representation of the neutralization reaction in self-adhesive resin cements. Under ideal conditions (*solid line*), when the cement is in contact with dentin and enamel, the neutralization reaction progresses as the acidic monomers are neutralized by the dental structures and the fillers, causing the pH to increase, thus turning the cement more hydrophobic and leaving no residual acidity. At the setting time for that particular cement (*square*), it cures to its maximum capacity and is hydrophobic, thus less prone to water sorption over time. Conversely, when conditions are not ideal (*dashed line*) for the neutralization to occur, such as when the cement is in contact with core build-up material, the pH rises more slowly because neutralization relies exclusively on the reaction with the fillers and it may never reach neutrality during the setting time and beyond (*triangle*). This leaves residual acidic monomers that can further compromise the curing, thus rendering a cement layer more prone to water sorption and its negative consequences on the properties of the cement.[a] The pH values are arbitrary and only show that neutralization of the acidic monomers raises the pH during the setting of the cement. Slight acidity may be expected even under ideal conditions after up to 24 hours for some cements.

materials may benefit from delayed light-activation, contrary to common belief and most manufacturer instructions.

Self-adhesive resin cements usually present a significant delayed initial polymerization rate because of the presence of acidic functional monomers, which can deactivate free radicals and compromise the curing reaction. This delayed polymerization can last from 24 hours to 7 days, depending on the product.[19] The amount/ratio of self-curing to light-curing components can vary considerably among different commercially available self-adhesive cements, and this may affect how well the material is expected to cure under conditions with less than ideal light exposure, such as under thick inlays or crowns. It is important, however, to highlight that the ability

Table 2
Functional acidic monomers commonly used in self-adhesive resin cements

Monomer Abbreviation	Complete Monomer Name
BMP	bis(2-methacryloxyethyl) acid phosphate
MDP	10-methacryloyloxydecyl dihydrogen phosphate
Penta-P	Dipentaerythritol penta-acrylate monophosphate
Phenyl-P	2-methacryl-oxyethyl phenyl hydrogen phosphate
PMGDM	Pyromellitic glycerol dimetracrylate
4-META	4-methacryloxyethyl trimellitic anhydride

of a self-adhesive resin cement to cure under clinical conditions depends on a multitude of factors. For instance, if the cementing substrate is mostly comprised of resin build-up material or amalgam or a metal casting, or any material other than dentin or enamel, the necessary neutralization of the acidic monomers can be significantly affected and, therefore, the amount of residual acidity may unbalance the setting reaction, likely reducing the curing rate, delaying final setting, and ultimately compromising the overall polymerization of the cement. These deleterious effects could result in a cement with increased water sorption. Unfortunately, most studies investigating bonding and curing of self-adhesive resin cements are conducted on dental substrates (mostly dentin), and the information on the behavior of the cements when in contact with other substrates is generally lacking.

Another aspect that directly affects the chemistry and curing of resin cements is storage temperature. Excessive (prolonged) heat during storage (>30°C) can have detrimental effects on the acidic monomers, and the components responsible for the self-curing reaction, and significantly alter working and setting time, either extending or reducing them depending on which component is more affected by heat.[20] It is recommended to store self-adhesive resin cements in a cool place (4°C–18°C) and to bring them to room temperature before using.

pH-NEUTRALIZATION, SORPTION, AND SOLUBILITY

Sorption of a resin cement has an important impact on the durability of the indirect restoration. Materials more prone to excessive water sorption are under increased risk of causing weakening and fracture of the indirect restoration.[21] In contrast, a slight water sorption may have a crucial role in compensating polymerization shrinkage, and possibly improving marginal seal.[22] Although sorption causes swelling and mass gain,[23] solubility reflects the released amount of unreacted monomers, and some filler particles and ions, resulting in loss of mass.[24,25] Different levels of sorption and solubility are observed in self-adhesive resin cements because of the differences in their chemical composition, mainly the organic matrices.[12,15,25] The amount of hydrophilic components,[25] cross-linking density and porosity,[26] and amount of acidic monomers or type of polar functional groups in the formulation have been shown to play an important role in these properties.[26–28] When self-adhesive resin cements are compared with conventional resin cements, the former are generally more prone to water sorption. The factor that determines the extent to which each material absorbs water is not the initial number of acidic groups, but the amount of remaining acidic groups that have not been neutralized during the setting reaction.[15] This supports the importance of neutralization of the acidic components to reduce water sorption and solubility, and further calls attention to situations when the prosthesis is cemented on materials other than dentin or enamel, when neutralization might be compromised.

It is clear that neutralization during setting plays a significant role in the performance of self-adhesive resin cements at multiple levels. Initially, a low pH and high hydrophilicity is desired in a self-adhesive resin cement to favor good wetting and bonding to the tooth substrate. During demineralization, functional acidic monomers are gradually neutralized by the reaction with the hydroxyapatite and fillers as previously described. Once adhesion is achieved, the pH would ideally increase,[10] and the material would turn more hydrophobic and, consequently, less susceptible to hydrolysis over time. Although the pH neutralization mechanism is considered a basic chemical setting process intrinsic to all self-adhesive resin cements, it varies significantly among available products.[29] A recent study found that self-adhesive resin cements with lower pH neutralization capacity displayed higher residual hydrophilicity and higher hygroscopic expansion.[14] Among the materials evaluated in the study, RelyX Unicem 2 (3M/ESPE, St. Paul, MN, USA), ICem (Heraeus-Kulzer, Hanau, Germany), and MaxCem Elite (Kerr, Orange, CA, USA) presented initial pHs of 3.8, 2.9, and 3.9, respectively. However, the pH increases over a period of 24 hours were significantly different, being 24.1% for RelyX Unicem 2, 11.7% for ICem, and 5.5% for MaxCem Elite, with the corresponding free expansion stresses observed as 14.5 MPa, 29.1 MPa, and 21.0 MPa, respectively. It is obvious that residual hydrophilicity can lead to water sorption and significant hygroscopic expansion stresses during and after the setting reaction. Thus, when a self-adhesive resin cement is the preferred clinical option, it is recommended to use cements with strong neutralization reactions, resulting in low hygroscopic expansion stresses.[14,30] One should keep in mind that these studies did not account for the additional neutralization that might occur when the cement is in contact with dentin or enamel. However, the results discussed previously provide an indication of what could happen when there is no dental substrate to help neutralization and the process relies exclusively on the intrinsic self-neutralization reaction of the cement.

MECHANICAL PROPERTIES

Improved properties is one of the reasons why clinicians have been shifting from conventional luting materials (zinc phosphate, zinc polycarboxylate, and glass-ionomer cements) to resin-based luting materials. Studies have demonstrated that self-adhesive resin cements are mechanically stronger than conventional, nonresin-based materials,[31] and some present flexural strength similar to conventional resin cements.[32] However, it has been observed that flexural properties and wear resistance can vary widely among commercial self-adhesive resin cements, and in general, self-adhesive cements have lower mechanical properties than conventional resin cements.[33] Nevertheless, self-adhesive resin cements are a viable clinical alternative concerning their mechanical properties, especially in cases when the benefits of a self-adhesive luting procedure surpass the need for maximum mechanical properties, such as cementation of fiber posts, monolithic zirconia crowns, and PFM crowns when moisture control is challenging for adhesive application.

BONDING TO RELEVANT SUBSTRATES

Self-adhesive resin cements do not require that a bonding agent or dental adhesive be placed before cementation. However, many self-adhesive resin cements can benefit from additional surface treatments before cementation to improve performance.[34–36] A complete understanding of how self-adhesive resin cements interact with the multiple bonding substrates present clinically can play a significant role in the decision-making process when selecting the best material for a particular clinical scenario. For a summary of clinical bonding protocols, please refer to **Table 3**.

Natural Dental Substrates: Enamel and Dentin

Self-adhesive resin cements are expected to simultaneously demineralize and infiltrate enamel and dentin. Even though micromechanical retention and chemical interaction between acidic groups and hydroxyapatite are expected, self-adhesive resin cements interact only superficially with dental hard tissues.[11,13,37]

Enamel bonding with self-adhesive resin cements can be compared with self-etching adhesive systems. The acidic monomers present in the composition of self-adhesive cements provide lower interprismatic hybridization and, consequently, weaker bond strengths compared with conventional hybridization techniques with

Table 3
Suggested surface treatment protocol before cementing with self-adhesive resin cements

Substrate	Suggested Procedures
Enamel	• Not suitable for direct bonding with self-adhesive resin cements • Phosphoric acid etch and bond of enamel is recommended if self-adhesive resin cements are used
Dentine	• Clean gross debris from temporary materials with hand instruments • Pumice the surface for complete surface cleaning; rinse well • Intraoral light sandblasting may be used to help cleaning • Polyacrylic acid (10%–25%) may also be used to clean and enhance bonding; do not use any chemical cleaning agent or strong acids • Do not overdry dentine before cementing
Core materials (resin build-up, metal cast, or amalgam core)	• Clean with hand instruments • Light intraoral sandblasting if available or slight bur roughening • Metal primers can be used as per manufacturer's instructions
Glass-matrix ceramics and lithium-disilicate ceramic	• Etch with hydrofluoric acid followed by silanization and bonding agent • Use proprietary, accompanying products of the cement brand if available • Follow respective manufacturer's instructions
Zirconia	• Light sandblasting followed by MDP-containing zirconia primer

the separate etching and bonding approach.[38] The functional acidic monomers are generally weaker when compared with traditional phosphoric acid etching and thus have reduced capacity to demineralize enamel. Bond strengths to enamel are usually low and make self-adhesive resin cements unsuitable for cementing veneers. For example, selective enamel etching is considered an alternative approach for creating increased bond strengths, producing results comparable with conventional resin cements.[36–38] Clinically, the selective enamel etch process has been proven to significantly increase retention and survival rate of partial ceramic crowns, particularly in complex restorations with extensive core build-ups or cavity linings, and reduced amount of exposed dentin and enamel available for bonding.[39]

Dentin bonding, conversely, does not benefit from phosphoric acid etching before self-adhesive resin cement application. Pre-etching has been shown to diminish the effectiveness of the bond, probably because of inadequate resin cement infiltration into the exposed collagen fibril network.[37,38] Some studies have demonstrated that the use of polyacrylic acid instead of phosphoric acid can have a positive impact on the bonding performance of self-adhesive resin cements to dentin,[35,40] but there are conflicting results. The optimal concentration of polyacrylic acid is not clearly established, but may vary from 10% up to 25%. It is assumed that there is a potential influence of the concentration of the polyacrylic acid and the respective acidity (pH). For instance, 20% polyacrylic acid has a reported pH of around 1.0,[41,42] whereas 10% polyacrylic acid is around 2.0.[43] These differences might account for rendering dentin surfaces more or less suitable for self-adhesive resin cements. More directed studies are required before the application of polyacrylic acid is routinely recommended before self-adhesive resin cements, and one should consider the benefit of the procedure against adding another step to the process.

In the clinical scenario, the presence of remnants of provisional cements can adversely affect the performance of self-adhesive resin cements. Application of different cleaning treatments to dentin before bonding can have effects ranging from simple removal of contaminants to total or partial removal of the smear layer.[44] A study found that the ideal cleaning treatment before bonding with RelyX Unicem was achieved by sandblasting the dentin surface. The same study demonstrated that either 0.12% chlorhexidine digluconate or 40% polyacrylic acid were not able to significantly increase shear bond strength when compared with a hand instrumentation cleaning protocol.[34] It is valid to highlight that the viscosity of some self-adhesive resin cements can also be partially responsible for a limited diffusion into the exposed dentinal tubules treated by the polyacrylic acid.[45] Cleaning the substrate before bonding with a self-adhesive resin cement seems a logical, required clinical procedure, but it is currently unclear as to the best approach to be used routinely. When additional retention to dentin is desirable, it seems that hand instrument cleaning followed by mild polyacrylic acid (ie, 10%–20%) or brief sandblasting are safe to use, but one should avoid strong acids (eg, phosphoric acid or highly concentrated polyacrylic acid) or other cleaning solutions with unknown interactions with the chemistry of self-adhesive resin cements.

Cementation of posts to radicular dentin is another clinical scenario that faces numerous challenges, especially when resinous materials are to be used. The main reason for failure of fiber posts is debonding of the resin cement from the radicular dentin.[46] Several aspects create challenges when using an adhesive system followed by conventional resin cements for luting posts, such as ideal moisture control, proper adhesive application, and subsequent light curing of the cement.[47] In this particular scenario, the use of self-adhesive resin cements seems to be a suitable and perhaps less technique-sensitive option than other luting strategies that may involve pretreating the difficult-to-access canals with adhesives.

A recent systematic review with meta-analysis of in vitro studies suggests that the use of self-adhesive resin cement could improve the retention of fiber posts into root canals.[48] Authors attributed the result to the bonding properties of self-adhesive resin cements, which create micromechanical retention and chemical bonding, greater moisture tolerance,[49] and lower polymerization stress compared with conventional resin cements.[50] Perhaps even more relevant clinically is the elimination of the technique sensitivity associated with intracanal bonding when conventional resin cements are used with separate adhesives.

Ceramic Substrates

Today, numerous ceramic products are available and a thorough understanding of the ideal luting material and surface treatment for each ceramic is crucial. More recently, new resin-matrix ceramic materials have been introduced, creating a new category of esthetic indirect restorative materials to which clinicians need to bond.[51] Even though dental ceramics are regarded as strong materials, it is well known that using a luting agent with bonding capability and enhanced mechanical properties is necessary for their durability because it significantly increases fracture resistance.[52] In general, resin cements meet those requirements and are the preferred choice as luting materials for all ceramic restorations.

Glass matrix ceramics are essentially nonmetallic inorganic ceramics containing a glass phase. They are represented by the traditional feldspathic ceramics; the synthetic ceramics, such as leucite, lithium disilicate, and fluorapatite ceramics; and the glass infiltrated ceramics, such as alumina (In-Ceram, Vita/Sirona, Bensheim, Germany). These ceramics allow for chemical treatment of the internal surface to improve retention, usually with hydrofluoric acid gels followed by silanization.[53] Recommended for all glass matrix ceramics, silanization has been shown to reduce the contact angle and increase the wettability of the ceramic surface,[54] making it a suitable substrate for resin cements. The combination of hydrofluoric acid etching and silanization is currently the standard, recommended procedure for bonding resin cements, including self-adhesive, to glass matrix ceramics.[55] Self-adhesive resin cements are not the best choice for cementing veneers. Although a good bond is accomplished to the veneer after hydrofluoric acid etching, silanization, and adhesive bonding, the bonding to the dental substrate (usually enamel) is weak and may result in early clinical dislodgment of the veneer. Light-cured-only cements remain the best option for cementing veneers. These cements do not contain certain amines required for the self-curing reaction that have been shown to discolor, and thus the light-cure-only cements are the most color stable.

Polycrystalline ceramics, which in general contain metal oxides, are represented by alumina ceramic (Procera All Ceram, Nobel Biocare Zurich, Switzerland) and stabilized zirconia (Procera Zr, Nobel Biocare; Lava Plus, 3M ESPE; In-Ceram Zr, Vita; IPS e-max ZirCad, Ivoclar Vivadent, Amherst, NY, USA).[51] It is known that the cement choice is less important to the clinical success when cementing zirconia prosthesis. The intaglio surface treatment, however, with light-pressure sandblasting combined with MDP-containing primers seems crucial for optimal long-term performance of conventional and self-adhesive resin cements.[56–59] In general, the application of universal primers (zirconia primers) alone, without prior airborne-particle abrasion (ie, light sandblasting), does not seem to improve adhesion of resin cements to zirconia.[60] The question, however, remains to be answered whether air-abrasion protocols exert detrimental effects on the fatigue strength of zirconia.[61] Recently, systematic reviews on adhesion to zirconia have demonstrated that the use of MDP-based self-adhesive cements after physicochemical conditioning of zirconia surface presented more favorable results.[56,58] Although water storage can affect the bond strength of resin cements to zirconia,[62] a meta-analysis found no difference among the cements for the aged-dataset, which may confirm that the cement choice is less essential to the durability of zirconia bonding, at least when resin cements are used.[58] The major reason for failures in porcelain-veneered zirconia crowns is chipping and fracture of the veneering ceramic.[61,63] As monolithic zirconia crowns become available and increasingly acceptable because of improvements in their optical appearance, chipping of the veneering ceramic may no longer be a clinical problem and, therefore, the clinical success of zirconia crowns will likely be more dependent on the retention capacity provided by the surface treatment and cement choice, leaving the clinician the responsibility of choosing the most appropriate, and evidence-based, cementation protocol.

Resin-matrix ceramics are essentially an organic matrix highly filled with ceramic particles (>50% by weight). Few studies have investigated the best resin cement and bonding protocol for this novel category of materials. The manufacturer's recommendations for each of these materials vary. Although hydrofluoric acid etching apparently is not the appropriate method for surface conditioning of resin-matrix ceramics, surface mechanical roughening followed by adhesive application seems promising.[64] A recent study found varied results for Vita Enamic (Vita Zahnfabrik, Langen, Germany) and Lava Ultimate (3M ESPE) resin-matrix ceramic blocks regarding optimal surface treatment and resin cement choice.[65] For Lava Ultimate, a composite formed of a resinous matrix highly filled with silica and zirconia particles, the most influential parameter was mechanical pretreatment; however, hydrofluoric acid (HF) acid etching had a significant positive effect on bond strength. Regarding the resin cement, the self-adhesive material presented significantly higher bond strengths to Lava Ultimate than the conventional resin cement.[65] Lava Ultimate is still indicated for inlays, onlays, and veneers; however, the manufacturer has removed the crown indication since June 2015 because of higher rates of premature debonding. In contrast, surface treatment had little impact when bonding to Vita Enamic, which is essentially a ceramic structure infiltrated with a resin. Optimal surface treatments were either silane application alone or HF followed by silane, as recommended by the manufacturer. However, the self-adhesive resin cement used presented overall lower bond strengths than the conventional resin cement within the same surface treatment group.[65] Because this category of indirect materials is new to the market, few studies are currently available to offer consistent guidance regarding the clinical protocol for bonding and cementing. Considering the studies available, it is clear that optimal cementation protocol (and consequently clinical retention) is material-dependent and closely following the respective manufacturer's instructions is warranted at this time.

CLINICAL PERFORMANCE OF SELF-ADHESIVE RESIN CEMENTS

RelyX Unicem is by far the most investigated product in clinical studies; however, long-term studies are still lacking.[66] Clinical studies have demonstrated that selective enamel etching before self-adhesive luting procedure with lithium disilicate inlays had no significant influence on marginal integrity when compared with the nonetched controls.[2,67] The authors, however, recognized that the findings were not conclusive and longer-term evaluation is still needed. A 12-month clinical evaluation of indirect resin composites luted with self-adhesive or conventional resin cements observed that both luting materials performed similarly, but this is not surprising because little or no difference between materials is what is usually expected at the early 1-year clinical evaluation.[68] When a self-adhesive resin cement was clinically compared with zinc phosphate for luting metal-based fixed partial dentures at a mean observation time of 3 years, none of the 49 prostheses was lost, regardless of the cement used,[69] suggesting that self-adhesive resin cements performed similarly to zinc phosphate luting materials within that 3-year time frame. Of clinical relevance was the finding that plaque accumulation and bleeding score were higher around prostheses cemented with the resin cement. Factors that possibly accounted for this finding were the content of resins and the resulting bacterial colonization on their surfaces; the bonding of the resin cement, which is not so easily removed from the sulcus; and the high solubility of zinc phosphate cement (ie, release of potentially antimicrobial zinc ions), which may be an advantage to repel microorganisms from the margins in the long term.[69] Conversely, other authors found less gingival inflammation around restorations cemented with self-adhesive resin cements.[70]

A recent review presented the current status of clinical studies on self-adhesive resin cements.[66] The review found only three studies comparing self-adhesive resin cements with traditional cements, none of them identifying retention loss either for self-adhesive resin cements or other traditional luting agents. Comparable clinical results were also found between conventional resin cements and self-adhesive resin cements as luting agent for inlays and onlays up to 4 years follow-up.[67,71] It is clear that more sophisticated clinical investigations of these new types of cements are required. The lack of consistent and relevant clinical studies on the performance of self-adhesive resin cements presents a limitation for a robust analysis of this category of resin cement. However, there is a good amount of sound laboratory investigations that can support clinicians in their decision.[66]

SUMMARY

Self-adhesive resin cements are considered as alternative luting cements with multiple applications in modern dentistry. However, one must consider the material's chemistry, bonding, and mechanical requirements for each particular clinical scenario, and the limitations that are intrinsic to the nature of the material. Clinical studies are still insufficient to completely understand the material clinical performance.

REFERENCES

1. Addison O, Marquis PM, Fleming GJ. Quantifying the strength of a resin-coated dental ceramic. J Dent Res 2008;87(6):542–7.
2. Peumans M, De Munck J, Van Landuyt K, et al. Two-year clinical evaluation of a self-adhesive luting agent for ceramic inlays. J Adhes Dent 2010;12(2):151–61.
3. Suh BI, Feng L, Pashley DH, et al. Factors contributing to the incompatibility between simplified-step adhesives and chemically-cured or dual-cured composites. Part III. Effect of acidic resin monomers. J Adhes Dent 2003;5(4):267–82.
4. Cheong C, King NM, Pashley DH, et al. Incompatibility of self-etch adhesives with chemical/dual-cured composites: two-step vs one-step systems. Oper Dent 2003;28(6):747–55.
5. Sanares AM, Itthagarun A, King NM, et al. Adverse surface interactions between one-bottle light-cured adhesives and chemical-cured composites. Dent Mater 2001;17(6):542–56.
6. Manso AP, Silva NR, Bonfante EA, et al. Cements and adhesives for all-ceramic restorations. Dent Clin North Am 2011;55(2):311–32, ix.
7. Diaz-Arnold AM, Vargas MA, Haselton DR. Current status of luting agents for fixed prosthodontics. J Prosthet Dent 1999;81(2):135–41.
8. Pegoraro TA, da Silva NR, Carvalho RM. Cements for use in esthetic dentistry. Dent Clin North Am 2007;51(2):453–71, x.
9. Ferracane JL, Stansbury JW, Burke FJ. Self-adhesive resin cements: chemistry, properties and clinical considerations. J Oral Rehabil 2011;38(4):295–314.
10. Madruga FC, Ogliari FA, Ramos TS, et al. Calcium hydroxide, pH-neutralization and formulation of model self-adhesive resin cements. Dent Mater 2013;29(4):413–8.
11. Gerth HU, Dammaschke T, Zuchner H, et al. Chemical analysis and bonding reaction of RelyX Unicem and Bifix composites: a comparative study. Dent Mater 2006;22(10):934–41.
12. Marghalani HY. Sorption and solubility characteristics of self-adhesive resin cements. Dent Mater 2012;28(10):e187–98.
13. Radovic I, Monticelli F, Goracci C, et al. Self-adhesive resin cements: a literature review. J Adhes Dent 2008;10(4):251–8.
14. Roedel L, Bednarzig V, Belli R, et al. Self-adhesive resin cements: pH-neutralization, hydrophilicity, and hygroscopic expansion stress. Clin Oral Investig 2016;21:1735–41.
15. Vrochari AD, Eliades G, Hellwig E, et al. Water sorption and solubility of four self-etching, self-adhesive resin luting agents. J Adhes Dent 2010;12(1):39–43.
16. Leprince JG, Palin WM, Hadis MA, et al. Progress in dimethacrylate-based dental composite technology and curing efficiency. Dent Mater 2013;29(2):139–56.
17. Meng X, Yoshida K, Atsuta M. Influence of ceramic thickness on mechanical properties and polymer structure of dual-cured resin luting agents. Dent Mater 2008;24(5):594–9.
18. Jang Y, Ferracane JL, Pfeifer CS, et al. Effect of insufficient light exposure on polymerization kinetics of conventional and self-adhesive dual-cure resin cements. Oper Dent 2016;42:E1–9.

19. Baena E, Fuentes MV, Garrido MA, et al. Influence of post-cure time on the micro-hardness of self-adhesive resin cements inside the root canal. Oper Dent 2012; 37(5):548–56.

20. Pegoraro TA, Fulgencio R, Butignon LE, et al. Effects of temperature and aging on working/setting time of dual-cured resin cements. Oper Dent 2015;40(6):E222–9.

21. Leevailoj C, Platt JA, Cochran MA, et al. In vitro study of fracture incidence and compressive fracture load of all-ceramic crowns cemented with resin-modified glass ionomer and other luting agents. J Prosthet Dent 1998;80(6):699–707.

22. Feilzer AJ, de Gee AJ, Davidson CL. Relaxation of polymerization contraction shear stress by hygroscopic expansion. J Dent Res 1990;69(1):36–9.

23. Ortengren U, Andersson F, Elgh U, et al. Influence of pH and storage time on the sorption and solubility behaviour of three composite resin materials. J Dent 2001; 29(1):35–41.

24. Ferracane JL. Hygroscopic and hydrolytic effects in dental polymer networks. Dent Mater 2006;22(3):211–22.

25. Ito S, Hashimoto M, Wadgaonkar B, et al. Effects of resin hydrophilicity on water sorption and changes in modulus of elasticity. Biomaterials 2005;26(33):6449–59.

26. Beatty MW, Swartz ML, Moore BK, et al. Effect of crosslinking agent content, monomer functionality, and repeat unit chemistry on properties of unfilled resins. J Biomed Mater Res 1993;27(3):403–13.

27. Kerby RE, Knobloch LA, Schricker S, et al. Synthesis and evaluation of modified urethane dimethacrylate resins with reduced water sorption and solubility. Dent Mater 2009;25(3):302–13.

28. Tanaka J, Hashimoto T, Stansbury JW, et al. Polymer properties on resins composed of UDMA and methacrylates with the carboxyl group. Dent Mater J 2001;20(3):206–15.

29. Zorzin J, Petschelt A, Ebert J, et al. pH neutralization and influence on mechanical strength in self-adhesive resin luting agents. Dent Mater 2012;28(6):672–9.

30. Sterzenbach G, Karajouli G, Tunjan R, et al. Damage of lithium-disilicate all-ceramic restorations by an experimental self-adhesive resin cement used as core build-ups. Clin Oral Investig 2015;19(2):281–8.

31. Piwowarczyk A, Lauer HC. Mechanical properties of luting cements after water storage. Oper Dent 2003;28(5):535–42.

32. Saskalauskaite E, Tam LE, McComb D. Flexural strength, elastic modulus, and pH profile of self-etch resin luting cements. J Prosthodont 2008;17(4):262–8.

33. Furuichi T, Takamizawa T, Tsujimoto A, et al. Mechanical properties and sliding-impact wear resistance of self-adhesive resin cements. Oper Dent 2016;41(3): E83–92.

34. Santos MJ, Bapoo H, Rizkalla AS, et al. Effect of dentin-cleaning techniques on the shear bond strength of self-adhesive resin luting cement to dentin. Oper Dent 2011;36(5):512–20.

35. Stona P, Borges GA, Montes MA, et al. Effect of polyacrylic acid on the interface and bond strength of self-adhesive resin cements to dentin. J Adhes Dent 2013; 15(3):221–7.

36. Benetti P, Fernandes VV, Torres CR, et al. Bonding efficacy of new self-etching, self-adhesive dual-curing resin cements to dental enamel. J Adhes Dent 2011; 13(3):231–4.

37. De Munck J, Vargas M, Van Landuyt K, et al. Bonding of an auto-adhesive luting material to enamel and dentin. Dent Mater 2004;20(10):963–71.

38. Hikita K, Van Meerbeek B, De Munck J, et al. Bonding effectiveness of adhesive luting agents to enamel and dentin. Dent Mater 2007;23(1):71–80.

39. Baader K, Hiller KA, Buchalla W, et al. Self-adhesive luting of partial ceramic crowns: selective enamel etching leads to higher survival after 6.5 years in vivo. J Adhes Dent 2016;18(1):69–79.

40. Pavan S, dos Santos PH, Berger S, et al. The effect of dentin pretreatment on the microtensile bond strength of self-adhesive resin cements. J Prosthet Dent 2010; 104(4):258–64.

41. Al-Assaf K, Chakmakchi M, Palaghias G, et al. Interfacial characteristics of adhesive luting resins and composites with dentin. Dent Mater 2007;23(7):829–39.

42. Gordan VV. Effect of conditioning times on resin-modified glass-ionomer bonding. Am J Dent 2000;13(1):13–6.

43. Tanumiharja M, Burrow MF, Tyas MJ. Microtensile bond strengths of glass ionomer (polyalkenoate) cements to dentin using four conditioners. J Dent 2000; 28(5):361–6.

44. Sarac D, Bulucu B, Sarac YS, et al. The effect of dentin-cleaning agents on resin cement bond strength to dentin. J Am Dent Assoc 2008;139(6):751–8.

45. Mazzitelli C, Monticelli F, Toledano M, et al. Dentin treatment effects on the bonding performance of self-adhesive resin cements. Eur J Oral Sci 2010; 118(1):80–6.

46. Rasimick BJ, Wan J, Musikant BL, et al. A review of failure modes in teeth restored with adhesively luted endodontic dowels. J Prosthodont 2010;19(8):639–46.

47. Naumann M, Koelpin M, Beuer F, et al. 10-year survival evaluation for glass-fiber-supported postendodontic restoration: a prospective observational clinical study. J Endod 2012;38(4):432–5.

48. Sarkis-Onofre R, Skupien JA, Cenci MS, et al. The role of resin cement on bond strength of glass-fiber posts luted into root canals: a systematic review and meta-analysis of in vitro studies. Oper Dent 2014;39(1):E31–44.

49. Bitter K, Aschendorff L, Neumann K, et al. Do chlorhexidine and ethanol improve bond strength and durability of adhesion of fiber posts inside the root canal? Clin Oral Investig 2014;18(3):927–34.

50. Frassetto A, Navarra CO, Marchesi G, et al. Kinetics of polymerization and contraction stress development in self-adhesive resin cements. Dent Mater 2012;28(9):1032–9.

51. Gracis S, Thompson VP, Ferencz JL, et al. A new classification system for all-ceramic and ceramic-like restorative materials. Int J Prosthodont 2015;28(3): 227–35.

52. Pagniano RP, Seghi RR, Rosenstiel SF, et al. The effect of a layer of resin luting agent on the biaxial flexure strength of two all-ceramic systems. J Prosthet Dent 2005;93(5):459–66.

53. Pattanaik S, Wadkar AP. Effect of etchant variability on shear bond strength of all ceramic restorations: an in vitro study. J Indian Prosthodont Soc 2011;11(1): 55–62.

54. Meng X, Yoshida K, Taira Y, et al. Effect of siloxane quantity and pH of silane coupling agents and contact angle of resin bonding agent on bond durability of resin cements to machinable ceramic. J Adhes Dent 2011;13(1):71–8.

55. Tian T, Tsoi JK, Matinlinna JP, et al. Aspects of bonding between resin luting cements and glass ceramic materials. Dent Mater 2014;30(7):e147–62.

56. Ozcan M, Bernasconi M. Adhesion to zirconia used for dental restorations: a systematic review and meta-analysis. J Adhes Dent 2015;17(1):7–26.

57. Yi YA, Ahn JS, Park YJ, et al. The effect of sandblasting and different primers on shear bond strength between yttria-tetragonal zirconia polycrystal ceramic and a self-adhesive resin cement. Oper Dent 2015;40(1):63–71.

58. Inokoshi M, De Munck J, Minakuchi S, et al. Meta-analysis of bonding effectiveness to zirconia ceramics. J Dent Res 2014;93(4):329–34.

59. Kern M, Barloi A, Yang B. Surface conditioning influences zirconia ceramic bonding. J Dent Res 2009;88(9):817–22.

60. Pereira Lde L, Campos F, Dal Piva AM, et al. Can application of universal primers alone be a substitute for airborne-particle abrasion to improve adhesion of resin cement to zirconia? J Adhes Dent 2015;17(2):169–74.

61. Guess PC, Zhang Y, Kim JW, et al. Damage and reliability of Y-TZP after cementation surface treatment. J Dent Res 2010;89(6):592–6.

62. de Sa Barbosa WF, Aguiar TR, Francescantonio MD, et al. Effect of water storage on bond strength of self-adhesive resin cements to zirconium oxide ceramic. J Adhes Dent 2013;15(2):145–50.

63. Swain MV. Unstable cracking (chipping) of veneering porcelain on all-ceramic dental crowns and fixed partial dentures. Acta Biomater 2009;5(5):1668–77.

64. Park JH, Choi YS. Microtensile bond strength and micromorphologic analysis of surface-treated resin nanoceramics. J Adv Prosthodont 2016;8(4):275–84.

65. Peumans M, Valjakova EB, De Munck J, et al. Bonding effectiveness of luting composites to different CAD/CAM materials. J Adhes Dent 2016;18(4):289–302.

66. Weiser F, Behr M. Self-adhesive resin cements: a clinical review. J Prosthodont 2015;24(2):100–8.

67. Peumans M, Voet M, De Munck J, et al. Four-year clinical evaluation of a self-adhesive luting agent for ceramic inlays. Clin Oral Investig 2013;17(3):739–50.

68. Marcondes M, Souza N, Manfroi FB, et al. Clinical evaluation of indirect composite resin restorations cemented with different resin cements. J Adhes Dent 2016;18(1):59–67.

69. Behr M, Rosentritt M, Wimmer J, et al. Self-adhesive resin cement versus zinc phosphate luting material: a prospective clinical trial begun 2003. Dent Mater 2009;25(5):601–4.

70. Piwowarczyk A, Schick K, Lauer HC. Metal-ceramic crowns cemented with two luting agents: short-term results of a prospective clinical study. Clin Oral Investig 2012;16(3):917–22.

71. Taschner M, Kramer N, Lohbauer U, et al. Leucite-reinforced glass ceramic inlays luted with self-adhesive resin cement: a 2-year in vivo study. Dent Mater 2012;28(5):535–40.

Biomaterials for Craniofacial Bone Regeneration

Greeshma Thrivikraman, PhD[a], Avathamsa Athirasala, MS[a],
Chelsea Twohig, DDS[a], Sunil Kumar Boda, PhD[b],
Luiz E. Bertassoni, DDS, PhD[a,c,d],*

KEYWORDS

- Tissue engineering • Stem cells • 3D bioprinting • Gene delivery
- Growth factor delivery • Bone regeneration • Calcium phosphate

KEY POINTS

- Calcium phosphate bioceramics remain some of the most widely used biomaterials for bone regeneration, particularly because of their long clinical track-record and well-studied mechanisms.
- Both natural and synthetic polymers, despite their comparatively low rigidity, offer a range of physical and biologic advantages over bioceramics, such as the possibility of controlling 3D cellular microenvironments for stem cell differentiation and tissue regeneration.
- Biomaterials are synthesized and/or manipulated to be used for growth factor, gene, and stem cell delivery applications with increasingly more successful outcomes.
- 3D printing and bioprinting have already revolutionized bone regeneration, and it is likely that the next generation of biomaterials for bone regeneration will take advantage of some method of 3D printing.

INTRODUCTION

Craniofacial bone regeneration has experienced tremendous expansion since the inception of the concept of tissue engineering[1] more than two decades ago. Research and development in the area of bone augmentation has contributed significantly to the

[a] Division of Biomaterials and Biomechanics, Department of Restorative Dentistry, OHSU School of Dentistry, 2730 SW Moody Avenue, Portland, OR 97201, USA; [b] Mary and Dick Holland Regenerative Medicine Program, Department of Surgery-Transplant, University of Nebraska Medical Center, Omaha, NE 68198-5965, USA; [c] Department of Biomedical Engineering, OHSU School of Medicine, 3303 SW Bond Avenue, Portland, OR 97239, USA; [d] OHSU Center for Regenerative Medicine, 3181 SW Sam Jackson Park Road, Portland, OR 97239, USA
* Corresponding author. Department of Restorative Dentistry, OHSU School of Dentistry, 2730 SW Moody Avenue, Portland, OR 97201.
E-mail address: bertasso@ohsu.edu

Dent Clin N Am 61 (2017) 835–856
http://dx.doi.org/10.1016/j.cden.2017.06.003
0011-8532/17/© 2017 Elsevier Inc. All rights reserved.

establishment of tissue engineering as a viable treatment option in medicine and dentistry.[2] Biomaterials represent a fundamental aspect of bone regeneration. It is widely recognized that biomaterials can be tailored to regulate the microenvironment in which cells reside during the process of new bone formation. This essentially means that the ability to manipulate the composition, architecture, and properties of different biomaterials allows one to control the rate of regeneration, and ideally enhance the process of new bone formation.[2,3]

Biomaterials are generally used as biocompatible scaffold systems that allow for the migration, proliferation, and differentiation of either resident or externally delivered cells, which are used to promote new bone formation. A wide variety of biomaterials have been used for craniofacial bone augmentation. These are typically divided into either organic or inorganic materials, where calcium phosphate (CaP) bioceramics represent most inorganic scaffolds, and natural or synthetic biopolymers form the most organic scaffolds. The basic rational behind such materials choice is based on a reductionist attempt to mimic the organic-inorganic composition of native bone, where collagen fibrils (a natural organic polymer) are reinforced with hydroxyapatite (HA) crystallites (a natural bioceramic) to form a strong and durable natural biomaterial.

This article reviews recent developments in the translation of biomaterials design and fabrication for clinical strategies of craniofacial bone augmentation. We describe recently reported aspects of CaP bioceramic regenerative materials, recent work on the synthesis and applications of natural and synthetic polymeric hydrogels, and protein delivery in the form of plasma rich fibrin, and hybrids of organic/inorganic scaffolds. Also discussed is the use of biomaterials as tools to enable the effective delivery of growth factors (GFs), stem cells, and gene therapy. Finally, we review recent developments in the three-dimensional (3D) printing of regenerative scaffold materials for craniofacial bone augmentation.

BIOCERAMICS
Calcium Phosphate Scaffolds and Cements

Bioceramics, such as CaP, calcium carbonates, calcium sulfates, bioactive glasses, and composite materials combining bioactive inorganic materials with biodegradable polymers are some of the most promising biomaterials for application in bone regeneration.[4] Research concerning the ability of CaP bioceramics to stimulate bone growth date back to the 1920s, when an aqueous slurry of "triple CaP" was used to enhance bone formation.[5] Especially since the establishment of tissue engineering as a viable treatment alternative in the late 1990s,[1] research around CaP materials for bone regeneration has expanded tremendously. These materials have received great attention in the bone regeneration community because of their ability to promote rapid bone formation on their surface (**Table 1**). Several reasons have been proposed to explain these advantageous properties, including the great compositional similarities of CaP materials to the main constituent of human bone, HA; the ability of osteoprogenitor cells to process and resorb CaP materials; and the complex yet highly effective intracellular signaling of osteogenesis that is triggered by the presence of soluble calcium and inorganic phosphates[6] resulting from byproducts of CaP crystal dissolution (**Fig. 1**).

Currently there exists a myriad of CaP materials that are commercially available for bone regeneration, and typically these include one or more phases of CaP in different mineral phases, crystal structures, and processing conditions (**Table 2**). Research has shown that the specific mineral phase constituting a CaP biomaterial plays a major role in determining the efficacy of the material for osteogenesis. Importantly, it has

Table 1
Calcium phosphate compounds and their solubility/degradation properties

Name	Chemical Formula	Symbol	Ca/P Ratio	$-\log(K_{sp})$ at 298 K
Monocalcium phosphate monohydrate	$Ca(H_2PO_4)_2 \cdot H_2O$	MCPM	0.5	1.14
Dicalcium phosphate anhydrous	$CaHPO_4$	DCPA	1.0	6.90
Dicalcium phosphate dihydrate	$CaHPO_4 \cdot 2H_2O$	DCPD	1.0	6.59
Octocalcium phosphate	$Ca_8H_2(PO_4)_6 \cdot 5H_2O$	OCP	1.33	96.6
Hydroxyapatite	$Ca_{10}(PO_4)_6(OH)_2$	HA	1.67	116.8
Fluorapatite	$Ca_{10}(PO_4)_6F_2$	FA	1.67	120.0
Monocalcium phosphate anhydrous	$Ca(H_2PO_4)_2$	MCPA	1.67	1.14
α-Tricalcium phosphate	α-$Ca_3(PO_4)_2$	α-TCP	1.5	25.5
β-Tricalcium phosphate	β-$Ca_3(PO_4)_2$	β-TCP	1.5	28.9
Tetracalcium phosphate	$Ca_4(PO_4)_2O$	TTCP	2.0	38.0

The parameter $-\log(K_{sp})$ denotes the solubility product. The lower the $-\log(K_{sp})$ value, the higher is the solubility. Similarly, it can also be noted that acidic products (MCPM) with lower Ca/P ratio have higher solubility compared with basic compounds, such as hydroxyapatite with higher Ca/P ratio. *Adapted from* Refs.[7–9]; with permission.

been demonstrated that the solubility of the CaP mineral phase is a key factor regulating osteoinduction.[10] Initial efforts to develop CaP scaffold materials focused on the synthesis of materials with a similar composition as the mineral found in natural bone, while ensuring high mechanical properties.[11] This was typically achieved by processing CaP grafts to form sintered HA or sintered β-tricalcium phosphate (β-TCP), or combinations thereof. However, the sintering process yields scaffold materials that are too brittle for load-bearing applications, have little injectability in bulk, and very low solubility, which hinders osteoclast-driven biodegradation and scaffold remodeling. The discovery of bone cements constituted of CaP phases that can be formed at room temperature (calcium-deficient HA, brushite, octacalcium phosphate, and monetite) opened up a wide range of possibilities in the manufacture of new CaP bone scaffolds.[11–14] Importantly, these materials have much lower solubility rates and have been shown to transform into a more stable HA phase on implantation.[15–17] It has been suggested that these less crystalline phases with lower solubility than sintered CaPs have superior biologic properties.[10]

Historically, CaP materials have commonly been found in particulate form, but have also been processed as blocks or porous blocks. These have posed relevant limitations on their clinical use, especially in dentistry, since injectable materials have improved handling and less invasive characteristics. Moreover, controlling shape and architecture using particulate materials is often difficult, in comparison with more user-friendly soft/moldable sponges and polymers, which has likely hindered their clinical use for craniofacial applications where larger reconstruction is necessary.

Although the mechanisms of CaP-induced bone formation are still incompletely understood, there currently exists a breadth of preclinical evidence demonstrating the efficacy of these materials for translational applications. A noteworthy study by Yuan and colleagues,[18] for instance, demonstrated that an osteoinductive TCP ceramic material yielded comparable results to an autograft scaffold and scaffolds loaded with a potent osteoinductive growth factor (recombinant human bone morphogenetic protein [rhBMP-2]), where bridging of an ovine critical sized defect was obtained with comparable results regardless of the material used. A series of clinical trials on various commercially available products also point to the promising use of CaP materials for orthopedic and craniofacial bone regeneration. Currently, according to clinicaltrials.gov there are more than 300 clinical trials being conducted in the world testing the effectiveness of CaP materials for bone applications, with 60 already completed in the United States alone, and an additional 58 in Europe.

In summary, although many phases and compositions of CaP have shown the ability to induce bone formation, studies comparing HA with TCP, or of HA with biphasic CaP (consisting of HA with TCP), have generally demonstrated that the presence of a more soluble phase enhances bone formation,[19–21] although some higher degree of stability

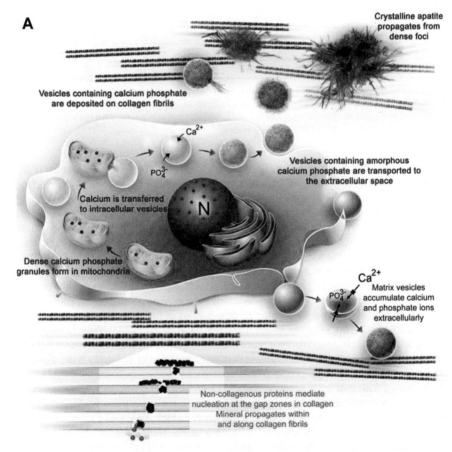

A

Crystalline apatite propagates from dense foci

Vesicles containing calcium phosphate are deposited on collagen fibrils

Ca^{2+}

PO_4^{3-}

Vesicles containing amorphous calcium phosphate are transported to the extracellular space

Calcium is transferred to intracellular vesicles

N

Dense calcium phosphate granules form in mitochondria

Ca^{2+}

PO_4^{3-}

Matrix vesicles accumulate calcium and phosphate ions extracellularly

Non-collagenous proteins mediate nucleation at the gap zones in collagen
Mineral propagates within and along collagen fibrils

Fig. 1. (*A*) Diagram outlining current models proposed for bone mineral formation. Bone apatite formation likely proceeds via several cooperative/redundant mechanisms. Calcium induces (*B*) cell proliferation and (*C*) bone morphogenetic protein-2 expression in human mesenchymal stem cells (hMSCs) treated with Ca^{2+}-enriched medium as compared with control medium. *p < 0.05; **p < 0.01; and ***p < 0.001. ([*A*] *From* Boonrungsiman S, Gentleman E, Carzaniga R, et al. The role of intracellular calcium phosphate in osteoblast-mediated bone apatite formation. Proc Natl Acad Sci U S A 2012;109(35):14174, with permission; and [*B, C*] *Adapted from* Barradas AM, Fernandes HA, Groen N, et al. A calcium-induced signaling cascade leading to osteogenic differentiation of human bone marrow-derived mesenchymal stromal cells. Biomaterials 2012;33(11):3206–8, with permission.)

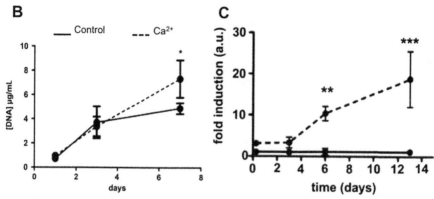

Fig. 1. (*continued*).

Table 2				
List of representative commercially available calcium orthophosphate cements				
Commercial Name	Formulations	End Product	Company Name	Applications
Biopex	75 wt% α-TCP, 18 wt% TTCP, 5 wt% DCPD and 2 wt% HA	Apatite	Mitsubishi Materials (Tokyo, Japan)	Bone defect repair, reinforcement of orthopedic screws and implants, filling gaps between cement-less artificial joints and bone
Norian SRS	MCPM + α-TCP + $CaCO_3$	Apatite	DePuy Synthes (Welwyn Garden City, United Kingdom)	Skeletal distal radius fractures, craniofacial
BoneSource	TTCP (73%), DCPD (27%)	Apatite	Stryker-Leibinger (Kalamazoo, MI)	Craniofacial
ChronOS	β-TCP (73%), MCPM (21%), $MgHPO_4 \cdot 3H_2O$ (5%)	Brushite	DePuy Synthes (West Chester, PA)	Metaphyseal bone defects, cranioplasty, onlay augmentations in the craniomaxillofacial area
α-BSM	ACP (50%), DCPD (50%)	Apatite	ETEX (Cambridge, MA)	Filling of bone defects and voids, dental, craniofacial
Cementek	α-TCP, TTCP	Apatite	Teknimed (Vic-en-Bigorre, France)	Filling of bone defects
Biocement D	58% α-TCP, 24% DCPA, 8.5% $CaCO_3$, 8.5% calcium-deficient HA	Apatite	Merck (GER) Biomet (Darmstadt, Germany)	Filling of bone defects in maxillary surgery
Mimix	TTCP, α-TCP	Apatite	Walter Lorenz Surgical (Jacksonville, FL)	Bony contouring of craniofacial skeleton, craniotomy cuts
Calcibon	α-TCP, DCPA, CaCO3, HA	Carbonated apatite	Biomet Inc (Warsaw, IN)	Filling of noninfected, metaphyseal, cancellous bone defects

in the mineral phase is generally required.[22] Moreover, it has been generally accepted that the surface structural properties of the CaP material, such as microporosity, grain size, and specific surface area for adsorption, play an important role in osteoinduction, perhaps even more so than internal porosity. Internal porosity has long been suggested to be more effective in the range of at least 100 μm,[23,24] although other literature has claimed that not only macrostructural porosity, but rather surface micropores in the range of 100 nm to 10 μm are as important to ensure fast scaffold resorption.[25]

An emerging area in the synthesis of CaP is the ability of ceramic materials to elicit not only osteogenic, but also vasculogenic properties, and it is relevant to highlight that it is unlikely that any regenerative material for bone formation will be successful without considering the challenges associated with bone vascularization. Novel methods of scaffold fabrication combining CaP materials with prefabricated blood vessels and capillaries present an interesting approach moving forward (**Fig. 2**).[26,27]

Bioinorganic Substitution of Calcium Phosphate Materials and Bioglasses

Another area of research involving CaP involves doping. Many trace elements are present in the mineral phase of natural bone. Cationic substitution with Mg or Sr on CaP scaffolds can influence the mechanical properties and biologic responses because of

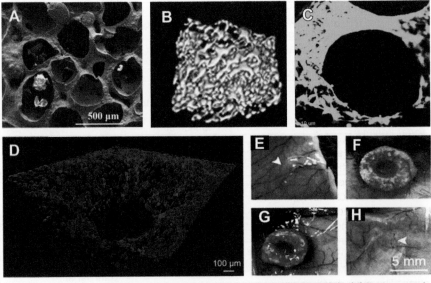

Fig. 2. Porous β-TCP scaffolds with angiogenic and osteogenic potentials. (*A*) Representative scanning electron microscopic image illustrating the 3D porous architecture of β-TCP scaffold. (*B*) Microcomputed tomography images showing interconnected pores of scaffold in 3D. (*C*) Fluorescent image showing the robust proliferation of human umbilical vein endothelial cells (HUVEC) after 7 days of culture. (*D*) Immunofluorescent image depicting the endothelium-lined microchannels of collagen-infiltrated, macroporous β-TCP scaffold. (*E–H*) Photographs showing the subcutaneous implantation of four types of implants: collagen/HUVEC (*E*), collagen/HUVEC/β-TCP (*F*), collagen/channel/β-TCP (*G*), and collagen/channel β-TCP-based grafts in nude mice (*H*). *White arrows* depicts the collagen gels. (*From [A–C]* Kang Y, Kim S, Fahrenholtz M, et al. Osteogenic and angiogenic potentials of monocultured and co-cultured hBMSCs and HUVECs on 3D porous β-TCP scaffold. Acta Biomater 2013;9(1):4909, with permission; and [*D–H*] Kang Y, Mochizuki N, Khademhosseini A, et al. Engineering a vascularized collagen-β-tricalcium phosphate graft using an electrochemical approach. Acta Biomater 2015;11:453–5, with permission.)

the changes in the physiochemical properties of CaPs, such as crystallinity, micro-structure, and solubility.[28] Tarafder and coworkers[28] investigated the influence of MgO and SrO doping of β-TCP scaffolds in an animal model and found increased early bone formation in the doped versus nondoped scaffolds. In addition to the CaPs, bioactive glass and glass-ceramics are materials that have been thoroughly studied for their potential for bone regeneration.[29] Since 1969 when Hench and colleagues[4] discovered that rat bone can bond chemically to certain silicate-based glass compo-sitions, bioactive glass has been investigated and used clinically for bone regeneration purposes. Bioactive glass has the ability to chemically react in physiologic body fluids resulting in the formation of a hydroxycarbonate apatite layer to which bone can bind.[4] Although bioactive glass and glass ceramics are still available in particulate form commercially, their limited strength and low fracture toughness have prevented their use for load-bearing implants, and therefore, the repair of larger bony defects at load-bearing anatomic sites remains a challenge.[4] However, because of the potential to improve the osteogenic cell response, bioactive glass is used as a filler or coating on polymer-based scaffolds. A few examples of clinically available materials for bone regeneration relying on the action of bioactive glass include GlassBone (Noraker Villeurbanne, France), BonAlive (BonAlive Biomaterials Ltd Turku, Finland), Vitoss (Stryker Kalamazoo, MI), and Perioglass (NovaBone Products LLC, Alachua, FL). Despite the promising results obtained from bioglass-based materials, and the claimed advantageous properties of this class of materials over typical CaP sintered ceramics, it is often the long-term clinical performance of these systems in vivo that determines their reliability and efficacy. Therefore, bioglass-based systems remain in their infancy as far as their craniofacial and orthopedic applications compared with other existing regenerative materials.

BIOPOLYMERS
Natural Polymers

Organic scaffolds, such as polymer hydrogels, find use in the delivery of cells and/or GFs for bone regeneration because of their cytocompatibility, ability to stimulate an appro-priate cellular response, porosity, and controlled degradability under physiologic condi-tions. Biopolymers of natural origin, such as collagen, gelatin, chitosan, and silk, are used for this purpose because they mimic the structure, chemical composition, and biochem-ical properties of the natural bone organic matrix; possess low immunogenic properties; and are able to stimulate appropriate cell response and function while supporting tissue remodeling.[30–36] Collagen, for instance, which is the most abundant protein in the extra-cellular matrix (ECM) of vertebrates, is a logical choice as a biomaterial for tissue regen-eration. The main drawback of pure collagen scaffolds remains their poor mechanical properties, which do not approach those of natural bone tissue. Additionally, collagen isolated from animal tissues poses a risk of infection and allergic reactions[37] and cannot be mass produced, although these concerns may be alleviated through the use of recom-binant collagen.[38] Natural polysaccharides, such as chitosan, agarose, and alginate, are other types of natural polymeric scaffolds. In addition to the desirable properties of all nat-ural polymers, these materials possesses positively charged amino groups on their sur-face that allow for interactions with anions, such as DNA, lipids, proteins, and even cell membranes. Particularly, the cationic nature of chitosan promotes interactions with gly-cosaminoglycans and proteoglycans, which are known to stimulate cytokines and GFs important for tissue regeneration.[39–41] This stimulatory effect has been evidenced in mul-tiple studies where chitosan-based scaffolds promoted new bone formation in in vivo models. Silk fibroin, another natural polymer, has also demonstrated ability to support cell proliferation,[42] induce osteogenesis in vitro, and bone formation in in vivo calvarial defect models.[43–49] Still, despite their biocompatibility and osteoconductive nature, silk-based scaffolds have been found to have low compressive strength, thus limiting their application to non-load-bearing bone tissue sites.[30]

Another category of natural bone substitutes that has been widely applied clinically is demineralized bone matrix (DBM), an allograft obtained by removing the mineral component of bone.[50,51] DBM is predominantly composed of type I collagen (~90%) along with various GFs (eg, bone sialoprotein, osteopontin, BMPs, insulin-like growth factor [IGF]-1), in addition to residues of calcium-based particles, inorganic phosphates, and some trace cell debris.[52,53] Although commercially available DBM products are well known for their osteoinductive and osteoconductive nature, each product exhibits large variability in terms of processing conditions, sterilization methods of storage, donor specifications, and so forth.[54] On comparing three different DBM products (Osteofil, Grafton, and Dynagraft) for reliability and efficacy, Wang and colleagues[55] reported differences in osteoinductive ability caused by the inconsistency in processing conditions. It was also reported that different DBM products had variability in handling properties, ultimately resulting in intraproduct differences during surgical procedure and after implantation.[56] For optimal surgical handling, DBM is often mixed with binders, such as glycerol (Grafton, Osteotech, Eatontown, NJ), poloxamer carrier (Dynagraft, Gensci Regeneration Sciences Inc., Toronto, Ontario, Canada), hyaluronan (DBX, Synthes USA, West Chester, PA), gelatin (Regenafil, Regeneration Technologies Inc., Alachua, FL), calcium sulfate (AlloMatrix, Wright Medical Technology Inc., Arlington, TN), lecithin (InterGro, Interpore Cross Inc., Irvine, CA), carboxymethyl cellulose (OsteoSelect, Bacterin International, Belgrade, MT), and bovine collagen with sodium alginate (PROGENIX Plus, Medtronic Sofamor Danek, Memphis, TN), among other examples. It is also available in the form of freeze-dried powder, granules, gel, putty, or strips.[56–58] Because DBM possess limited structural support and mechanical strength, it has been commonly used as a bone graft extender in well-supported, stable skeletal defects.[59] Nonetheless, DBM is considered advantageous over standard autografts because it revascularizes rapidly and facilitates the local endogenous release of GFs and therapeutic agents to induce new bone formation.

The osteoinductive and vasculogenic potential of scaffolds may be further enhanced by the introduction of appropriate GFs that induce chemotaxis, proliferation, and differentiation of the encapsulated and surrounding cells. Platelet-rich plasma, blood concentrated for thrombocytes, is an autologous source of physiologic concentrations of platelet-derived growth factor (PDGF), transforming growth factor (TGF)-ß1, TGF-ß2, IGF-I, IGF-II, and vascular endothelial growth factor (VEGF)[60] that has been successfully used in bone repair and regeneration.[61,62] However, the lack of standardization in the method of preparation of platelet-rich plasma has led to discrepancies in the results.[63] Recently, a second-generation platelet-rich biomaterial, platelet-rich fibrin, has been developed, which is simpler to produce because it does not require the use of the coagulating agents thrombin and calcium chloride.[64] This material has been demonstrably successful individually and in concert with other scaffold materials in promoting osteogenic differentiation and augmenting bone formation.[65,66] In addition to the GFs previously enumerated, platelet-rich fibrin is rich in leukocytes, cytokines, and glycoproteins that participate in wound healing, matrix remodeling, immune activity, and stimulation of GFs.[67]

Synthetic Polymers

Several synthetic polymer-based scaffold materials have been developed, including poly (ε-caprolactone) (PCL), polylactic acid (PLA), polyglycolide (PGA), poly (lactide-co-glycolide) (PLGA), poly(propylene fumarate), and polyhydroxyalkanoates. These have been designed to enable better control over a wider range of mechanical properties of the scaffold through variations in the concentrations and degrees of cross-linking of the polymers, or even through copolymerization of two or more of them. These polymers can be synthesized in large quantities under controlled conditions thus ensuring uniform and reproducible properties while negating risks of infections and immunogenicity. The poly (α hydroxyl) esters PCL, PLA, PGA, and their copolymer PLGA are the most commonly used synthetic polymers for tissue engineering because of their mechanical stability, cytocompatibility, and resorbability.[68] Although PLA and PGA are unsuitable as scaffolds for bone tissue because of their low osteoconductivity and compressive strength, respectively, PLGA copolymers with varying ratios of PLA and PGA are more soluble, and provide a wider range of mechanical properties, enhanced osteoconductivity, and controlled rates of degradation.[69,70] PCL is yet another aliphatic polyester scaffold that is preferred for its flexibility and controlled rate of degradation. In vivo, these scaffolds undergo hydrolytic degradation wherein their monomeric degradation products are removed through natural pathways and are hence approved by the Food and Drug Administration (FDA) for use in tissue engineering.[68] However, their degradation products are often acidic in nature causing undesirable local changes in pH. Furthermore, their hydrophobic nature is not conducive to cell attachment, and the absence of functional groups results in inferior osteoinduction.[68] These shortcomings may be somewhat diminished in composite scaffolds with hydrophilic polymers, such as polyethylene glycol (PEG), and by coating with natural biomaterials, such as collagen.[71–76] Recent advances in scaffolds for bone regeneration involve the use of hybrid natural and synthetic biomaterials to take advantage of the benefits of each. Inclusion of PCL or PCL-PEG-PCL copolymer nanofibers in collagen[77,78] or chitosan[79] serves to combine the biomimicry and stimulatory effects of natural polymers with the structural and mechanical stability of synthetic polymers, thus offering viable scaffold options with superior osteogenic potential.

BIOMATERIALS FOR CONTROLLED DELIVERY

A synergistic combination of cells, proteins, genes, and biophysical signals is critical to trigger functional bone regeneration. In the native tissue milieu, the local presentation and spatiotemporal distribution of these combinatorial factors are highly orchestrated by ECM components. This native complex microenvironment has inspired the design and development of biomimetic and biodegradable material carriers possessing ECM-like properties for the controlled delivery and retention of regenerative factors at the injury site over a prolonged period. In light of the tremendous advantage of biomaterials for the targeted and sustained release of therapeutic agents, this section discusses some of the recent developments in biomaterial-based delivery formulations, from a clinical and translational perspective.

Growth Factor Delivery

Many GFs have been clinically proven to play a key role in craniofacial growth and development, including TGF-β, fibroblast growth factor, VEGF, PDGF, IGFs, and BMPs (BMP-2 and BMP-7).[80–82] For example, rhBMPs,[83] one of the widely investigated FDA-approved GFs, are involved in various developmental processes critical for the formation of soft and hard callus, cranial neural crest, facial primordia, tooth, lip, and palate.[84,85] BMPs act in concert with TGF-β to modulate mesenchymal stem cell (MSC) differentiation during skeletal development, bone formation, and bone homeostasis via the activation of the Smad-dependent signaling pathway or

MAPK pathway. Likewise, fibroblast growth factor signaling is known to exhibit multiple functions in craniofacial skeletogenesis,[86] whereas PDGFs are potent mediators involved in wound healing, bone repair, and remodeling during trauma/infection by inducing proliferation of osteoblastic precursor cells.[87] Similarly, IGFs have an important role in general growth and maintenance of the body skeleton. VEGF, apart from its role in proliferation, vascularization, and ossification during bone formation is known to influence calvarial ossification and maxillary and palatal mesenchyme.[88] Altogether, an imbalance of these GFs is associated with severe craniofacial anomalies. Thus, they can be used widely in clinical settings as potential therapeutic agents to augment the healing process.[89,90]

Although direct administration of GFs into damaged/degenerated tissues is considered an obvious strategy, often large doses and multiple injections are required to achieve specific biologic responses in humans because of its shorter half-life in circulation, slow diffusion, rapid degradation, and cleavage.[91] However in vivo, GFs are protected and stabilized by their binding to different ECM molecules. Hence, selecting a suitable biomaterial carrier system has long been considered to be of critical importance to tailor the localized and sustained release of single or multiple GFs.[92]

Currently, a plethora of delivery vehicles based on natural and synthetic polymers, inorganic biomaterials, and their composites have been designed in the form of sponges, nanofibrous membranes, micro/nanoparticles, and hydrogels, to either chemically or physically entrap GFs into or onto the substrate.[93] For instance, dual delivery of VEGF and BMP-2 has shown great capacity for nearly complete regeneration of a critical size defect in rats (**Fig. 3**).[94] Depending on the mode of immobilization, the release rate of the GFs may be regulated by processes including diffusion; flow; erosion or degradation; surface charge; charge density; swelling; wettability;

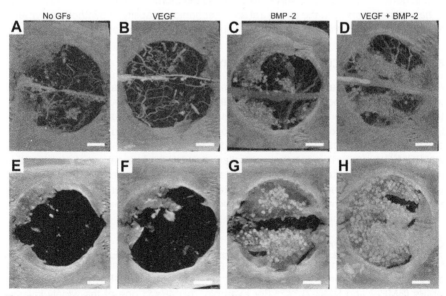

Fig. 3. Microcomputed tomography images of bone regeneration in rat calvarial critical size defect at 4 (*top*) and 12 (*bottom*) weeks with no growth factor delivery (*A, E*), VEGF delivery only (*B, F*), BMP-2 delivery only (*C, G*), and VEGF/BMP-2 dual delivery (*D, H*). Scale bars = 200 μm. (*From* Patel ZS, Young S, Tabata Y, et al. Dual delivery of an angiogenic and an osteogenic growth factor for bone regeneration in a critical size defect model. Bone 2008;43(5):937; with permission.)

dissolution; or via an on-demand triggering mechanism including pH, temperature, enzymes, light, electric/magnetic field, and ultrasound.[95] Despite these extensive in vitro studies, the efficacy and safety of these delivery systems are not well established in preclinical and clinical stages.

Notably, some of the commercially available products that are available for clinical use are based on rhBMPs. For instance, rhBMP-2 infiltrated within absorbable collagen sponge (Infuse, Medtronic, Memphis, TN) has FDA approval for various bone defects including sinus lift and localized alveolar ridge augmentation.[96] Similarly, OP-1 Putty (Stryker Biotech, Hopkinton, MA), comprised of bovine-derived collagen incorporating rhBMP-7, is another commercially available graft material for nonunion fractures. Other carrier-based grafts recognized for clinical applications in the United States include β-TCP porous carrier infused with rhPDGF (GEM 21S, Osteohealth, Norristown, PA) to treat periodontally related bone defects and associated gingival recession.[97] Therefore, the inclusion of GFs within biomaterials not only sustains the release kinetics but also provides a porous osteoconductive framework for the bone ingrowth to occur.

Another interesting concept for accelerated bone regeneration is the combined or sequential delivery of multiple GFs. Although this approach seems extremely challenging because of difficulties in choosing the appropriate concentrations of GF cocktails, tailoring the release profiles, controlling the gradients and timings, and so forth, these dual or multiple delivery vehicles are proven to be effective in stimulating angiogenesis and bone healing.[98–100] For example, a phase I/II human clinical trial displayed the efficacy and safety of a combination of PDGF/IGF-I in eliciting increased defect fill in periodontal lesions, when codelivered in a methylcellulose gel vehicle.[101]

Stem Cell Delivery

Another promising application of biomaterials is their use as stem cell-delivery vehicles. Preclinical studies have shown poor engraftment and survival of cells that are directly administered only in saline or media, because of their immediate encounter with harsh conditions, such as hypoxia, inflammation, and reactive oxygen species.[102] Biomaterials can function as a substitute to native ECM, conferring a conducive framework for the attachment and growth of encapsulated cells, and thereby preventing anoikis, a form of apoptosis. Moreover, biomaterials can be optimized to offer protection against host immune attack, and they can be manipulated to induce major cellular processes necessary for tissue regeneration.[103,104] Most of all, the attractive approach of using hydrogels as minimally invasive stem cell delivery vehicles opens exciting avenues to reconstruct craniofacial defects resulting from trauma, disease, or congenital abnormalities, without the need for extensive invasive surgeries. For instance, the regenerative potential of injectable composite hydrogels for MSC delivery was demonstrated in a rat critical size cranial defect.[105] However, a drawback of this injectable hydrogel system in craniofacial regeneration is a lack of ability to provide 3D architecture and mechanical stability, especially in cases involving significant bone loss, such as in traumatic injury or oncologic surgery.

The cells that have been predominantly investigated under clinical trials to date include adult stem/progenitor cells from limbus, adipose tissue, bone marrow, placenta, dental pulp, and periodontal ligament.[106] Because of the limitation of the clinical use of pluripotent stem cells (embryonic stem cells (ESCs) and induced pluripotent stem cells (iPSCs)), the alternate choice for bone and cartilage repair is MSC therapies. This work continues despite a few reports on clinical trial failures in the treatment of ulcerative colitis, ischemic stroke, cardiac repair, acute kidney injury, ischemic stroke, acute respiratory distress syndrome, and critical limb ischemia.[106] At this time there are a limited number of commercially available bone graft materials incorporating MSCs for clinical use and these graft materials are all centered on DBM. The products include Allostem (AlloSource, Centennial, CO), Map3 (rti surgical, Alachua, Fl), Osteocel Plus (NuVasive, San Diego, CA), and Trinity Evolution Matrix (Orthofix, Lewisville, TX).[107] It is noteworthy to mention that some of the other commercially available bone grafts are also envisioned as carrier systems for MSC delivery, including collagen sponge (CopiOs sponge, Zimmer, Austin, TX), β-TCP (Vitoss, Stryker, Kalamazoo, MI), collagen-β-TCP composite (Collage Putty, Orthofix, Lewisville, TX), and nano-HA-collagen carrier (nanOss Bioactive, rti surgical, Alachua, Fl).[107,108] Another noninvasive source of stem cells is the dental pulp and the inclusion of dental pulp stem/progenitor cells within collagen sponge was clinically established to restore human mandibular bone defects caused by the extraction of third molars.[109] In summary, biomaterial-mediated stem cell delivery has significant potency to regenerate oral and maxillofacial structures, although its long-term clinical safety and efficacy is yet to be determined.

Gene Delivery

Because of the limited bioactivity, in vivo instability, and high hepatic/renal clearance rates of GFs, gene therapy has been proposed as an alternative to achieve localized and sustained gene expression at the defect site to achieve spatiotemporally coordinated protein synthesis.[110,111] Although a variety of viral vector systems (adenovirus, adeno-associated virus, lentivirus, and retrovirus)[112] have been considered effective because of their high transfection efficiency, biomaterials are often preferred in terms of immunogenicity, safety, ease of manipulation, and mutagenesis.[113] To date, several material-based systems (lipid-, peptide-, and polymer-based systems) and various gene transfer approaches (microinjection, the "gene gun," and electroporation) have been evaluated for gene delivery.[113] Nevertheless, the rational design of a suitable biomaterial-based vector for human clinical trials remains elusive, because the vectors have to bypass a series of systemic, extracellular, and subcellular barriers including blood serum proteins/enzymes, cell membrane, endosomes, and the nuclear membrane.[114–116] All the gene therapy clinical trials reported thus far for a range of disorders (eg, SCID-X1, cancer, cardiovascular disease, AIDS, cystic fibrosis, muscular dystrophy) were mostly based on viral vectors.[117,118] Despite encouraging results of nonviral-biomaterial-based gene delivery in in vitro and in vivo studies, no significant progress has been made toward attaining clinical success. Nevertheless, well-studied biomaterial-mediated gene delivery approaches involve the use of gene-activated matrices, composed of porous collagen sponges for the site-specific delivery of plasmid DNA directly to the fracture site.[112] Bonadio and colleagues established the potency of physically entrapping PTH 1-34/BMP-4 encoding cDNAs in these gene-activated matrices for new bone formation in a beagle tibia critical defect model.[119–127] Thus, direct delivery of pure DNA complexes using biomaterial carrier systems offers the flexibility of integrating cells, drugs, and groups of other interacting factors to achieve multifunctional therapeutic benefits. Hence, it is believed that biomaterial-mediated gene delivery technologies that are currently under development will eventually be used clinically to treat difficult bone loss problems.

3D PRINTING AND BIOPRINTING

The rapid expansion of 3D printing in the past 5 years has had a considerable and immediate impact in the area of craniofacial bone augmentation. 3D printing addresses a series of significant challenges that up to now have prevented bone tissue engineering from being translated into clinical practice. The benefits of 3D printing include the ability to control the internal and external 3D architecture of scaffold systems, the ease of fabrication of scaffolds that precisely match patient-specific needs, the possibility of fabricating scaffolds with multiple materials, and the ability to control cell behavior and mechanical response by predefining scaffold architecture.[128,129] We have addressed the characteristics of 3D printing that make this method especially relevant for craniofacial regeneration in a recent review.[128]

Although 3D printing and 3D bioprinting are concepts that often have been used interchangeably, they involve different requirements as far as the materials and printing capabilities are concerned. 3D printing is often used to describe the fabrication of inert or bioactive scaffold materials without the presence of living cells, whereas 3D bioprinting generally refers to printing of cells and scaffolds together (cell-laden biomaterials) or dense aggregates of cells free from scaffold support.[128] Although there has been immense growth in the number of printing methods available in the past 5 years, the more well established 3D printing modalities for tissue engineering applications are typically categorized as extrusion printing, inkjet printing, laser printing, and to a lesser some extent lithography printing (which shares similarities with the laser 3D printing modality). Extrusion 3D printers/bioprinters have been the most relevant for bone augmentation research because, compared with other printers, they allow rapid fabrication of the larger scale constructs required for clinically relevant tissue constructs. Moreover, depending on the materials and hardware characteristics, extrusion 3D printers can be tailored to dispense a wide range of materials that have proven osteoinductive capacity, including CaP injectable pastes, ceramic bases, cell-laden hydrogels, and other types of FDA-approved medical-grade polymers, such as PCL.[130–135]

There are noteworthy examples that exemplify how 3D printers can revolutionize the manner in which craniofacial/long bone augmentation is conducted in the clinic. Recent work by Atala's group demonstrated that a large mandibular bone defect could be regenerated using a sizable multitypic tissue construct 3D bioprinted with cell-laden hydrogels and a supporting scaffold having controlled porosity to stimulate new vasculature formation (**Fig. 4**).[129] Another recent example of the successful application of 3D-printed scaffolds for bone regeneration was the use of a 3D-printed medical-grade PCL with TCP combined with rhBMP-7, which has been reported to enable bridging of a 30-mm-long bone defect in a sheep model with superior results compared with the gold standard of autologous bone.[136] Postsurgical biomechanical and microcomputed tomography analyses after 12 months showed significantly greater bone formation and bone quality for the printed scaffolds compared with a bone autograft material.

Examples of how these 3D printing technologies will be introduced to the market remain uncertain, because the FDA has yet to standardize a series of questions that relate to the process of 3D tissue/scaffold fabrication that go beyond simple validation of the printing material itself. Nevertheless, examples of companies commercializing pre-3D-printed scaffold systems for craniofacial regeneration are already commercially available, such as OsteoFlux (Vivos Dental AG, Villaz-Saint-Pierre, Switzerland), a 3D-printed CaP osteoinductive material. Despite the uncertainty that is common for the early adoption of a new technology, the current literature presents countless examples of how 3D printing methods can facilitate the fabrication of scaffolds with controlled structure architecture and porosity, of prevascularized tissue constructs,[137] patient-specific characteristics,[138] enhanced mechanical properties,[136] and many other advantages. Therefore, one may argue that the future of craniofacial bone augmentation will most certainly cross paths with the next generation of 3D-printed materials.[128]

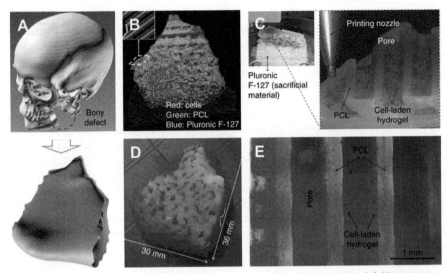

Fig. 4. 3D bioprinted human-scale mandible and calvarial bone constructs. (*A*) 3D computer-aided design model of mandible bony defect obtained by converting the medical computed tomography scan data. (*B*) Visualized motion program depicting the required dispensing paths of cell-laden hydrogel (*red*); a mixture of PCL and tricalcium phosphate (*green*) as a scaffold; and Pluronic F127 (*blue*), which is used as a temporary support structure. (*C*) 3D patterning of cell-laden hydrogel on PCL platform. (*D*) Macroscopic image of the 3D-printed mandible bone defect construct, grown in osteogenic medium for 28 days. (*E*) Alizarin red S staining indicates terminal osteogenic induction and mineral deposition in human amniotic fluid–derived stem cell. (*From* Kang HW, Lee SJ, Ko IK, et al. A 3D bioprinting system to produce human-scale tissue constructs with structural integrity. Nat Biotechnol 2016;34(3):314; with permission.)

SUMMARY

Several decades of intense research have yielded a new generation of biomaterials and novel design strategies with limitless benefits of incorporating cells, drugs, and other biochemical signals to promote the formation of engineered bone tissue. With the latest advent of 3D biofabrication technologies, the future of craniofacial reconstruction will witness patient-specific surgical implants for large-volume bone defects that can fully vascularize and rapidly integrate with the supporting host tissue. Furthermore, the innovative approach of engineering the inherent biomaterial properties to regulate stem cell fate decisions in the host will not only have important implications in fostering bone regeneration but also will nullify the side effects of using biochemical inducers or soluble factors. Apart from the promise of replacing intricate craniofacial deformities with synthetic materials, biomaterials also envisions additional breakthrough approaches involving a combination of physical, chemical, biologic, and engineering processes to stimulate accelerated bone regeneration.

ACKNOWLEDGMENTS

The authors acknowledge funding from the National Institute of Dental and Craniofacial Research, National Institutes of Health (R01DE026170 to LEB), and the Medical Research Foundation of Oregon (to LEB).

REFERENCES

1. Langer R, Vacanti JP. Tissue engineering. Science 1993;260(5110):920–6.
2. Bertassoni LE, Coelho PG. Engineering mineralized and load bearing tissues. New York: Springer; 2015.
3. Annabi N, Tamayol A, Uquillas JA, et al. 25th anniversary article: rational design and applications of hydrogels in regenerative medicine. Adv Mater 2014;26(1): 85–123.
4. Gerhardt LC, Boccaccini AR. Bioactive glass and glass-ceramic scaffolds for bone tissue engineering. Materials 2010;3(7):3867.
5. Albee FH. Studies in bone growth: triple calcium phosphate as a stimulus to osteogenesis. Ann Surg 1920;71(1):32–9.
6. Boonrungsiman S, Gentleman E, Carzaniga R, et al. The role of intracellular calcium phosphate in osteoblast-mediated bone apatite formation. Proc Natl Acad Sci U S A 2012;109(35):14170–5.
7. Dorozhkin SV. Calcium orthophosphates: occurrence, properties, biomineralization, pathological calcification and biomimetic applications. Biomatter 2011; 1(2):121–64.
8. Habraken W, Habibovic P, Epple M, et al. Calcium phosphates in biomedical applications: materials for the future? Mater Today 2016;19(2):69–87.
9. Chow LC. Solubility of calcium phosphates. In: Chow LC, Eanes ED, editors. Octacalcium phosphate, vol 18. Basel: Karger Publishers; 2001. p. 94–111.
10. Kamakura S, Sasano Y, Shimizu T, et al. Implanted octacalcium phosphate is more resorbable than beta-tricalcium phosphate and hydroxyapatite. J Biomed Mater Res 2002;59(1):29–34.
11. Galea LG, Bohner M, Lemaître J, et al. Bone substitute: transforming beta-tricalcium phosphate porous scaffolds into monetite. Biomaterials 2008; 29(24–25):3400–7.
12. Steffen T, Stoll T, Arvinte T, et al. Porous tricalcium phosphate and transforming growth factor used for anterior spine surgery. Eur Spine J 2001;10(2):S132–40.
13. Kasten P, Luginbühl R, van Griensven M, et al. Comparison of human bone marrow stromal cells seeded on calcium-deficient hydroxyapatite, β-tricalcium phosphate and demineralized bone matrix. Biomaterials 2003;24(15):2593–603.
14. Munting E, Mirtchi AA, Lemaitre J. Bone repair of defects filled with a phospho-calcic hydraulic cement: an in vivo study. J Mater Sci Mater Med 1993;4(3): 337–44.
15. Constantz BR, Barr BM, Ison IC, et al. Histological, chemical, and crystallographic analysis of four calcium phosphate cements in different rabbit osseous sites. J Biomed Mater Res 1998;43(4):451–61.
16. Bohner M, Theiss F, Apelt D, et al. Compositional changes of a dicalcium phosphate dihydrate cement after implantation in sheep. Biomaterials 2003;24(20): 3463–74.
17. Suzuki O, Nakamura M, Miyasaka Y, et al. Bone formation on synthetic precursors of hydroxyapatite. Tohoku J Exp Med 1991;164(1):37–50.
18. Yuan H, Fernandes H, Habibovic P, et al. Osteoinductive ceramics as a synthetic alternative to autologous bone grafting. Proc Natl Acad Sci U S A 2010; 107(31):13614–9.
19. Yuan H, van Blitterswijk CA, de Groot K, et al. A comparison of bone formation in biphasic calcium phosphate (BCP) and hydroxyapatite (HA) implanted in muscle and bone of dogs at different time periods. J Biomed Mater Res A 2006; 78A(1):139–47.

20. Yuan H, van Blitterswijk CA, de Groot K, et al. Cross-species comparison of ectopic bone formation in biphasic calcium phosphate (BCP) and hydroxyapatite (HA) scaffolds. Tissue Eng 2006;12(6):1607–15.

21. Habibovic P, Yuan H, van der Valk CM, et al. 3D microenvironment as essential element for osteoinduction by biomaterials. Biomaterials 2005;26(17):3565–75.

22. Habibovic P, Kruyt MC, Juhl MV, et al. Comparative in vivo study of six hydroxyapatite-based bone graft substitutes. J Orthop Res 2008;26(10): 1363–70.

23. Hulbert SF, Young FA, Mathews RS, et al. Potential of ceramic materials as permanently implantable skeletal prostheses. J Biomed Mater Res 1970;4(3): 433–56.

24. Klawitter JJ, Hulbert SF. Application of porous ceramics for the attachment of load bearing internal orthopedic applications. J Biomed Mater Res 1971;5(6): 161–229.

25. Klein CP, de Groot K, Driessen AA, et al. Interaction of biodegradable β-whitlockite ceramics with bone tissue: an in vivo study. Biomaterials 1985;6(3): 189–92.

26. Kang Y, Mochizuki N, Khademhosseini A, et al. Engineering a vascularized collagen-β-tricalcium phosphate graft using an electrochemical approach. Acta Biomater 2015;11:449–58.

27. Kang Y, Kim S, Fahrenholtz M, et al. Osteogenic and angiogenic potentials of monocultured and co-cultured human-bone-marrow-derived mesenchymal stem cells and human-umbilical-vein endothelial cells on three-dimensional porous beta-tricalcium phosphate scaffold. Acta Biomater 2013;9(1):4906–15.

28. Tarafder S, Davies NM, Bandyopadhyay A, et al. 3D printed tricalcium phosphate scaffolds: effect of SrO and MgO doping on in vivo osteogenesis in a rat distal femoral defect model. Biomater Sci 2013;1(12):1250–9.

29. Kaur G, Pandey OP, Singh K, et al. A review of bioactive glasses: their structure, properties, fabrication and apatite formation. J Biomed Mater Res A 2014; 102(1):254–74.

30. Stoppel WL, Ghezzi CE, McNamara SL, et al. Clinical applications of naturally derived biopolymer-based scaffolds for regenerative medicine. Ann Biomed Eng 2015;43(3):657–80.

31. Tsai KS, Kao SY, Wang CY, et al. Type I collagen promotes proliferation and osteogenesis of human mesenchymal stem cells via activation of ERK and Akt pathways. J Biomed Mater Res A 2010;94A(3):673–82.

32. Themistocleous GS, Katopodis HA, Khaldi L, et al. Implants of type I collagen gel containing MG-63 osteoblast-like cells can act as stable scaffolds stimulating the bone healing process at the sites of the surgically-produced segmental diaphyseal defects in male rabbits. In Vivo 2007;21(1):69–76.

33. Shih YR, Chen CN, Tsai SW, et al. Growth of mesenchymal stem cells on electrospun type I collagen nanofibers. Stem Cells 2006;24(11):2391–7.

34. O'brien FJ. Biomaterials & scaffolds for tissue engineering. Mater Today 2011; 14(3):88–95.

35. Yoshioka SA, Goissis G. Thermal and spectrophotometric studies of new crosslinking method for collagen matrix with glutaraldehyde acetals. J Mater Sci Mater Med 2008;19(3):1215–23.

36. Yunoki S, Matsuda T. Simultaneous processing of fibril formation and crosslinking improves mechanical properties of collagen. Biomacromolecules 2008; 9(3):879–85.

37. Lynn AK, Yannas IV, Bonfield W. Antigenicity and immunogenicity of collagen. J Biomed Mater Res B Appl Biomater 2004;71(2):343–54.
38. Adachi T, Tomita M, Shimizu K, et al. Generation of hybrid transgenic silkworms that express bombyx mori prolyl-hydroxylase alpha-subunits and human collagens in posterior silk glands: production of cocoons that contained collagens with hydroxylated proline residues. J Biotechnol 2006;126(2):205–19.
39. Costa-Pinto AR, Reis RL, Neves NM. Scaffolds based bone tissue engineering: the role of chitosan. Tissue Eng Part B Rev 2011;17(5):331–47.
40. Wang L, Stegemann JP. Thermogelling chitosan and collagen composite hydrogels initiated with beta-glycerophosphate for bone tissue engineering. Biomaterials 2010;31(14):3976–85.
41. Costa-Pinto AR, Correlo VM, Sol PC, et al. Chitosan-poly(butylene succinate) scaffolds and human bone marrow stromal cells induce bone repair in a mouse calvaria model. J Tissue Eng Regen Med 2012;6(1):21–8.
42. Meechaisue C, Wutticharoenmongkol P, Waraput R, et al. Preparation of electrospun silk fibroin fiber mats as bone scaffolds: a preliminary study. Biomed Mater 2007;2(3):181–8.
43. Uebersax L, Apfel T, Nuss KM, et al. Biocompatibility and osteoconduction of macroporous silk fibroin implants in cortical defects in sheep. Eur J Pharm Biopharm 2013;85(1):107–18.
44. Zhang Y, Wu C, Friis T, et al. The osteogenic properties of CaP/silk composite scaffolds. Biomaterials 2010;31(10):2848–56.
45. Mata A, Geng Y, Henrikson KJ, et al. Bone regeneration mediated by biomimetic mineralization of a nanofiber matrix. Biomaterials 2010;31(23):6004–12.
46. Holmes TC. Novel peptide-based biomaterial scaffolds for tissue engineering. Trends Biotechnol 2002;20(1):16–21.
47. Hartgerink JD, Beniash E, Stupp SI. Self-assembly and mineralization of peptide-amphiphile nanofibers. Science 2001;294(5547):1684–8.
48. Kantlehner M, Schaffner P, Finsinger D, et al. Surface coating with cyclic RGD peptides stimulates osteoblast adhesion and proliferation as well as bone formation. Chembiochem 2000;1(2):107–14.
49. Gandavarapu NR, Mariner PD, Schwartz MP, et al. Extracellular matrix protein adsorption to phosphate-functionalized gels from serum promotes osteogenic differentiation of human mesenchymal stem cells. Acta Biomater 2013;9(1):4525–34.
50. Sawkins MJ, Bowen W, Dhadda P, et al. Hydrogels derived from demineralized and decellularized bone extracellular matrix. Acta Biomater 2013;9(8):7865–73.
51. Kolk A, Handschel J, Drescher W, et al. Current trends and future perspectives of bone substitute materials: from space holders to innovative biomaterials. J Craniomaxillofac Surg 2012;40(8):706–18.
52. Gruskin E, Doll BA, Futrell FW, et al. Demineralized bone matrix in bone repair: history and use. Adv Drug Deliv Rev 2012;64(12):1063–77.
53. Holt DJ, Grainger DW. Demineralized bone matrix as a vehicle for delivering endogenous and exogenous therapeutics in bone repair. Adv Drug Deliv Rev 2012;64(12):1123–8.
54. Kinney RC, Ziran BH, Hirshorn K, et al. Demineralized bone matrix for fracture healing: fact or fiction? J Orthop Trauma 2010;24(Suppl 1):S52–5.
55. Wang JC, Alanay A, Mark D, et al. A comparison of commercially available demineralized bone matrix for spinal fusion. Eur Spine J 2007;16(8):1233–40.

56. Acarturk TO, Hollinger JO. Commercially available demineralized bone matrix compositions to regenerate calvarial critical-sized bone defects. Plast Reconstr Surg 2006;118(4):862–73.

57. Matassi F, Nistri L, Chicon Paez D, et al. New biomaterials for bone regeneration. Clin Cases Miner Bone Metab 2011;8(1):21–4.

58. Drosos GI, Touzopoulos P, Ververidis A, et al. Use of demineralized bone matrix in the extremities. World J Orthop 2015;6(2):269–77.

59. Lieberman JR, Friedlaender GE. Bone regeneration and repair: biology and clinical applications. New Jersey: Humana Press; 2007.

60. Weibrich G, Kleis WK, Hafner G. Growth factor levels in the platelet-rich plasma produced by 2 different methods: curasan-type PRP kit versus PCCS PRP system. Int J Oral Maxillofac Implants 2002;17(2):184–90.

61. Nash TJ, Howlett CR, Martin C, et al. Effect of platelet-derived growth factor on tibial osteotomies in rabbits. Bone 1994;15(2):203–8.

62. Aghaloo TL, Moy PK, Freymiller EG. Investigation of platelet-rich plasma in rabbit cranial defects: a pilot study. J Oral Maxillofac Surg 2002;60(10):1176–81.

63. Sanchez AR, Sheridan PJ, Kupp LI. Is platelet-rich plasma the perfect enhancement factor? A current review. Int J Oral Maxillofac Implants 2003;18(1):93–103.

64. Choukroun J, Diss A, Simonpieri A, et al. Platelet-rich fibrin (PRF): a second-generation platelet concentrate. Part V: histologic evaluations of PRF effects on bone allograft maturation in sinus lift. Oral Surg Oral Med Oral Pathol Oral Radiol Endod 2006;101(3):299–303.

65. Lee EH, Kim JY, Kweon HY, et al. A combination graft of low-molecular-weight silk fibroin with Choukroun platelet-rich fibrin for rabbit calvarial defect. Oral Surg Oral Med Oral Pathol Oral Radiol Endod 2010;109(5):e33–8.

66. Wang Z, Weng Y, Lu S, et al. Osteoblastic mesenchymal stem cell sheet combined with Choukroun platelet-rich fibrin induces bone formation at an ectopic site. J Biomed Mater Res B Appl Biomater 2015;103(6):1204–16.

67. Anitua E, Sánchez M, Nurden AT, et al. New insights into and novel applications for platelet-rich fibrin therapies. Trends Biotechnol 2006;24(5):227–34.

68. Gunatillake PA, Adhikari R. Biodegradable synthetic polymers for tissue engineering. Eur Cell Mater 2003;5:1–16 [discussion: 16].

69. Gentile P, Chiono V, Carmagnola I, et al. An overview of poly(lactic-co-glycolic) acid (PLGA)-based biomaterials for bone tissue engineering. Int J Mol Sci 2014; 15(3):3640–59.

70. Remya KR, Joseph J, Mani S, et al. Nanohydroxyapatite incorporated electrospun polycaprolactone/polycaprolactone-polyethyleneglycol-polycaprolactone blend scaffold for bone tissue engineering applications. J Biomed Nanotechnol 2013;9(9):1483–94.

71. Wang T, Yang X, Qi X, et al. Osteoinduction and proliferation of bone-marrow stromal cells in three-dimensional poly (epsilon-caprolactone)/hydroxyapatite/ collagen scaffolds. J Transl Med 2015;13:152.

72. Chen GQ, Wu Q. The application of polyhydroxyalkanoates as tissue engineering materials. Biomaterials 2005;26(33):6565–78.

73. Cool SM, Kenny B, Wu A, et al. Poly(3-hydroxybutyrate-co-3-hydroxyvalerate) composite biomaterials for bone tissue regeneration: in vitro performance assessed by osteoblast proliferation, osteoclast adhesion and resorption, and macrophage proinflammatory response. J Biomed Mater Res A 2007;82(3): 599–610.

74. Doyle C, Tanner ET, Bonfield W. In vitro and in vivo evaluation of polyhydroxybutyrate and of polyhydroxybutyrate reinforced with hydroxyapatite. Biomaterials 1991;12(9):841–7.

75. Timmer MD, Carter C, Ambrose CG, et al. Fabrication of poly(propylene fumarate)-based orthopaedic implants by photo-crosslinking through transparent silicone molds. Biomaterials 2003;24(25):4707–14.

76. Fisher JP, Vehof JW, Dean D, et al. Soft and hard tissue response to photocrosslinked poly(propylene fumarate) scaffolds in a rabbit model. J Biomed Mater Res 2002;59(3):547–56.

77. Baylan N, Bhat S, Ditto M, et al. Polycaprolactone nanofiber interspersed collagen type-I scaffold for bone regeneration: a unique injectable osteogenic scaffold. Biomed Mater 2013;8(4):045011.

78. Fu S, Ni P, Wang B, et al. Injectable and thermo-sensitive PEG-PCL-PEG copolymer/collagen/n-HA hydrogel composite for guided bone regeneration. Biomaterials 2012;33(19):4801–9.

79. Yang X, Chen X, Wang H. Acceleration of osteogenic differentiation of preosteoblastic cells by chitosan containing nanofibrous scaffolds. Biomacromolecules 2009;10(10):2772–8.

80. Tollemar V, Collier ZJ, Mohammed MK, et al. Stem cells, growth factors and scaffolds in craniofacial regenerative medicine. Genes Dis 2016;3(1):56–71.

81. van Hout WM, Mink van der Molen AB, Breugem CC, et al. Reconstruction of the alveolar cleft: can growth factor-aided tissue engineering replace autologous bone grafting? A literature review and systematic review of results obtained with bone morphogenetic protein-2. Clin Oral Investig 2011;15(3):297–303.

82. Sukul M, Nguyen TB, Min YK, et al. Effect of local sustainable release of BMP2-VEGF from nano-cellulose loaded in sponge biphasic calcium phosphate on bone regeneration. Tissue Eng Part A 2015;21(11–12):1822–36.

83. Gautschi OP, Frey SP, Zellweger R. Bone morphogenetic proteins in clinical applications. ANZ J Surg 2007;77(8):626–31.

84. Oryan A, Alidadi S, Moshiri A, et al. Bone morphogenetic proteins: a powerful osteoinductive compound with non-negligible side effects and limitations. Biofactors 2014;40(5):459–81.

85. Nie X, Luukko K, Kettunen P. BMP signalling in craniofacial development. Int J Dev Biol 2006;50(6):511–21.

86. Nie X, Luukko K, Kettunen P. FGF signalling in craniofacial development and developmental disorders. Oral Dis 2006;12(2):102–11.

87. Caplan AI, Correa D. PDGF in bone formation and regeneration: new insights into a novel mechanism involving MSCs. J Orthop Res 2011;29(12):1795–803.

88. Duan X, Bradbury SR, Olsen BR, et al. VEGF stimulates intramembranous bone formation during craniofacial skeletal development. Matrix Biol 2016;52–54:127–40.

89. Schilephake H. Bone growth factors in maxillofacial skeletal reconstruction. Int J Oral Maxillofac Surg 2002;31(5):469–84.

90. Francis CS, Mobin SS, Lypka MA, et al. rhBMP-2 with a demineralized bone matrix scaffold versus autologous iliac crest bone graft for alveolar cleft reconstruction. Plast Reconstr Surg 2013;131(5):1107–15.

91. Lee K, Silva EA, Mooney DJ. Growth factor delivery-based tissue engineering: general approaches and a review of recent developments. J R Soc Interface 2011;8(55):153–70.

92. Azevedo HS, Pashkuleva I. Biomimetic supramolecular designs for the controlled release of growth factors in bone regeneration. Adv Drug Deliv Rev 2015;94:63–76.

93. Lee SH, Shin H. Matrices and scaffolds for delivery of bioactive molecules in bone and cartilage tissue engineering. Adv Drug Deliv Rev 2007;59(4–5): 339–59.

94. Patel ZS, Young S, Tabata Y, et al. Dual delivery of an angiogenic and an osteogenic growth factor for bone regeneration in a critical size defect model. Bone 2008;43(5):931–40.

95. King WJ, Krebsbach PH. Growth factor delivery: how surface interactions modulate release in vitro and in vivo. Adv Drug Deliv Rev 2012;64(12):1239–56.

96. Triplett RG, Nevins M, Marx RE, et al. Pivotal, randomized, parallel evaluation of recombinant human bone morphogenetic protein-2/absorbable collagen sponge and autogenous bone graft for maxillary sinus floor augmentation. J Oral Maxillofac Surg 2009;67(9):1947–60.

97. Kretlow JD, Young S, Klouda L, et al. Injectable biomaterials for regenerating complex craniofacial tissues. Adv Mater 2009;21(32–33):3368–93.

98. Richardson TP, Peters MC, Ennett AB, et al. Polymeric system for dual growth factor delivery. Nat Biotechnol 2001;19(11):1029–34.

99. Strobel C, Bormann N, Kadow-Romacker A, et al. Sequential release kinetics of two (gentamicin and BMP-2) or three (gentamicin, IGF-I and BMP-2) substances from a one-component polymeric coating on implants. J Control Release 2011; 156(1):37–45.

100. Mehta M, Schmidt-Bleek K, Duda GN, et al. Biomaterial delivery of morphogens to mimic the natural healing cascade in bone. Adv Drug Deliv Rev 2012;64(12): 1257–76.

101. Howell TH, Fiorellini JP, Paquette DW, et al. A phase I/II clinical trial to evaluate a combination of recombinant human platelet-derived growth factor-BB and recombinant human insulin-like growth factor-I in patients with periodontal disease. J Periodontol 1997;68(12):1186–93.

102. O'Neill HS, Gallagher LB, O'Sullivan J, et al. Biomaterial-enhanced cell and drug delivery: lessons learned in the cardiac field and future perspectives. Adv Mater 2016;28(27):5648–61.

103. Qi C, Yan X, Huang C, et al. Biomaterials as carrier, barrier and reactor for cell-based regenerative medicine. Protein Cell 2015;6(9):638–53.

104. Mooney DJ, Vandenburgh H. Cell delivery mechanisms for tissue repair. Cell Stem Cell 2008;2(3):205–13.

105. Vo TN, Shah SR, Lu S, et al. Injectable dual-gelling cell-laden composite hydrogels for bone tissue engineering. Biomaterials 2016;83:1–11.

106. Trounson A, McDonald C. Stem cell therapies in clinical trials: progress and challenges. Cell Stem Cell 2015;17(1):11–22.

107. Temple HT, Malinin TI. Orthobiologics in the foot and ankle. Foot Ankle Clin 2016; 21(4):809–23.

108. Nandi SK, Roy S, Mukherjee P, et al. Orthopaedic applications of bone graft & graft substitutes: a review. Indian J Med Res 2010;132:15–30.

109. d'Aquino R, De Rosa A, Lanza V, et al. Human mandible bone defect repair by the grafting of dental pulp stem/progenitor cells and collagen sponge biocomplexes. Eur Cell Mater 2009;18:75–83.

110. Ito H, Koefoed M, Tiyapatanaputi P, et al. Remodeling of cortical bone allografts mediated by adherent rAAV-RANKL and VEGF gene therapy. Nat Med 2005; 11(3):291–7.

111. Scheller EL, Villa-Diaz LG, Krebsbach PH. Gene therapy: implications for cranio-facial regeneration. J Craniofac Surg 2012;23(1):333–7.
112. Winn SR, Hu Y, Sfeir C, et al. Gene therapy approaches for modulating bone regeneration. Adv Drug Deliv Rev 2000;42(1–2):121–38.
113. Han S, Mahato RI, Sung YK, et al. Development of biomaterials for gene therapy. Mol Ther 2000;2(4):302–17.
114. Park TG, Jeong JH, Kim SW. Current status of polymeric gene delivery systems. Adv Drug Deliv Rev 2006;58(4):467–86.
115. Dang JM, Leong KW. Natural polymers for gene delivery and tissue engineering. Adv Drug Deliv Rev 2006;58(4):487–99.
116. Franceschi RT. Biological approaches to bone regeneration by gene therapy. J Dent Res 2005;84(12):1093–103.
117. Kohn DB. Gene therapy for XSCID: the first success of gene therapy. Pediatr Res 2000;48(5):578.
118. Kumar SR, Markusic DM, Biswas M, et al. Clinical development of gene therapy: results and lessons from recent successes. Mol Ther Methods Clin Dev 2016;3: 16034.
119. Baltzer AW, Lieberman JR. Regional gene therapy to enhance bone repair. Gene Ther 2004;11(4):344–50.
120. Bonadio J, Smiley E, Patil P, et al. Localized, direct plasmid gene delivery in vivo: prolonged therapy results in reproducible tissue regeneration. Nat Med 1999;5(7):753–9.
121. Breitbart AS, Grande DA, Mason JM, et al. Gene-enhanced tissue engineering: applications for bone healing using cultured periosteal cells transduced retrovir-ally with the BMP-7 gene. Ann Plast Surg 1999;42(5):488–95.
122. Schek RM, Taboas JM, Hollister SJ, et al. Tissue engineering osteochondral im-plants for temporomandibular joint repair. Orthod Craniofac Res 2005;8(4): 313–9.
123. Chang SC, Wei FC, Chuang H, et al. Ex vivo gene therapy in autologous critical-size craniofacial bone regeneration. Plast Reconstr Surg 2003;112(7):1841–50.
124. D'Mello SR, Elangovan S, Hong L, et al. A pilot study evaluating combinatorial and simultaneous delivery of polyethylenimine-plasmid DNA complexes encod-ing for VEGF and PDGF for bone regeneration in calvarial bone defects. Curr Pharm Biotechnol 2015;16(7):655–60.
125. Kushibiki T, Tabata Y. Future direction of gene therapy in tissue engineering. Top Tissue Eng 2005;1–33.
126. Santos JL, Pandita D, Rodrigues J, et al. Non-viral gene delivery to mesen-chymal stem cells: methods, strategies and application in bone tissue engineer-ing and regeneration. Curr Gene Ther 2011;11(1):46–57.
127. Tokatlian T, Cam C, Siegman SN, et al. Design and characterization of micropo-rous hyaluronic acid hydrogels for in vitro gene transfer to mMSCs. Acta Bio-mater 2012;8(11):3921–31.
128. Obregon F, Vaquette C, Ivanovski S, et al. Three-dimensional bioprinting for regenerative dentistry and craniofacial tissue engineering. J Dent Res 2015; 94(9 Suppl):143S–52S.
129. Kang HW, Lee SJ, Ko IK, et al. A 3D bioprinting system to produce human-scale tissue constructs with structural integrity. Nat Biotechnol 2016;34(3):312–9.
130. Trombetta R, Inzana JA, Schwarz EM, et al. 3D printing of calcium phosphate ceramics for bone tissue engineering and drug delivery. Ann Biomed Eng 2017;45(1):23–44.

131. Inzana JA, Olvera D, Fuller SM, et al. 3D printing of composite calcium phosphate and collagen scaffolds for bone regeneration. Biomaterials 2014;35(13): 4026–34.
132. Do AV, Khorsand B, Geary SM, et al. 3D printing of scaffolds for tissue regeneration applications. Adv Healthc Mater 2015;4(12):1742–62.
133. Shim JH, Won JY, Sung SJ, et al. Comparative efficacies of a 3D-printed PCL/PLGA/β-TCP membrane and a titanium membrane for guided bone regeneration in beagle dogs. Polymers 2015;7(10):1500.
134. Wu Z, Su X, Xu Y, et al. Bioprinting three-dimensional cell-laden tissue constructs with controllable degradation. Sci Rep 2016;6:24474.
135. Ozbolat IT, Hospodiuk M. Current advances and future perspectives in extrusion-based bioprinting. Biomaterials 2016;76:321–43.
136. Reichert JC, Cipitria A, Epari DR, et al. A tissue engineering solution for segmental defect regeneration in load-bearing long bones. Sci Transl Med 2012;4(141):141ra93.
137. Bertassoni LE, Cecconi M, Manoharan V, et al. Hydrogel bioprinted microchannel networks for vascularization of tissue engineering constructs. Lab Chip 2014;14(13):2202–11.
138. Morrison RJ, Hollister SJ, Niedner MF, et al. Mitigation of tracheobronchomalacia with 3D-printed personalized medical devices in pediatric patients. Sci Transl Med 2015;7(285):285ra64.

Dental Implants

Jason A. Griggs, PhD, FADM

KEYWORDS

- Cumulative survival rate • Bone augmentation • Implant design • Platform switching
- Implant abutment • Surface roughness • Surface coatings • rhBMP-2

KEY POINTS

- The actual failure rates of dental implants are likely to be higher than the rates published in the clinical literature.
- Roughened implant collars, microthreads, and platform switching are all effective in bone maintenance.
- Bone augmentation is effective at increasing functional surface area but does not significantly increase implant success rates.
- Reduced-diameter implants have higher probability of failure, especially when the diameter is 3.75 mm or narrower.
- Implant bodies made from zirconia have performed well clinically when their surfaces were smooth, but this material may not be able to withstand the application of roughened surfaces or sharp structural features.

INTRODUCTION

The literature on dental implants has advanced tremendously over the past 10 years. **Fig. 1** shows the results of a search in Scopus using the Boolean phrase ("dental implant" OR "dental implants") AND (failure OR replaced OR survival OR success OR fracture). The annual publication rate on success/failure of dental implants suddenly accelerated beginning in 1988, and it continued to increase at a rate of 22 manuscripts/year/year almost up to the present. **Fig. 2** shows the types of publications in the dental implant literature. It consists of 11.0% review articles, a proportion that remains unchanged to the present. The recent rate of publication has provided a wealth of systematic reviews. This search captured 748 reviews between 2008 and the present. After screening their abstracts, 599 of them were subsequently excluded on the basis of being studies of superstructures, studies limited to interventions for previously failing implants, studies that were concluded before abutment placement, in vitro studies, and studies regarding complex facial reconstruction (such as the placement of implants in a mandible constructed from the fibula). The remaining publications

Conflicts of Interest: None.
Biomedical Materials Science, The University of Mississippi Medical Center School of Dentistry, 2500 North State Street, Room D528, Jackson, MS 39216-4505, USA
E-mail address: jgriggs@umc.edu

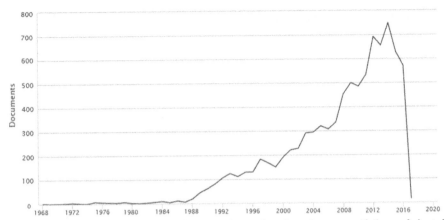

Fig. 1. Publication rate over time of manuscripts related to the success/failure of dental implants.

were analyzed in detail, and their results were compiled to produce the guidance in later discussion. This guidance is based on evidence from clinical studies whenever possible, although for some topics the earliest systematic reviews included only animal models.

INFLATED SUCCESS RATES

A word of caution is needed before reviewing the dental implant literature. Recent clinical studies regularly report success rates upwards of 95%. These reports provides the appearance that the challenges in dental implantology have mostly been resolved, but that is a false impression. The "cumulative survival rate" (CSR) for those studies is often much lower than the reported "success rate." There is an important difference between these 2 measures of success.[1] If 60 implants are followed over a 2-year period and 5 of them fail (**Fig. 3**), then the typical study would report a 92% success rate. However, some of those implants should probably be censored data points (dropouts, deaths, relocations, and so forth). A simple success rate would erroneously

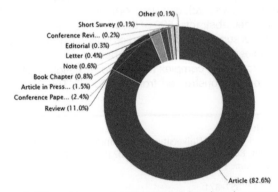

Fig. 2. Proportions of different types of publications related to the success/failure of dental implants.

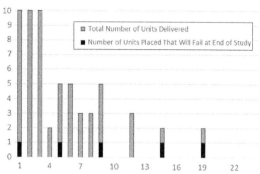

Fig. 3. Hypothetical data for a 2-year clinical study. (*Adapted from* Kelly JR. Dental ceramics: current thinking and trends. Dent Clin North Am 2004;48(2):523; with permission.)

include the censored implants in the denominator of the failure rate calculation, whereas CSR would (more appropriately) eliminate censored implants from the denominator. In addition, some of the implants would be placed after the first month of the study, and those would not be followed for the entire 2 years. A simple success rate assumes that all implants were followed for 2 years even though that is often not the case. Kelly has shown that in such cases the corresponding CSR could easily be as low as 83% (**Fig. 4**).[1] If many of the implants were placed toward the end of the study, then a 92% success rate could possibly correspond to a CSR of only 33% at 2 years! It is important to report the CSR, but few studies do. It is hoped that more investigators will report CSR instead of simple success rates in future literature. Another factor is sponsorship bias. Dental implant studies sponsored by manufacturers report significantly lower failure rates (4.8 times lower on average) than nonsponsored studies.[2] Likewise, prospective studies (more likely to be sponsored) report higher

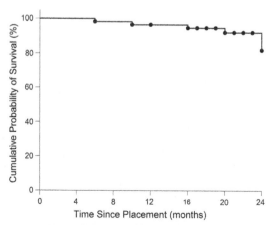

Fig. 4. Kaplan-Meier survival analysis of data from **Fig. 3**. Circles indicate censored data points. Downward steps in the line indicate failures. For this analysis, a best case scenario where all of the failures occurred in the final month of the study was assumed. (*Adapted from* Kelly JR. Dental ceramics: current thinking and trends. Dent Clin North Am 2004;48(2):524; with permission.)

success rates than retrospective studies. For example, Lee and colleagues[3] conducted a meta-analysis on 11 retrospective studies and 8 prospective studies. Prospective studies had failure rates 3.3 times lower on average. It is also more common for investigators to have a financial conflict of interest regarding intellectual property in prospective studies. A third factor is that follow-up times in most publications are not long enough to observe some modes of failure, especially mechanical complications due to screw loosening and/or fatigue fracture. Despite these concerns and limitations, a review of the current literature still reveals some interesting effects of the factors controlling the success or failure of dental implants.

TOOTH LOCATION

The maxilla typically has less bone mass than the mandible, and one might intuitively expect this to lead to higher failure rates for implants placed in the maxilla. Studies appear to support this expectation. One meta-analysis of the literature sought to determine the effects of implant length on failure rates. They examined 29 clinical studies containing 2611 implants. The meta-analysis revealed that failure rates in the maxilla were 3 times greater than in the mandible.[4] An even larger meta-analysis of 54 studies containing 19,083 implants found that the risk of failure for smooth, short implants placed in the maxilla is much higher than for rough, short implants. The risk ratio is 5.4 in the anterior maxilla and 3.4 in posterior maxilla.[5] Del Fabbro and colleagues[6] focused on implants that were either tilted with angulated abutments or were upright across 10 clinical studies (1992 implants) and found that 96% of the implants that failed within the first year had been placed in the maxilla.

INSERTION TORQUE

A higher insertion torque is associated by many investigators with greater bone-implant contact area and possibly with increased bone density. Therefore, one might intuitively expect insertion torque to be correlated with success. However, a meta-analysis of 6 studies investigating this variable showed no significant correlation between insertion torque and marginal bone loss.[7]

NECK DESIGN

Roughened surfaces on implant collars have the potential to attract plaque, so one might wonder whether the bone maintenance benefit derived from rough surfaces is significant enough to offset the risk of possible future peri-implantitis. Niu and colleagues[8] conducted a systematic review and meta-analysis of 5 randomized clinical trials on implants with or without microthreads on the necks. Four of the 5 trials reported less marginal bone loss for the cases where microthreaded implants were used, and the meta-analysis showed this difference to be statistically significant ($P = .03$). One might wonder whether the threaded shape of the microthreads is important, or does the collar in these implants simply act as a roughened surface? Two additional systematic reviews attempted to separate the effect of collar roughness from that of microthreads. Aloy-Prósper and colleagues[9] reviewed 11 clinical studies, which included 626 smooth collar implants, 499 rough collars without microthreads, and 177 rough collars with microthreads. Over a follow-up period of 12 to 60 months, there were similar success rates for implants without microthreads having smooth (87% to 98% success) and rough (94% to 100%) collars, but implants with microthreads had success rates of 100% in every study. Likewise, Koodaryan and Hafezeqoran[10] analyzed 12 clinical studies (1163 implants) and found that rough collars resulted in significantly less marginal bone loss than smooth collars (mean difference = 0.32 mm, $P<.01$) and that rough, microthreaded collars resulted in even less marginal bone loss than rough collars without microthreads (mean difference = 0.83 mm, $P<.01$). In summary, there is overwhelming evidence that a rough collar and microthreads play important roles in bone maintenance.

Because the reviews discussed above have shown the importance of surface roughness for bone maintenance, one may wonder how far above or below the original bone level is the optimal location for the roughened portion of the implant surface to terminate. Schwarz and colleagues[11] conducted a meta-analysis of 13 studies to determine the effects of implant collar height and implant-abutment connection height relative to the bone level. They found that supracrestal positioning of the rough-smooth transition line resulted in 0.835 mm less marginal bone loss than subcrestal positioning, and this effect was statistically significant ($P<.001$). Furthermore, the treatment groups that were deeply subcrestal lost more marginal bone than the groups with a more superficial subcrestal position. In addition, it was revealed that a subcrestal position of the implant-abutment connection resulted in 0.479 mm less marginal bone loss on average compared with a supracrestal position ($P<.001$).

SHORT IMPLANTS

In many cases, especially in the maxillary sinus, there is insufficient bone to place an implant of average length. The consequences of using an implant that is shorter has been a major topic of interest and is related to the study of bone augmentation methods, each of them being the subject of 20 literature reviews over the past 10 years. Kotsovilis and colleagues[12] conducted a meta-analysis of 22 clinical studies and found that treatment with short (8–10 mm) implants having roughened surfaces was as successful on average as treatment with implants longer than 10 mm. Pommer and colleagues[5] found that short implants with smooth surfaces had significantly higher failure rates than long implants, but that short implants with rough surfaces had failure rates that were not significantly different from long implants. Annibali and colleagues[13] reviewed short (less than 10 mm) implants exclusively and reported that a roughened surface was associated with higher success rates. However, Menchero-Cantalejo and colleagues[14] went farther and concluded that, regardless of surface finish, implants shorter than 10 mm had similar failure rates compared with longer implants. Monje and colleagues[15,16] conducted a systematic review of implants shorter versus longer than 10 mm and a meta-analysis of short versus very short implants. They found no difference in failure rates between short and long implants ($P = .63$) and significantly lower risk for very short implants ($P<.001$). Sun and colleagues[17] conducted a large meta-analysis that included 35 studies (14,722 implants) and found no clear trend relating the failure rate and implant length (**Fig. 5**). The lack of importance of length is underscored by the fact that 58% of the failures occurred before loading, and hence before the length coming into play. Likewise, Atieh and colleagues[18] performed a systematic review of 33 clinical studies and reported that 75% of failures occurred before loading, with similar failure rates for short and long implants. In addition, 9 other small reviews of the implant literature concluded that short implants have similar success rates as long implants.[19–27] Several of these also reported a greater incidence of complications associated with long implants when bone augmentation was performed to accommodate the greater length, and so they recommended short implants over long implants when the bone height is insufficient.[21–23,26,27]

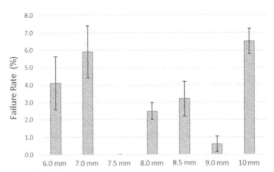

Fig. 5. Results of a large-scale meta-analysis regarding the possible effect of implant length on failure rate. Bars indicate the actual proportion that failed for each size group. Whiskers indicate the 95% confidence interval for predicting performance in future studies. There were no implants with lengths of 6.5 mm or 9.5 mm. There were only 66 implants with a length of 7.5 mm, and none of them failed during the observation period. (*Adapted from* Sun HL, Huang C, Wu YR, et al. Failure rates of short (≤10 mm) dental implants and factors influencing their failure: a systematic review. Int J Oral Maxillofac Implants 2011;26(4):821; with permission.)

However, the opinions regarding implant length are not unanimous. Telleman and colleagues[4] conducted a meta-analysis that included a smaller number of implants (2611 implants in 29 studies) and found that among those implants the shorter ones (5 mm) had slightly lower probability of survival (93.1%) than the longer (9.5 mm) ones (98.6%). Another small meta-analysis (with only 762 short implants) reported higher failure rates among implants shorter than 8 mm compared with longer implants (P<.01).[28] One systematic review by Karthikeyan and colleagues[29] provided an interesting perspective on the changes over time in the use of short implants. Over a 20-year period, the success rates gradually increased from 80% to 90% and then suddenly leapt to nearly 100%. In summary, for the past 10 years, the placement of short implants has been a topic of great concern and caution, but reviews of the clinical literature overwhelmingly support the currently available short implants as a safe and effective alternative to long implants in combination with bone augmentation. As confidence with placing shorter implants has been bolstered over time, the threshold for defining a short implant has progressed from 10 mm to 8 mm and then to 5 mm.

BONE AUGMENTATION

Given the amount of attention that has been focused on the consequences of using short implants in locations with a lack of bone, it should not be surprising that methods of bone augmentation is also a topic of intense study. As of 2008, the clinical studies on bone augmentation were not numerous and homogeneous enough to draw solid conclusions, but that database has expanded over the past decade. An early attempt to review the literature (that included only 4 clinical studies) concluded that there was possibly no effect of lateral ridge augmentation.[30] A slightly larger review included 17 studies with 455 patients but was unable to rank various methods of bone augmentation.[31] They were able to conclude that synthetic bone scaffolds performed equally well as autogenous bone for both sinus floor augmentation and ridge augmentation. Also in 2008, Del Fabbro and colleagues[32] reviewed 59 studies, but they were unable to differentiate the effects of rough implant surfaces and nonautogenous bone augmentation because 90% of cases in the literature confounded these 2 factors together. However, the trend suggested that nonautogenous bone was not inferior to autogenous bone. Whether nonautogenous bone produces inferior results compared to autogenous bone is an important question that was tested many times because the ability to use nonautogenous bone or synthetic bone scaffolds avoids the possibility of comorbidity at the donor site. In 2009, Nkenke and Stelzle[33] reviewed 21 studies and concluded that bone substitutes were not inferior to autogenous bone for sinus floor augmentation. Waasdorp and Reynolds[34] reviewed 9 studies and found insufficient data to draw a conclusion about the effectiveness of alveolar ridge augmentation. By 2012, the literature contained 3975 cases related to sinus augmentation alone. These data permitted a meta-analysis that concluded sinus augmentation is effective (94.3% overall survival rate) and that there is no difference in success rate between synthetic materials and autogenous bone.[35] Another meta-analysis compared the effectiveness of several scaffolding materials including beta-tricalcium phosphate (beta-TCP) versus autogenous bone neat or with additions of animal bone, growth factors, Bioglass, or hydroxyapatite.[36] Five-month results showed that beta-TCP was inferior to the other materials in terms of bone formation ($P = .036$), but 12-month results showed no difference in failure rates. By 2013, an immense meta-analysis of 122 studies (16,268 implants) was able to demonstrate that there is no significant difference between scaffolding materials used for sinus augmentation.[37] However, there was significantly reduced risk of complications when membranes were also used. Several reviews having smaller databases concurred with Duttenhoefer and colleagues.[38–41] A recent meta-analysis used Bayesian probabilities and was able to rank several materials for ridge augmentation, which included no graft (control), calcium sulfate, calcium phosphosilicate putty, porcine bone, porcine bone plus membrane, bovine bone, freeze dried bone, and autogenous bone.[42] Regarding ridge height, the best material was freeze-dried bone, and autogenous bone was the best regarding ridge width. Ridge augmentation was successful in terms of preserving both bone height ($P<.001$) and width ($P<.000001$). However, bone augmentation may seldom be necessary given the comparatively equal success of short implants described above.

Another question regarding bone augmentation is whether growth factors should be incorporated with the scaffolding material. A systematic review of 7 clinical studies revealed that recombinant human bone morphogenetic protein (rhBMP-2) had a positive effect on bone growth in both ridge and sinus augmentation.[43] In fact, meta-analysis of these studies showed a dose-dependent positive response. However, rhBMP-2 was also associated with increased facial edema with a dose-dependent response of this side effect. Recombinant human platelet-derived growth factor and plasma-rich growth factor showed a trend that suggested beneficial effects of lower magnitude than the effect of rhBMP-2.[43]

IMPLANT WIDTH

Functional surface area is related to the square of implant diameter but only linearly related to implant length. This relation raises the question of whether clinical success is significantly influenced by implant width. In addition, the moment of inertia, which helps an implant to resist bending, is related to the square of implant diameter. Therefore, one would intuitively expect the incidence of mechanical complications to be affected by implant width. It is surprising that this topic has received little attention. One meta-analysis of 19 clinical studies showed that implants wider than 6 mm have significantly lower failure rates compared with 5- to 6-mm-diameter implants ($P<.001$).[3] Another meta-analysis of 16 studies revealed that implants less than

3.3 mm in diameter had an average failure rate of 25%, which was significantly greater than the failure rate for wider implants (13%) over the same follow-up periods.[44] Andersen and colleagues[45] followed 32 implants that were 3.25 mm in diameter and 30 implants that were 3.75 mm and reported 2 failures (both in the 3.25-mm group), but there was insufficient statistical power to conclude whether this was a significant difference. Baqain and colleagues[46] reported 399 implants with an 8% failure rate. There was a significant effect of implant width ($P = .035$) with 7 failures in implants narrower than 3.5 mm, 7 failures in implants measuring 3.5 to 4.5 mm, and only one failure among the implants wider than 4.5 mm. The effect of implant length was not significant ($P = .78$). Olate and colleagues[47] followed a large group of implants (1649) and reported failure rates of 5.1% for narrow implants, 3.8% for regular implants, and 2.7% for wide implants. However, there were 2 systematic reviews that failed to observe an effect of implant width. One of these reviews only included 4 studies in which narrow implants were included.[48] One of these 4 studies reported only one failure among all of the implants followed and was unable to discriminate based on width.[49] Another study contained only one narrow implant, and implant width was confounded with radiation treatment of the patient.[50] Another study only included 3 failures,[51] and among these, 2 were narrow implants, and only one was standard diameter; yet the systematic review cited the study as showing a lack of effect of implant width as well as citing a study that did not have any narrow implants.[52] Finally, despite the fact that Peleg and colleagues[53] did not report which category (narrow or regular) failed implants were classified, this study was still cited regarding implant width.[48] The other review on this side of the issue included 38 short-term studies and calculated a relative risk failure of 1.1 between narrow and regular implants, which was not statistically significant.[54] Klein and colleagues[54] judged the studies in the meta-analysis to be of low quality with high risk of bias. In summary, implant width appears to strongly affect failure rate, but relatively little research has been performed on this topic so far. The increasing rate of failure with decreasing implant diameter appears to more sharply increase at a size threshold near 3.75 mm. Caution is recommended when placing implants of narrow diameter, and further research should be conducted on designing narrow implants having improved performance.

TAPERED IMPLANT WIDTH

Tapered implants are often used in bone that has low density and/or a thin cortical layer, especially in the posterior maxilla. The rationale for using a tapered implant in this situation is that the screw threads around the widest portion (near the implant collar) will engage bone that has not yet been damaged by the apical screw threads. This strategy is aimed at achieving better primary stability. However, a systematic review of 5 clinical studies (72 implants) placed in the posterior maxilla without sinus augmentation was not able to detect a difference in success rate between using tapered implants versus implants with constant cross-section.[55]

PLATFORM SWITCHING

Platform switching is the practice of placing a smaller-diameter abutment and smaller prosthesis on a wider implant body (**Fig. 6**). In theory, this should provide a greater functional surface area as well as a wider platform and a large moment of inertia to resist forces without increasing the moment arm through which eccentric loading is multiplied. Systematic reviews and meta-analyses over the past decade have shown that there is a real benefit to platform switching. In 2008, a

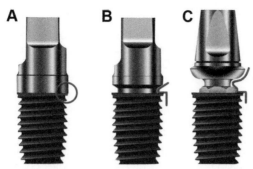

Fig. 6. Comparison between silhouettes of implants with (*A*) platform-matched abutment, (*B*) platform-switched abutment having an internal connection, and (*C*) platform-switched abutment having an external connection.

systematic review of 9 clinical studies and 3 animal studies concluded that platform switching is effective in reducing marginal bone loss.[56] Another review that included a meta-analysis surveyed 10 clinical studies (1239 implants) and found platform-switched implants to have 0.39-mm lower marginal bone loss on average, which may or may not be considered clinically significant but is highly statistically significant ($P<.0001$) given the large sample size.[57] However, there was no significant difference in risk of failure (relative risk 0.93, $P = .89$). By 2011, the literature contained 19 clinical studies, and a systematic review found 100% support for the benefit of platform switching on preserving bone height.[58] Several smaller reviews concurred with Atieh and colleagues.[13,16,59–63] Finally, a large meta-analysis of 28 clinical studies (2373 implants) provided some additional details.[64] Marginal bone loss was lower for platform-switched implants compared with platform-matched implants ($P<.00001$). This difference increased with increasing follow-up time ($P<.0001$), and it increased with increasing degree of mismatch between abutment and platform ($P<.0001$). In summary, it is clear that platform matching preserves bone by a measurable degree. However, it is not clear whether this bone preservation reduces the risk of implant failure.

INTERNAL VERSUS EXTERNAL CONNECTION

Although the adoption of the external implant-abutment connection and then the internal Morse taper connection were inspired by perceived improvements in stability in vitro, systematic reviews of clinical studies do not clearly favor one side of this issue or the other. This lack of clinical evidence may be a case where effects observed in vitro during overstress testing are not actually present in the clinic. A review of 27 clinical studies showed risk of connector screw loosening over 3 years to be 2.4% for internal connections and 2.7% for external connections.[65] Another review of 14 studies included both titanium and zirconia abutments.[66] In this case, connector screw loosening was significantly more common among external connections. For both titanium and zirconia abutments, there was no difference in risk of abutment fracture between internal and external connections. Finally, a review of 17 studies containing 2708 implants concluded that internal connections are associated with less marginal bone loss.[67] However, platform switching is more commonly used with internal connections, and platform switching is associated with reduced marginal bone loss (as discussed above), so the difference found could have been caused by platform switching instead of a difference in connection type.

CERAMIC IMPLANTS/ABUTMENTS

Although titanium has a greater Young's modulus of elasticity (100–105 GPa) compared with bone (15–30 GPa), ceramic materials tend to be far stiffer than both (alumina 390 GPa, zirconia 160–240 GPa). This difference in stiffness raises a question as to whether implants fabricated from these ceramics will be mechanically compatible with bone. The brittleness of ceramics further raises a question regarding their mechanical durability over time. There is also the question of plaque accumulation on ceramic surfaces. Is it different from plaque accumulation on titanium, and will it lead to a greater incidence of peri-implantitis? In light of these questions, it is not surprising that ceramic dental implants were the subject of 10 literature reviews in the past 10 years. In 2008, a systematic review of 7 animal studies concluded that zirconia implants achieved the same degree of bone-implant contact as titanium implants.[68] Another review compared implant abutments made from alumina, zirconia, titanium, or gold alloy in 6 clinical studies and 3 animal studies.[69] They found that the abutment material had no effect on marginal bone loss when implant bodies were all manufactured from titanium. In 2009, Andreiotelli and colleagues[70] published a systematic review of ceramic implant bodies in 25 clinical studies and concluded that alumina was not as successful as titanium for use in implants. However, the literature to that point did not yet contain sufficient information on zirconia dental implants to draw a conclusion. By 2010, the literature confirmed that zirconia implants were sufficiently fracture resistant and had a low level of plaque accumulation.[71] A later meta-analysis of 24 clinical studies showed no difference between zirconia implants and titanium implants, respectively, regarding 5-year failure rates (2.5% and 2.4%), technical complications (11.8% and 12.0%), and biological complications (6.4% and 6.1%).[72] A smaller systematic review concurred.[73] However, beginning in 2015, the reviews became less positive regarding zirconia implants. Vohra and colleagues[74] found failure rates from 0% to 32.4% and greater marginal bone loss than around titanium implants. Vechiato-Filho and colleagues[75] found twice as much marginal bone loss around zirconia implants (only 0.40 mm of loss). In 2016, Hashim and colleagues[76] performed a meta-analysis of 14 articles and found a mean failure rate of 8% at only 12 months for zirconia implants. In summary, alumina (having a stiffness 13–26 times that of bone) was shown early on to be a poor choice of material for dental implants. The literature was favorable regarding the performance of zirconia implants until the past 2 years. It is possible that new implant designs were introduced having geometry or rough surface coatings that were incompatible with the brittleness of zirconia. This deleterious effect of surface treatment on durability seems to be the case for at least one zirconia implant line that the author is currently conducting failure analysis on.

SURFACE ROUGHNESS/COATINGS

Although the surface roughness and surface coatings applied to dental implants have been topics of intense in vitro research, it is disappointing that the clinical literature still contains few studies with specific information about the surfaces of implants. It is also disappointing that the little information that is available is confounded with other observational factors instead of being part of well-controlled experimental studies.[77] Because in vitro results often do not translate to clinical results, it is difficult to draw specific conclusions, but it is clear that an average surface roughness of at least 1 micron has a beneficial effect overall on bone maintenance and implant survival. This general conclusion is supported by 9 systematic reviews over the past 10 years.[3,5,10,11,13,14,32,78,79] Regarding surface coatings, the clinical literature does provide a few more specific details. A meta-analysis of 19 Large-animal models revealed that implant coatings significantly improve bone-implant contact area (BIC) relative to uncoated implants. Inorganic coatings (14.7% more BIC than for uncoated) outperformed extracellular matrix coatings (10.0% more BIC), peptide coatings (7.1% more BIC), and rhBMP-2 coatings (3.3% less BIC).[80] However, meta-analysis of clinical studies found hydroxyapatite coatings to have no significant effect on implant survival.[81,82]

REFERENCES

1. Kelly JR. Dental ceramics: current thinking and trends. Dent Clin North Am 2004; 48:513–30.
2. Popelut A, Valet F, Fromentin O, et al. Relationship between sponsorship and failure rate of dental implants: a systematic approach. PLoS One 2010;5:e10274.
3. Lee C-T, Chen Y-W, Starr JR, et al. Survival analysis of wide dental implant: systematic review and meta-analysis. Clin Oral Implants Res 2016;27(10):1251–64.
4. Telleman G, Raghoebar GM, Vissink A, et al. A systematic review of the prognosis of short (10 mm) dental implants placed in the partially edentulous patient. J Clin Periodontol 2011;38:667–76.
5. Pommer B, Frantal S, Willer J, et al. Impact of dental implant length on early failure rates: a meta-analysis of observational studies. J Clin Periodontol 2011;38: 856–63.
6. Del Fabbro M, Bellini CM, Romeo D, et al. Tilted implants for the rehabilitation of edentulous jaws: a systematic review. Clin Implant Dent Relat Res 2012;14: 612–21.
7. Li H, Liang Y, Zheng Q. Meta-analysis of correlations between marginal bone resorption and high insertion torque of dental implants. Int J Oral Maxillofac Implants 2015;30:767–72.
8. Niu W, Wang P, Zhu S, et al. Marginal bone loss around dental implants with and without microthreads in the neck: a systematic review and meta-analysis. J Prosthet Dent 2017;117:34–40.
9. Aloy-Prósper A, Maestre-Ferrín L, Peñarrocha-Oltra D, et al. Marginal bone loss in relation to the implant neck surface: an update. Med Oral Patol Oral Cir Bucal 2011;16:365–8.
10. Koodaryan R, Hafezeqoran A. Evaluation of implant collar surfaces for marginal bone loss: a systematic review and meta-analysis. Biomed Res Int 2016;2016: 1–10.
11. Schwarz F, Hegewald A, Becker J. Impact of implant-abutment connection and positioning of the machined collar/microgap on crestal bone level changes: a systematic review. Clin Oral Implants Res 2014;25:417–25.
12. Kotsovilis S, Fourmousis I, Karoussis IK, et al. A systematic review and meta-analysis on the effect of implant length on the survival of rough-surface dental implants. J Periodontol 2009;80:1700–18.
13. Annibali S, Bignozzi I, Cristalli MP, et al. Peri-implant marginal bone level: a systematic review and meta-analysis of studies comparing platform switching versus conventionally restored implants. J Clin Periodontol 2012;39:1097–113.
14. Menchero-Cantalejo E, Barona-Dorado C, Cantero-Álvarez M, et al. Meta-analysis on the survival of short implants. Med Oral Patol Oral Cir Bucal 2011;16: e546–51.
15. Monje A, Fu J-H, Chan H-L, et al. Do implant length and width matter for short dental implants (10 mm)? A meta-analysis of prospective studies. J Periodontol 2013;84:1783–91.

16. Monje A, Suarez F, Galindo-Moreno P, et al. A systematic review on marginal bone loss around short dental implants (10 mm) for implant-supported fixed prostheses. Clin Oral Implants Res 2014;25:1119–24.
17. Sun HL, Huang C, Wu YR, et al. Failure rates of short ($\leq$ 10 mm) dental implants and factors influencing their failure: a systematic review. Int J Oral Maxillofac Implants 2011;26:816–25.
18. Atieh MA, Zadeh H, Stanford CM, et al. Survival of short dental implants for treatment of posterior partial edentulism: a systematic review. Int J Oral Maxillofac Implants 2012;27:1323–31.
19. Al-Hashedi AA, Taiyeb Ali TB, Yunus N. Short dental implants: an emerging concept in implant treatment. Quintessence Int 2014;45:499–514.
20. Lee S-A, Lee C-T, Fu MM, et al. Systematic review and meta-analysis of randomized controlled trials for the management of limited vertical height in the posterior region: short implants (5 to 8 mm) vs longer implants (>8 mm) in vertically augmented sites. Int J Oral Maxillofac Implants 2014;29:1085–97.
21. Aloy-Prósper A, Peñarrocha-Oltra D, Peñarrocha-Diago M, et al. The outcome of intraoral onlay block bone grafts on alveolar ridge augmentations: a systematic review. Med Oral Patol Oral Cir Bucal 2015;20:e251–8.
22. Nisand D, Picard N, Rocchietta I. Short implants compared to implants in vertically augmented bone: a systematic review. Clin Oral Implants Res 2015;26: 170–9.
23. Fan T, Li Y, Deng W-W, et al. Short implants (5 to 8 mm) versus longer implants (>8 mm) with sinus lifting in atrophic posterior maxilla: a meta-analysis of RCTs. Clin Implant Dent Relat Res 2017;19(1):207–15.
24. Lemos CAA, Ferro-Alves ML, Okamoto R, et al. Short dental implants versus standard dental implants placed in the posterior jaws: a systematic review and meta-analysis. J Dent 2016;47:8–17.
25. Sierra-Sánchez J-L, García-Sala-Bonmatí F, Martínez-González A, et al. Predictability of short implants (<10 mm) as a treatment option for the rehabilitation of atrophic maxillae. A systematic review. Med Oral Patol Oral Cir Bucal 2016;21: e392–402.
26. Alqutaibi AY, Altaib F. Short dental implant is considered as a reliable treatment option for patients with atrophic posterior maxilla. J Evid Based Dent Pract 2016;16:173–5.
27. Camps-Font O, Burgueño-Barris G, Figueiredo R, et al. Interventions for dental implant placement in atrophic edentulous mandibles: vertical bone augmentation and alternative treatments. A meta-analysis of randomized clinical trials. J Periodontol 2016;87:1444–57.
28. Mezzomo LA, Miller R, Triches D, et al. Meta-analysis of single crowns supported by short (<10 mm) implants in the posterior region. J Clin Periodontol 2014;41: 191–213.
29. Karthikeyan I, Desai SR, Singh R. Short implants: a systematic review. J Indian Soc Periodontol 2012;16:302–12.
30. Donos N, Mardas N, Chadha V. Clinical outcomes of implants following lateral bone augmentation: systematic assessment of available options (barrier membranes, bone grafts, split osteotomy). J Clin Periodontol 2008;35:173–202.
31. Esposito M, Grusovin MG, Kwan S, et al. Interventions for replacing missing teeth: bone augmentation techniques for dental implant treatment. Aust Dental J 2009;54:70–1.
32. Del Fabbro M, Rosano G, Taschieri S. Implant survival rates after maxillary sinus augmentation. Eur J Oral Sci 2008;116:497–506.

33. Nkenke E, Stelzle F. Clinical outcomes of sinus floor augmentation for implant placement using autogenous bone or bone substitutes: a systematic review. Clin Oral Implants Res 2009;20:124–33.

34. Waasdorp J, Reynolds MA. Allogeneic bone onlay grafts for alveolar ridge augmentation: a systematic review. Int J Oral Maxillofac Implants 2010;25: 525–31.

35. Cabezas-Mojón J, Barona-Dorado C, Gómez-Moreno G, et al. Meta-analytic study of implant survival following sinus augmentation. Med Oral Patol Oral Cir Bucal 2012;17:e135–9.

36. Rickert D, Slater JJRH, Meijer HJA, et al. Maxillary sinus lift with solely autogenous bone compared to a combination of autogenous bone and growth factors or (solely) bone substitutes. A systematic review. Int J Oral Maxillofac Surg 2012;41:160–7.

37. Duttenhoefer F, Souren C, Menne D, et al. Long-term survival of dental implants placed in the grafted maxillary sinus: systematic review and meta-analysis of treatment modalities. PLoS One 2013;8:e75357.

38. Al-Nawas B, Schiegnitz E. Augmentation procedures using bone substitute materials or autogenous bone - a systematic review and meta-analysis. Eur J Oral Implantol 2014;7:S1–16.

39. Sanz-Sánchez I, Ortiz-Vigón A, Sanz-Martín I, et al. Effectiveness of lateral bone augmentation on the alveolar crest dimension. J Dent Res 2015;94:128S–42S.

40. Ioannou AL, Kotsakis GA, Kumar T, et al. Evaluation of the bone regeneration potential of bioactive glass in implant site development surgeries: a systematic review of the literature. Clin Oral Investig 2015;19:181–91.

41. Wu J, Li B, Lin X. Histological outcomes of sinus augmentation for dental implants with calcium phosphate or deproteinized bovine bone: a systematic review and meta-analysis. Int J Oral Maxillofac Surg 2016;45:1471–7.

42. Iocca O, Farcomeni A, Pardiñas Lopez S, et al. Alveolar ridge preservation after tooth extraction: a Bayesian network meta-analysis of grafting materials efficacy on prevention of bone height and width reduction. J Clin Periodontol 2017;44: 104–14.

43. Shimono K, Oshima M, Arakawa H, et al. The effect of growth factors for bone augmentation to enable dental implant placement: a systematic review. Jpn Dental Sci Rev 2010;46:43–53.

44. Ortega-Oller I, Suárez F, Galindo-Moreno P, et al. The influence of implant diameter on its survival: a meta-analysis based on prospective clinical trials. J Periodontol 2014;85:569–80.

45. Andersen E, Saxegaard E, Knutsen BM, et al. A prospective clinical study evaluating the safety and effectiveness of narrow-diameter threaded implants in the anterior region of the maxilla. Int J Oral Maxillofac Implants 2001;16:217–24.

46. Baqain ZH, Moqbel WY, Sawair FA. Early dental implant failure: risk factors. Br J Oral Maxillofac Surg 2012;50:239–43.

47. Olate S, Lyrio MC, de Moraes M, et al. Influence of diameter and length of implant on early dental implant failure. J Oral Maxillofac Surg 2010;68:414–9.

48. Javed F, Romanos GE. Role of implant diameter on long-term survival of dental implants placed in posterior maxilla: a systematic review. Clin Oral Investig 2014;19:1–10.

49. Ormianer Z, Piek D, Livne S, et al. Retrospective clinical evaluation of tapered implants: 10-year follow-up of delayed and immediate placement of maxillary implants. Implant Dent 2012;21:350–6.

50. Buddula A, Assad DA, Salinas TJ, et al. Survival of dental implants in irradiated head and neck cancer patients: a retrospective analysis. Clin Implant Dent Relat Res 2012;14:716–22.
51. Simion M, Fontana F, Rasperini G, et al. Long-term evaluation of osseointegrated implants placed in sites augmented with sinus floor elevation associated with vertical ridge augmentation: a retrospective study of 38 consecutive implants with 1- to 7-year follow-up. Int J Periodontics Restorative Dent 2004;24:208–21.
52. Attard NJ, Zarb GA. Implant prosthodontic management of partially edentulous patients missing posterior teeth: the Toronto experience. J Prosthet Dent 2003; 89:352–9.
53. Peleg M, Garg AK, Mazor Z. Predictability of simultaneous implant placement in the severely atrophic posterior maxilla: a 9-year longitudinal experience study of 2,132 implants placed into 731 human sinus grafts. Int J Oral Maxillofac Implants 2006;21:94–102.
54. Klein MO, Schiegnitz E, Al-Nawas B. Systematic review on success of narrow-diameter dental implants. Int J Oral Maxillofac Implants 2014;29:43–54.
55. Alshehri M, Alshehri F. Influence of implant shape (tapered vs cylindrical) on the survival of dental implants placed in the posterior maxilla: a systematic review. Implant Dent 2016;25:855–60.
56. López-Marí L, Calvo-Guirado JL, Martín-Castellote B, et al. Implant platform switching concept: an updated review. Med Oral Patol Oral Cir Bucal 2009;14: e450–4.
57. Atieh MA, Ibrahim HM, Atieh AH. Platform switching for marginal bone preservation around dental implants: a systematic review and meta-analysis. J Periodontol 2010;81:1350–66.
58. Serrano-Sánchez P, Calvo-Guirado JL, Manzanera-Pastor E, et al. The influence of platform switching in dental implants. A literature review. Med Oral Patol Oral Cir Bucal 2011;16:400–5.
59. Al-Nsour MM, Chan H-L, Wang H-L. Effect of the platform-switching technique on preservation of peri-implant marginal bone: a systematic review. Int J Oral Maxillofac Implants 2012;27:138–45.
60. Herekar M, Sethi M, Mulani S, et al. Influence of platform switching on periimplant bone loss: a systematic review and meta-analysis. Implant Dent 2014;23:439–50.
61. Romanos GE, Javed F. Platform switching minimizes crestal bone loss around dental implants: truth or myth? J Oral Rehabil 2014;41:700–8.
62. Di Girolamo M, Calcaterra R, Di Gianfilippo R, et al. Bone level changes around platform switching and platform matching implants: a systematic review with meta-analysis. Oral Implantol 2016;9:1–10.
63. Santiago JF, De Souza Batista VE, Verri FR, et al. Platform-switching implants and bone preservation: a systematic review and meta-analysis. Int J Oral Maxillofac Surg 2016;45:332–45.
64. Chrcanovic BR, Albrektsson T, Wennerberg A. Tilted versus axially placed dental implants: a meta-analysis. J Dent 2015;43:149–70.
65. Theoharidou A, Petridis HP, Tzannas K, et al. Abutment screw loosening in single-implant restorations: a systematic review. Int J Oral Maxillofac Implants 2008;23: 681–90.
66. Gracis S, Michalakis K, Vigolo P, et al. Internal vs. external connections for abutments/reconstructions: a systematic review. Clin Oral Implants Res 2012;23: 202–16.

67. de Medeiros RA, Pellizzer EP, Vechiato Filho AJ, et al. Evaluation of marginal bone loss of dental implants with internal or external connections and its association with other variables: a systematic review. J Prosthet Dent 2016;116:501–6.
68. Wenz HJ, Bartsch J, Wolfart S, et al. Osseointegration and clinical success of zirconia dental implants: a systematic review. Int J Prosthodont 2008;21:27–36.
69. Linkevicius T, Apse P. Influence of abutment material on stability of peri-implant tissues: a systematic review. Int J Oral Maxillofac Implants 2008;23:449–56.
70. Andreiotelli M, Wenz HJ, Kohal R-J. Are ceramic implants a viable alternative to titanium implants? A systematic literature review. Clin Oral Implants Res 2009;20: 32–47.
71. Nakamura K, Kanno T, Milleding P, et al. Zirconia as a dental implant abutment material: a systematic review. Int J Prosthodont 2010;23:299–309.
72. Zembic A, Kim S, Zwahlen M, et al. Systematic review of the survival rate and incidence of biologic, technical, and esthetic complications of single implant abutments supporting fixed prostheses. Int J Oral Maxillofac Implants 2014;29: 99–116.
73. Kapos T, Evans C. CAD/CAM technology for implant abutments, crowns, and superstructures. Int J Oral Maxillofac Implants 2014;29:117–36.
74. Vohra F, Al-Kheraif AA, Ab Ghani SM, et al. Crestal bone loss and periimplant inflammatory parameters around zirconia implants: a systematic review. J Prosthet Dent 2015;114:351–7.
75. Vechiato-Filho AJ, Pesqueira AA, De Souza GM, et al. Are zirconia implant abutments safe and predictable in posterior regions? A systematic review and meta-analysis. Int J Prosthodont 2016;29:233–44.
76. Hashim D, Cionca N, Courvoisier DS, et al. A systematic review of the clinical survival of zirconia implants. Clin Oral Investig 2016;20:1403–17.
77. Wennerberg A, Albrektsson T. Effects of titanium surface topography on bone integration: a systematic review. Clin Oral Implants Res 2009;20:172–84.
78. Pattanaik B, Pawar S, Pattanaik S. Biocompatible implant surface treatments. Indian J Dent Res 2012;23:398–406.
79. Doornewaard R, Christiaens V, De Bruyn H, et al. Long-term effect of surface roughness and patients' factors on crestal bone loss at dental implants. A systematic review and meta-analysis. Clin Implant Dent Relat Res 2017;19(2): 372–99.
80. Jenny G, Jauernik J, Bierbaum S, et al. A systematic review and meta-analysis on the influence of biological implant surface coatings on periimplant bone formation. J Biomed Mater Res A 2016;104(11):2898–910.
81. Alsabeeha NHM, Ma S, Atieh MA. Hydroxyapatite-coated oral implants: a systematic review and meta-analysis. Int J Oral Maxillofac Implants 2012;27: 1123–30.
82. van Oirschot BAJA, Bronkhorst EM, van den Beucken JJJP, et al. Long-term survival of calcium phosphate-coated dental implants: a meta-analytical approach to the clinical literature. Clin Oral Implants Res 2013;24:355–62.

Moving?

Make sure your subscription moves with you!

To notify us of your new address, find your **Clinics Account Number** (located on your mailing label above your name), and contact customer service at:

Email: journalscustomerservice-usa@elsevier.com

800-654-2452 (subscribers in the U.S. & Canada)
314-447-8871 (subscribers outside of the U.S. & Canada)

Fax number: 314-447-8029

**Elsevier Health Sciences Division
Subscription Customer Service
3251 Riverport Lane
Maryland Heights, MO 63043**

*To ensure uninterrupted delivery of your subscription, please notify us at least 4 weeks in advance of move.

Printed and bound by CPI Group (UK) Ltd, Croydon, CR0 4YY

07/10/2024

01040505-0003